I0477322

ARABS IN TREATMENT:

ARABS IN TREATMENT:

DEVELOPMENT OF MENTAL HEALTH SYSTEM AND PSYCHOANALYSIS IN THE ARABO-ISLAMIC WORLD

YANA KOROBKO

Copyright © 2016 by Yana Korobko.

The cover image is the photo of Yana Korobko's
psychoanalytic office

Library of Congress Control Number:		2016911657
ISBN:	Hardcover	978-1-5245-2633-7
	Softcover	978-1-5245-2632-0
	eBook	978-1-5245-2631-3

All rights reserved. No part of this book may be reproduced or transmitted
in any form or by any means, electronic or mechanical, including photocopying,
recording, or by any information storage and retrieval system,
without permission in writing from the copyright owner.

Any people depicted in stock imagery provided by Thinkstock are models,
and such images are being used for illustrative purposes only.
Certain stock imagery © Thinkstock.

Print information available on the last page.

Rev. date: 08/19/2016

To order additional copies of this book, contact:
Xlibris
1-888-795-4274
www.Xlibris.com
Orders@Xlibris.com
746515

CONTENTS

PART I
HISTORICAL INTERACTIONS BETWEEN
PSYCHOANALYSIS AND ISLAM

PART II
THE STRUCTURE OF MUSLIM PSYCHE

PART III
MENTAL DISORDERS IN THE CONTEMPORARY
ARAB WORLD

ABSTRACT

"There is no God in this book," such were the last words of Freud before his death. And somewhat earlier, Nietzsche proclaimed that God had died. Were they both the precursors of the apocalypse, or, conversely, of a relief for the nihilistic Europe? Nobody knew that. However, when looking back into the epoch of denial, Europe was found soaking in the abyss of moral dissolution, all-permissiveness and, at once, desperately looking for its lost object. For Europe God is dead. And its place has been gradually taken by the objects of material wealth, luxury, and enjoyment. In contrast to the Muslim world, which stands as the total opposite of the Freud`s enunciation. It experienced a wholly different exposure. In Islam, God is ubiquitous and it is the central signifier of the Muslim psyche. If God cannot be personified, which Islam forbids, He can also not become part of history or die.[1] God is thus omnipresent, humankind can never be alone in the world, every movement is watched by God.[2] Islam is the last phase of a long development of Revelation in history. Two principal phases preceded Islam, Judaism, and Christianity. The Islamic world, which has its concrete term in Arabic ummah, is more than 30% of the world's population and this number is constantly growing.[3] The Muslim world lives now in its fifteenth century. The stagnation period started in the end of the fourteenth century and continued until the eighteenth.[4] During

---

[1]   https://en.qantara.de/content/islam-and-psychoanalysis-a-tale-of-mutual-ignorance, consulted on 01.07.2016

[2]   *Ibid*

[3]   http://www.pewforum.org/2011/01/27/the-future-of-the-global-muslim-population, consulted on 01.07.2016

[4]   Dwairy M., *Counseling and psychotherapy with Arabs and Muslims: a culturally sensitive approach*, New York: Teachers College Press, 2006, p.4.

---

the stagnation period, the Arabs became divided between loyalty to the Muslim non-Arab rulers in their fight against the European Crusaders and opposition to these rulers.[5] For the first time in Arab history, however, the Arabic identity became distinct from the Islamic.[6] At the end of that period the pan-Arabic movement emerged, and Arabic and Islamic identities became distinct one from another.[7] Today the Arab states comprise Algeria, Bahrain, Comoros, Djibouti, Egypt, Iraq, Jordan, Kuwait, Lebanon, Libya, Mauritania, Morocco, Oman, Palestine, Qatar, Saudi Arabia, Somalia, Sudan, Syria, Tunisia, United Arab Emirates and Yemen. And among the Muslim states there are Afghanistan, Albania, Azerbaijan, Bangladesh, Benin, Brunei, Burkina Faso, Cameroon, Cote d'Ivoire, Maldives, Chad, Gabon, Gambia, Guinea, Guinea-Bissau, Guyana, Indonesia, Iran, Kazakhstan, Kyrgyzstan, Malaysia, Mali, Mozambique, Niger, Nigeria, Pakistan, Senegal, Sierra Leone, Suriname, Togo, Turkey, Turkmenistan, Uganda and Uzbekistan. As shown above, the question of the Muslim is not only that of religion but also of identity. When dealing with identity, here the Islamic will be often intertwined with the Arabic. Since it is a double identity, specifically this standpoint gives a broader and fuller grasp of understanding of the core of the contemporary Muslim mind. Also, the reader might be contemplating upon the differences between the Muslim and the Islamic, which are distinct concepts, applied in this book. "Islamic", grammatically speaking, refers to the religion or the acts done in the name of that religion, and not a person who practices that religion. Consequently, it can be referred to the Islamic community or Islamic art. And "Muslim" is used to describe all people of the Islamic faith but not the faith itself. You will find this book mentioning the religion of Muslims, but not the Muslim religion. In such a way, we have gradually approached the original query, which stood at the roots of the idea of creating this book. So, why there ever arose a need of writing separately about the Muslim consciousness? Cannot the same metapsychological discourse apply productively to Muslims as well as to non-Muslims? Actually, the very idea of this book came up as a result of constant reflections upon the issues, which, among others, also include:

- Whether, psychoanalysis is possible and needed in the Muslim world?
- What challenges might psychoanalysis face in the Muslim world?

---

[5]   *Ibid*

[6]   *Ibid*

[7]   *Ibid, p.5.*

- What can be considered as the sufficient knowledge about the functioning of the Islamic mind so that to work effectively with the Muslim patient?

This is a book about the other psycholinguistic and sensuously perceptive structure, which is also an attempt to:

1) Fill in the existing gap of information about:
   a) the interaction between Islam and psychoanalysis;
   b) the up-to-date psychological treatment, which would respect the tradition and recognize the modern changes at once;
2) Find analytical explanation to the metapsychological occurrences in the Muslim life;
3) Explain and establish the correlation between the prevalent mental conditions in the Arab region and its cultural specificities.

The difficulties encountered in the course of the research about the psychoanalysis in the Muslim world have prompted me to envisage the presentation of this work not only in a form of portrayal of the range of problems, but also through attaching of more significance to the particular conditions of reception of the analytical practice in the Muslim world, and illustrating the still existing limits of psychoanalysis in the context of the modern Muslim society. Hopefully, this research will inspire more discussion and raise more questions.

Abbreviations

ADHD:	Attention Deficit Hyperactivity Disorder
AH:	Anno Hegirae
AS:	Autism Spectrum
DASS:	Depression, Anxiety and Stress Scale
DBT:	Dialectical Behavioral Therapy
ECT:	Electro-Convulsive Therapy
GAD:	Generalised Anxiety Disorder
GP:	General Practitioner
ICD:	International Classification of Diseases
IOMS:	Islamic Organisation for Medical Science
MBT:	Mentalization Based Therapy
MDD:	Major Depressive Disorder
MENA:	the Middle East and North Africa
MHPSS:	Mental Health and Psycho-Social Support
MOH:	Ministry of Health
MSF:	Médecins Sans Frontières (Doctors Without Borders)
NCDC:	National Center for Disease Control
OCD:	Obsessive-Compulsive Disorder
PHC:	Primary Health Care
PTSD:	Post-Traumatic Stress Disorder

UNRWA:	United Nations Relief and Work Agency for Palestine Refugees in the Near East
WHO:	World Health Organization
WIAT:	Wechsler Individual Achievement Test

TABLES AND CHARTS

Tables:

QUOTATIONS

"Do not give your property which God assigned you to manage to the insane:
but feed and clothe the insane with this property and tell splendid words to them."

Quran (sura 4, ayat 5)

"[Metaphysics] surpasses all other sciences, except for divine science [...] and so we must hold that the science of the soul comes before the other sciences; and for this reason, we placed it in a position of priority among all subjects of inquiry."

Averroes (Ibn Rushd)

"A great religion and a pagan life!"

Naguib Mahfouz

"The one who sent down the disease sent down the remedy."

The Prophetic Hadith

"What you seek is seeking you."

Rumi

"Immorality, no less than morality, has at all times found support in religion."

Sigmund Freud

"How old is the habit of denial? We keep secrets from ourselves that all along we know...For perhaps we are like stones; our own history and the history of the world embedded in us, we hold a sorrow deep within and cannot weep until that history is sung."

Susan Griffin

"I'm one of the growing number of psychological counselors who believe that psychological healing did not ever belong to the realm of medicine. The focus of all counseling is to help us learn to change our relationship with ourselves and others. I believe this kind of learning is really no different than any other deliberate learning."

Tom Rusk

"Sunshine all the time makes a desert."

Arabic Proverb

GLOSSARY

Asabiya (tribalism) is an Arabic term for "social solidarity", designating the clan spirit and tribal unity. The term was popularized by Ibn Khaldun in the book "The Muqaddima".

Association in psychoanalysis means a liaison between two or more psychic elements, which collectively form an associative chain.

Castration anxiety is the universal unconscious fear of being emasculated. In the symbolic sense, castration anxiety refers to the fear of being undervalued, dominated or made insignificant.

Complex is literally a grouping of parts around some central emotional theme. In Jung's terminology, it is a system of related thoughts and emotions tied together by a psychologically powerful event, which unconsciously influences the human behavior.

Dar Al Shifaa literally means "house of cure", which is an Islamic health hospital. Synonymous terms for this type of building are the Persian words "Bimaristan", "Moristan", "Bimarkhana", "Šifakhana", or "Timarkhana".

Defense Mechanisms are used by the ego as a way to deal with the inner conflict. Operating at an unconscious level, defense mechanisms help to reduce negative feelings (e.g. anxiety and guilt). Common defense mechanisms include repression, denial, and projection.

Disavowal is a splitting of an ego confronted by some distressing demand from the outer world.

Ethnoconsciousness (Ethnic Consciousness) is the awareness of belonging to a particular racial and ethnic family, which settles the perception of the self and of the environment, shapes the identity and determines the behavioural patterns.

Family Romance is the tendency to defensively glamorize one's family of origin in order to avoid hating them.

Forensic Prisoner – a person with mental disorder(s) who is in jail.

Imaginary is a part of the Lacanian imaginary-real-symbolic module of the psyche structure. The imaginary becomes the internalized image of this ideal, whole, self and is situated around the notion of coherence rather than fragmentation.

Jouissance in French means enjoyment. It also denotes the excessive kind of pleasure linked to the division and splitting of the subject. Thus jouissance is suffering.

Maaqaba is a concept of Islamic psychology, which means to punish oneself for wrong deeds and forcefully restraining the self from it, which is alike self – cleaning, keeping oneself clean.

Maataba is a concept of Islamic psychology, which means to protect oneself from getting into bad habit again and avoid such situations. It is like self- governing, controlling actions and behaviors.

Marabout\muttawa is a traditional healer in the Arab world.

Maraqaba is a concept of Islamic psychology, which means to guard oneself from the evil and bad things.

Masharqa is a concept of Islamic psychology, which means to keep oneself on a straight path.

Mujahida is a concept of Islamic psychology, which means to express the self fully and properly and not keep anything hidden. It is like self-analysis.

Mental Health Legislation denotes legal clauses regarding the protection of the basic human and civil rights of people with mental disorders.

Mental Health Policy–a formal document issued by the Government or Ministry of Health, which sets the specific goals for the amelioration of the national mental health care domain and provides the main directions to achieve them.

Mental Health System is the entire complex of mental health institutions, clinics, hospitals, organizations, research centers, rehabilitation services and individual professionals, who support and treat people with mental health disorders on the country level.

Mundus Imaginalis (or imaginal world) is a term coined by Ibn Arabi, which is thought to go beyond the unconscious and include the superconscious.

National Mental Health Programme is a national plan of actions in the mental health field.

Name-of-the-Father is a metaphorical operator of the presence of the father, which installs the symbolic order for a child.

Noetics is a branch of metaphysical philosophy related to the study of mind and intellect.

Oedipus Complex is used by Freud as an illustration to a childhood developmental stage, occurring between the ages of three and six, when a child desires to have the parent of the opposite sex all to him/herself, to the exclusion of the other parent. In the myth, Oedipus kills Laius, who he does not realize is his father, and then marries his widow, Jokasta, who is actually Oedipus's mother.

Phallic Symbolism in psychoanalysis does not refer so much to the male reproductive organ as to the signifier of the desire (in accordance to Lacan).

Psychiatrist is a medical doctor who has had at least two years of post-graduate training in psychiatry at a recognized teaching institution.

Psychoanalysis is (1) a system of theories concerning the relation between the conscious and unconscious psychological processes. (2) a method of exploring the unconscious conflicts through the techniques of free associations, interpretations of dreams and lapsus, recovery of repressed child memories, etc. for the purpose of releasing the inner tension and bringing psychological relief.

Psychologist Working in Mental Health is a graduate from a recognized institution with a specialization in clinical psychology, who works in the mental health field.

Real–a part of the Lacanian imaginary-real-symbolic module of psyche structure. In the Lacanian theory, the real becomes that which resists representation, what is pre-mirror, pre-imaginary, pre-symbolic – what cannot be symbolized – what loses its "reality" once it is symbolized (made conscious) through language.

Resistance refers to a patient's unconscious opposition to the unveiling and exploration of painful memories during psychoanalysis.

Signified is the concept indicated by the signifier, which has an internal meaning to the perceiver. Whilst the signifier is more stable, the signified varies between people and contexts.

Signifier is the phonological element of the sign; not the actual sound itself, but the mental image of such a sound.

Substance Abuse Policy is a formal document issued by the Government or Ministry of Health, which sets the strategic goals of preventing the substance abuse at the country level.

Symbolic is a part of the Lacanian imaginary-real-symbolic module of psyche structure. The symbolic is about language and narrative. The symbolic is made possible because of the child's acceptance of the Name-of-the-Father, those laws and restrictions that control both the desire and the rules of communication.

Transference is the projection onto another person (e.g. the analyst) of feelings, past associations, or experiences.

Umma is the Muslim community throughout the world.

Unconscious is the part of the mind that stores feelings, thoughts, and urges unaware to the individual.

CHAPTER 1

INTRODUCTION

Gustav Jung taught that remnants of the past are strong determining factors of reaction patterns to stresses, symptomatology of mental illnesses and the way a people look at disease, treatment, life, death, human emotions and the like. History and mythology are living determinants for psychiatry and mental health. Thence, to comprehend better the state of psychoanalysis in the Islamic world, we should look closer at the evolutionary stages, it has gone through, starting from the pre-Islamic era and proceeding until the present days. Islam and psychoanalysis are not a so-called "tale of mutual ignorance". Certain elements of psychoanalytic treatment existed in Muslim world even earlier before they were introduced in Europe by Freud. Hegel called Islam "the religion of sublimity". In Hegel's "passion for abstraction" narrative from the Philosophy of History (1837), Islam appears an abstraction that vanquished the imaginary.

Religion, history, culture, language and climate, which such vast territories, as the Islamic world shares, are at the same time common uniting and disuniting factors. The divergences lay in different approaches to the interpretation of key historic events and cultural customs; the existence of a huge number of spoken dialects, as well as concepts of health and illness. Even in the religious domain, which is a part of shared identity, the disparities happen (e.g. sunnits and shiites). Islam is more than just a religion, it has become a way of life. Throughout the history, the national cultures and traditions have left such a deep impact on the practice of Islam, that nowadays an average Muslim finds it difficult to tell apart one from another. Moreover, the permanent interactions with the outside world (via trade) have brought in the elements of foreign, oftentimes, opposite cultures into the region, therefore, enabling the coexistence of numerous autochthonous worldviews on one land. And this is another phenomenon that constitutes a Muslim identity. Medicine along with psychiatry, in particular, was the first one to benefit from this synthesis.

The interest in the psychoanalysis in the Muslim world is a relatively recent fact, which can be dated to the period 1970-1990. The reasons for this late reception shall be sought for at once in the status of the developing countries and their difficulties in the domain of education of human resources after the independence, rather than in the specificities of relations maintained between the Muslim world and the West.

Overview of the Book

The book is divided into three main parts in addition to an introduction and a conclusion.

Part I (Historical Interactions between Psychoanalysis and Islam) introduces the historical background, on the basis of which the book is organized. The chronological timeline begins with the jahiliya epoch and extends until nowadays. The analytical element comprises various theories, hypothetical reflections and conceptual equations regarding the events, which occurred in the Arab history and influenced the formation of the collective mind. All good things need not come together — so, the synopsis of the strengths and the weaknesses of the mental health systems in the Arab region is also included. It also contains the in-depth country examples with inclusive statistics provided by WHO and other stakeholders.

Part II (The Structure of Muslim Psyche) introduces the identification for the main signifiers of the Muslim psyche and comprehensively provides the cultural underpinning for each of them. The conceptual grounds are supported by the practical experience of the world influential psychoanalysts.

Part III (Mental Health Disorders in the Contemporary Arab World) shifts the focus from the broad macro-dynamical survey to the specifics of mental dysfunctions of modern Arabs less as ends in themselves than as means to address the prevalent symptomatology and the therapeutic constraints of the region.

The conclusion to the book seeks to draw out lessons from the glorious past of the Arab medicine and apply its principles to the modern Muslim mental health care system. It also reviews the actual problematics of the relation between psychoanalysis and Islam and seeks a way to overcome the underlying challenges.

PART I

HISTORICAL INTERACTIONS BETWEEN PSYCHOANALYSIS AND ISLAM

CHAPTER 2

JAHILIYA PERIOD

Arabs belong to the sinton race. And in order to understand Muslims, one should study the two main bases that form their identity: a) Islam, and b) the desert. For the desert environment explains the special mentality of the Bedouin, his conception of existence, his qualities and his weaknesses. Consequently, it explains Islam, a secretion of the Arab brain; and finally, it explains the Muslim that Islam has run into its rigid mold.[1] The integral essence of a Muslim comprises the following signifiers: the Desert — the Bedouin — Nomadism — the Warrior — Fatalism — Endurance — the Tribe — Sensuality — the Ideal — Religion.

The term Jahiliya derives from the Arabic word *jahala*, which stands for ignorance. Quran, in sura al-Maida, describes the pre-Islamic society using the term jahiliya. They are a society plagued with ignorance, rejected Allah guidance, had no moral values, had no civilization, could not read or write and were disobedient to the laws of Allah.[2] Jahiliya followed soon after the falling down of Saba kingdom around 300 BC and lasted for

---

[1]   Servier, Andre. Islam and the Psychology of the Musulman. New York: Scribner, 1923, p.14.
       *This Quranic verse summarized Islam's attitudes towards the mentally ill, who were considered unfit to manage property but must be treated humanely and be kept under care by either a guardian or the state.

[2]   Syakir, Mahmud. Al-Tarikh al-Islamiy Qabl al-Bi'thah. Beirut: Al-Maktab al-Islamiy. 1991, p. 10.

three centuries (310 years) until the revelation of Quran in 610M. The Holy Book describes jahiliya as follows:

"Or like darkness on a deep sea obscure, covered by a wave, above which is a wave, above which is a cloud. Layers of darkness one upon the other. When he holds out his hand, well-nigh he cannot see it. And he for whom God has assigned no light, for him there is no light."

(sura 24, ayat 40)

Jahiliya time is attributed to the following features:

1) No prophecies (guidance);
2) No civilization;
3) No good manner;
4) Illiteracy.

Definitely, the elements of jahilya are left as a hardened residue in an Arab psyche. Just to mention a few archaic affects: rage, anger, ferocity, savagery, etc. The study of the pre-Islamic livelihood allows the broader understanding of what is inexplicable about the modern Arabic complexity.

Historical Context

Long before the appearance of Christianity and Islam, Arabs lived in Najd (Arabia) and the Syrian deserts. And Arab geographers divide Arabia into five regions:

1. Hijaz extending from Aila (al-Aqaba) to Yemen. It was so named because the range of mountains running parallel to the Western coast separates the low coastal belt of Tihama from Najd;
2. Tihama inside the inkier range is a plateau extending to the foothills;
3. Yemen, south of Hijaz, occupies the southwest corner of Arabia;
4. Najd, the north central plateau, extends from the mountain ranges of Hijaz in the west to the deserts of Bahrain in the east and encompasses a number of deserts and mountain ranges;
5. Aruz which is bounded by Bahrain to its east and Hijaz to its west. Lying between Yemen and Najd it was also known as Yamama.

On this huge territory, one common language has been spoken, which is Arabic. Arabic has been the common lingua franca of the desert bedouins as well as of the sedentary populations like the Qahtan and Adnan. Despite a huge variety of local dialects, which were marking the geographical location of a tribe, Arabic has always been understandable to any Arab.

Political Conditions

In Arabia neither government nor law was ever existent before an advent of Islam, with the exception of Yemen in the southwest. Tribes were the primary and only structure of a communal organization. The authority of the tribal leaders was rather informal, granted for the outstanding personal moral qualities, and did not have any particular election tradition. Tribal chiefs were considered as the wisest members of the community, and, therefore, entitled to "administer" justice in a capacity of police, courts, and even, judges. It was the tribe's duty to protect its people even if they had committed crimes. Tribalism or asabiya (the clan spirit) still remains a powerful part of Muslim consciousness. At that time ethics was not known to Arabs, whereas, war, on the contrary, took a place of a leading ideology. Sometimes war, or vendetta were turning into the preferable manner to dispute solving. Literally speaking vendetta meant "you kill one of ours, we will kill one of yours". Killing per se was not considered immoral, even though killing a member of one's own clan was condemned. Another common practice was ghazu raids. When tribes were in conflict with each other they would raid an enemy tribe and appropriate their camels and other goods.

Economic Conditions

Probably, after the war, trading was the most exciting pastime for Arabs. At that time Arabia was inhabited by various populations, and Jews played there an imminent role. They were the monopolistic owners of the top arable lands in Hijaz, as well as savvy agricultural experts.

One of the particularities of jahiliya was the institution of slavery. Male and female slaves were considered to be the property of their owners, alongside with husbandry and one's own material possessions. Slaves formed the lowest rank of the Arab society. Whereas the most influential class was made up by money-lender entrepreneurs. They were charging excessively high rates on loan interests, which was purposefully intended to make them even richer, and the borrowers poorer. Nonetheless, Mecca was notorious for practicing riba and did not cease it until Quran banned it. The core trade centers were Mecca and Yathrib, both in the Hijaz region. Merchants were sending their caravans in summer to Syria and in winter to Yemen. They were also commercial ways to Bahrain in the east and to Iraq in the northeast. The caravans were a prototype of nowadays economic relations in Mecca. Almost everyone in Mecca invested in the merchandises carried by camels, including raisins, silver, oils, perfumes and others.[3] For this reason, it was a well-expected event for the Meccans to meet and see them off.

Social Conditions

The pre-Islamic society consisted of the settled people (hadari), who were dwelling in the oases and the Bedouin nomads, who were residing in rural areas. Arabia was a patriarchal society, meaning that women there had no status at all. To cite an example, a number of women, a man could marry, was unlimited. And even when a man died, his son "inherited" all his wives except his own mother. Arabs were infamously known for an ill ritual to bury newly born females alive. Even if a father did not wish, he was obliged to do so under the social pressure.

To mention a few other evils, which struck jahiliya society: drunkenness, gambling and prostitution. Many women were forced to sell their bodies since it was the only way for them to make a living. For these means, they flew flags on their houses and were called "ladies of the flags" (dhat-er-rayyat).

Foreign Relations

In this period practically all innovations were coming from outside. Thus, maintenance of relations with near and far neighbors was beneficial in different aspects. Mecca, Hira, Yaman, Oman, and Bahrain were supporting diplomatic and trade relations between each other. Moreover, they were regarded as strategic trade routes, through which many religions spread. Mecca then was serving as a central idol worshipping place.

Arabs' Origins

The first mentioning of Arabs dates back to the mid 9th century BC, as a reference to Arabian tribal people. Ibn Khaldun was among the first, who drew a line between sedentary Arabian Muslims and nomadic Arab

---

[3]   Bodley, Ronald. The Messenger: The Life of Mohammed. New York: Doubleday Incorporated. 1946, p.31.

Bedouins.[4] Initially, a term Arab signified Bedouins of the desert who were opposing Muhammad`s mission, i.e. ayat 9.97 says: "al arabu asaddu kufran wa nifaqan", which means "Bedouins are the worst in disbelief and hypocrisy". According to Abu Ishaq, with the spread of Islam, Bedouin`s language was chosen as a basis for the common Arab language, since its grammar was considered the purest. Mainly for this reason, understanding of the Islamic mentality directs us to its primary sources, which are the Bedouin culture and the Arabic language.

The Nabataeans, who were also nomadic people, and whose language was Aramaic, gradually switched into Arabic. And since they had the writing, it was they who made the first inscriptions in Arabic. The Nabataean alphabet was adopted by Arabs of the south and evolved into modern Arabic script around the 4th century.

So, we can see that a Muslim identity is rigidly interconnected with an Arab identity, making it, in a certain sense, a double identity. Sometimes it can be very confusing since the Bedouin rituals are still actively practiced in parallel with Islamic worshipping. Bedouin`s origins are an archaic part of a Muslim "I", which did not succeed in being totally absorbed by an Islamic identity. And this causes massive neuroses of Arab societies.

To track the origins of the Bedouin identity, first of all, we should refer to the specificity of their genesis (see Chart 2.1.) Like many other successful lineages from the Middle East, J1 holagroup, which all Arabs possess, is thought to have undergone a major population expansion during the Neolithic period.[5] Chiaroni found that the greatest genetic diversity of J1 haplotypes was found in eastern Anatolia, near Lake Van in central Kurdistan[6].Neolithic J1 goat herders were almost certainly not homogenous tribes consisting exclusively of J1 lineages but in all likelihood a blend of J1 and T1 lineages. So much is evident from the presence of both J1 and T1 in north-east Africa, Yemen, Saudi Arabia, but also in the Fertile Crescent, the Caucasus and the mountainous parts of southern Europe.[7]

J1-P58, the Central Semitic branch of J1, appears to have expanded from the southern Levant (Israel, Palestine, Jordan) across the Arabian peninsula during the Bronze Age, from approximately 3,500 to 2,500

---

4   Ibn Khaldun, The Muqaddimah : an introduction to history, Princeton University Press, 1989, p.43.

5   http://www.ncbi.nlm.nih.gov/pmc/articles/PMC2987219, consulted on 30.04.2016

6   http://www.eupedia.com/europe/Haplogroup_J1_Y-DNA.shtml, consulted on 01.05.2016

7   *Ibid*

BCE. Camels were domesticated in Somalia and southern Arabia c. 3,000 BCE, but did not become widely used in the southern Levant before approximately 1,100 BCE. Camels played a significant role in the further diffusion of J1-P58 lineages, notably with the Bedouins in the desertic parts of the Middle East and North Africa. Bedouins now make up a substantial percentage of the population of Sudan (33%), Libya (15%), the United Arab Emirates (8%) and Saudi Arabia (5%)[8].In Arabic countries, J1 climaxes among the Marsh Arabs of South Iraq (81%), the Sudanese Arabs (73%), the Yemeni (72%), the Bedouins (63%), the Qatari (58%), the Saudi (40%), the Omani (38%) and the Palestinian Arabs (38%). High percentages are also observed in the United Arab Emirates (35%), coastal Algeria (35%), Jordan (31%), Syria (30%), Tunisia (30%), Egypt (21%) and Lebanon (20%). Most of the Arabic J1 belongs to the J1-P858 variety.[9]

J1-P58 (J1a2b on the ISOGG tree, formerly known as J1e, then as J1c3) is by far the most widespread subclade of J1. It is a typically Semitic haplogroup, making up most of the population of the Arabian peninsula, where it accounts for approximately 40% to 75% of male lineages.[10]

J1-P58 is thought to have expanded from eastern Anatolia and the southern Caucasus to the Taurus and Zagros mountains, then Mesopotamia, and eventually the Arabian peninsula at the end of the last Ice Age (12,000 years ago) with the seasonal migrations of goat and sheep pastoralists. It is during the Neolithic that subclades like L860 and L93 would have reached the mountainous parts of the southern Arabian peninsula (Yemen, Oman), whereas L816 and L862 remained in the Fertile Crescent. Arabic speakers recolonised the Arabian peninsula in the Bronze Age from the north-west of the peninsula, close to present-day Jordan. The rise of Islam in the 7th century CE played a major part in the re-expansion of J1 from Arabia throughout the Middle East, as well as to North Africa, and to a lower extent to Sicily, Spain and Portugal.[11] L93 is restricted to Saudi Arabia, Yemen and Oman, while L386 was found chiefly the United Arab Emirates. J1-L1279 corresponds to DYS497=16. A rare subclade identified in the United Arab Emirates. J1-Z640 (aka Z641 or Z644) is particularly common in Syria and Lebanon, but also has been found also in Turkey, Israel and in the Arabian peninsula, as well as well as in many European countries, particularly Spain. It was very probably found among the ancient Phoenicians. Z640+ members typically have DYS561=14.

---

[8]   *Ibid*

[9]   *Ibid*

[10] *Ibid*

[11] *Ibid*

Its subclade L174.1 can be identified by the STR value DYS594=11[12]. J1-L444 is a small Arabic subclade defined by DYS531=12. Both L615 (found in the United Arab Emirates) and L859 (found in Iraq and Saudi Arabia) share an STR value for DYS485 around 14[13]. It is easy to assume that P58 is a marker of Arabic ancestry because it reaches its maximum frequency in and around the Arabian peninsula. Most present-day Arabic speakers outside the Arabian Peninsula are likewise only very partially or not all Arabic genetically. In the northern half of the Middle East, most of the people who call themselves Arabs of today are in fact mainly descendants of other historic peoples, such as the Phoenicians, Assyrians, Babylonians, or even the Hurrians. The confusion comes from the fact that the Arabic language, which appeared a little more than 1,500 years ago, is much more recent than the haplogroup J1 (31,000 years old) or even the P58 subclade (14,000 years old). Even the J1-L858 subclade (5,000 years old), associated with Southwest Asian people, very clearly predates the Arabic language. The common ancestor of the J1-L858 men alive today dates back to approximately 4500 years ago, a time that corresponds to the development of the oldest Semitic languages, like Akkadian and Amorite. In fact, L858 is not specific to the Arabian peninsula[14]. E1b1b-M34 is another important Arabic lineage, being found in 25% of Jordanians and 10% of Saudis.

---

[12] *Ibid*

[13] http://www.eupedia.com/europe/Haplogroup_J1_Y-DNA.shtml, consulted on 30.04.2016

[14] *Ibid*

Chart 2.1 Phylogenetic Tree of Haplogroup J2
(as of August 2013)

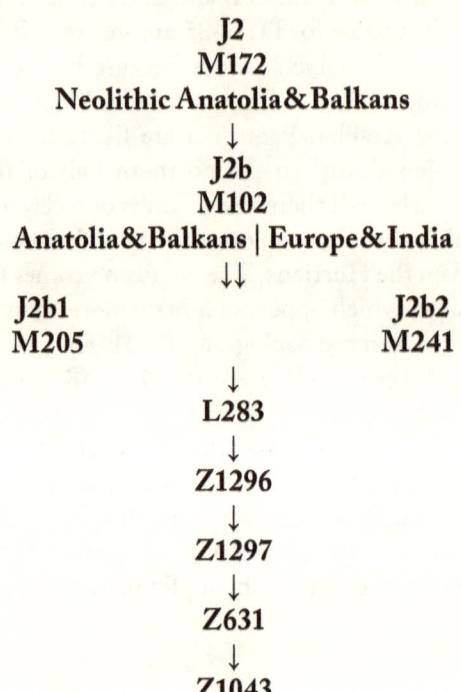

J2
M172
Neolithic Anatolia & Balkans
↓
J2b
M102
Anatolia & Balkans | Europe & India
⇓⇓

J2b1	**J2b2**
M205	**M241**

↓
L283
↓
Z1296
↓
Z1297
↓
Z631
↓
Z1043

Thus, tracing the primary source of nomadism in the Middle East from its inception until the Golden Age of Islam, which is the period of the most rapid spread of Islamic culture all around the world, has significance for understanding the development of the Arab civilization. According to Sadek Jawad Sulaiman, the former Ambassador of Oman to the United States:[15] "The Arabs are defined by their culture, not by race; and their culture is defined by its essential twin constituents of Arabism and Islam. To most of the Arabs, Islam is their indigenous religion; to all of the Arabs, Islam is their indigenous civilization. The Arab identity, as such, is a culturally defined identity, which means being Arab is being someone whose mother culture, or dominant culture, is Arabism. Beyond that, he or she might be of any ancestry, of any religion or philosophical persuasion, and a citizen of any country in the world. Being Arab does not

---

[15] Sadek Jawad Sulaiman, The Arab Identity, Al-Hewar/The Arab-American Dialogue, Winter 2007

contradict with being non-Muslim or non-Semitic or not being a citizen of an Arab state."

Appearance of Tribes and Ruling Clans

The historical evolution of an Arab tribe bears a particular interest because an Islamic society has remained fundamentally intact ever since.

The geographical conditions and necessity of survival in the desert environment prompted the process of tribes formation on the Arabian peninsula. Bedouin and Hadhari Arabs complied with the primitive administering system called Kabilah. Tribes were constantly competing for control over the territory, distribution of goods, and power one with another. The defeated tribe became enslaved by a winner. Therefore, neighbors were considered as potential enemies. Consequently, in conditions of austere rebelliousness and tribal perverseness, the clan system was set and solidified.

Women, at that period, did not have rights and were considered as objects. The whole organization of a tribal system led to a number of negative effects[16]. Asabiya, which is a feeling of extreme closeness to one's own clan, is, probably, the most contradictory one, since it has resulted in the onset of many unceasing wars within the Arab society. Asabiya was also fueled up by a principle "one is all, all is one", so, an individual as such could not exist. If a member of a tribe suffered, the whole tribe would come to his succor. To get the full benefit of this mutual support, the group or hay must not only fight together but as far as possible move together.[17] So, self-sacrifice was expected from everyone. And giving life for one's own tribe was considered as an act of honour. Tribes were ready to commit revenge so that to safeguard their self-respect and dignity. Arabs were living a chaotic and disordered life. The war between clans could have flared up even on trivial grounds. The al-Basus war between the Bakr and Rabiah clans demonstrated an odious trait of the Jahiliya society, such as fighting for pleasure principle.

Later, the rulers of Arabia would be divided into two categories: crowned kings, who were not, in fact, independent; and the chiefs of tribes and clans, who were as much privileged, as the crowned kings, and independent at the same time. The crowned kings were only in Yemen,

---

16 Shukri H., From Jahiliyyah To Islamic Worldview: In A Search Of An Islamic Educational Philosophy, International Journal of Humanities and Social Science Vol. 3 No. 2, Special Issue – January 2013, p.216.

17 William S., Kinship and Marriage in Early Arabia, Oxford Press, 2014, p.17.

Hira and Ghassan. All other rulers of Arabia were non-crowned. The former ones were choosing from animal names their own forms of the appellation, like Panthers, Dogs, Lizards, Spotted Snakes (Anmar, Kilab, Dibab, Aracima), which are exactly similar to the Totem names found in so many parts of the world[18].

[18] *Ibid*

CHAPTER 3

PRIMAL CULTURAL WORLDVIEW

As Burkert noted, that studying the formation of private rituals, the sociological-functional approach provides a necessary complement to psychology[19].Therefore, archaic beliefs (including, deities worshipping and the cult of dead), messages of early prophets, as well as poetry all together form the primary source of Islamic unconscious. This is only an initial, however, an essential step towards the understanding of a modern Muslim.

Early Arabs, who lived more than four millennia before Islam, were venerating a pantheon of gods and goddesses. Some other inhabitants of the Arabian Peninsula were observing Christianity, Judaism, Iranian religions, etc. Arab polytheism comprised god Hubal, goddesses Al-Lat, Al-Uzza, Manat and others. Frank Peters interprets that the Quran argues that these three goddesses and others were angels whose identities have been corrupted into female goddesses. So, Manaf became just another Meccan god. The Meccans were accustomed to name their children in the name of their gods, i.e. Abd Manaf. For example, Muhammad's great-great-grandfather's name was Abd Manaf which means "slave of Manaf".

Arab`s gods were worshiped at local temples, such as the Kaaba. In Mecca there were represented over 360 idols, which, supposedly, corresponded to days of the year. Kaaba, a cube-like roofless structure

---

[19]   Burkert, Walter. Homo Necans.Berkeley: University of California Press. 1983, p. 25.

that has housed a black stone, was venerated as a fetish. It is believed that Kaaba was dedicated to Hubal at the epoch. According to some traditions, the Kaaba contained no statues, but its interior was decorated with images of Mary and Jesus, of prophets, angels, and trees[20]. Spring water acquired a sacred character in Arabia early on and Islamic sources state that the well of Zamzam became holy long before the Islamic era.[21]

The religious practices of the nomadic bedouins were distinct from those of the settled Arabs. Bedouins were mostly concerned with their day-to-day life, and their practices are believed to have included fetishism, totemism, and ancestor worship. Alan Jones infers from Bedouin poetry that the gods, even Allah, were less important to the Bedouins than Fate. They did not worry about the afterlife, in contrast to the settled Arabs, who, are thought to have believed in a great variety of deities. According to F. Peters, "one of the characteristics of Arab paganism as it has come down to us is the absence of a mythology, narratives that might serve to explain the origin or history of the gods." The Bedouins established a code of honour, which guided them in matters of ethics. This code treated such issues as bravery, hospitality, respecting one's promises and agreements, and vengeance. Numerous mentions of jinn in the Quran and testimony of both pre-Islamic and Islamic literature indicate that the belief in spirits was prominent in pre-Islamic Bedouin religion. Bedouin religious experience also included an apparently indigenous cult of ancestors.

As the history shows, the word Allah was used even long before Islam, in both pagan and Christian pre-Islamic inscriptions. Pre-Islamic Christians, Jews, and the monotheistic Arabs stated that Hanifs used the term Bismillah ("in the name of Allah") and the name Allah to refer to their main god. That is what becomes evident from Arabic stone inscriptions made centuries before Islam. Muhammad's father's name was Abd-Allah meaning "the servant of Allah".

In this context, the religions of the pre-Islamic Arab Peninsula can be categorized as:

- Zoroastrianism;
- Judaism;
- Christianity;
- Hanif religion;
- Wathani religion;

---

[20] Robin C., Arabia and Ethiopia, In The Oxford Handbook of Late Antiquity, OUP USA, 2012, pp. 304–305.

[21] Irving M. Zeitlin, The Historical Muhammad, Polity, 19 March 2007, p. 31.

- Manichaeism;
- Sabines;
- Animism;

Zoroaster is originated from Persia. This is a religion without holy books, or prophets, mainly venerated in the region of Oman, Yemen, and Bahrain.

Judaism was sent with Torah, the holy book, revealed to the Prophet Moses. People of Banu Israel from the northern Arabian Peninsula were its main followers. Moreover, the peninsula had been subject to Jewish migration since Roman times, which had resulted in a diaspora community supplemented by local converts. However, the original Moses`s teachings were falsified and the Torah`s message was altered.

Christianity derives from the teaching of Prophet Jesus (Isa), which are preserved in Injil (the Bible). The Christians also originated from Banu Israel, who also altered the teaching of Prophet Jesus. This religion spread out throughout the northern region of Arabian Peninsula by the Ghassan and Hirah people and Habsyah (Ethiopia) at the southern side. They were also in Mecca, and Waraqah Ibn Naufal is one of the examples. With the exception of Nestorianism in the northeast and the Persian Gulf, the dominant form of Christianity was Monophysitism.

Hanif religion was professed by the Prophet Abraham. Quran emphasized that Ibrahim is Hunafa People, who embraced Hanif religion, did not worship idols, gamble, drink alcohol, or behave unlawfully. It is believed that Prophet`s Mohamed family observed Hanif religion.

Wathani is the cult of idols worshipping. According to Ibn Kalbi, the idol worshipping was originally brought by Umar bin Luai after his visit to Syria. He saw the Balqa tribes worshipping idols, therefore, imported the ritual to Mecca.

Zindiqs believed in good and evil, a common creed of Persian people. They maintained that there existed only two gods representing two opposing forces of light and darkness, which were constantly struggling one against the other. There is also evidence that Manichaeism (the religion of zindiqs) was practiced in Mecca.

Sabines worshiped the stars.

Some of the Arabs did not have religion at all, and some were animists. Palmyra and Petra worshiped sun and Maeen people worshiped the moon. Many of Arabs believed in superstitions and black magic.

For the most part, all pre-Islamic beliefs described here, express that at the rise of Islam the old ideals did not necessarily die. Some part of them survived and exist even nowadays. Among them, there are Madh, Karama, and Hija. Whilst some others were actually purified and restored.

Beliefs

Monotheism was present in Arabia even before the annunciation of Muhamad`s mission. William Muir writes that knowledge of the Abrahamic roots of Mecca and the Kaaba was widely accepted long before the coming of Muhamed. Michaël Cook quotes Islamic traditions in depicting this narrative with the story of Ibrahim and Ismail and their establishing of the holy altar for the One God. Thus, the Arabs were familiar with the monotheist faith. However, for certain reasons, and the influence of newcomers worshipping practices, is among them, the Arab society fell into idolatry. Monotheism was replaced by polytheism and superstitions, awaiting the coming of a Prophet who can be seen to be a "messenger sent to restore" the Arabian birthright of monotheism,[22] an answer from God to the call of Ibrahim to "send among them a messenger of their own."[23] It is no surprise then that the Quran praises Ibrahim on numerous accounts as a model for the Arabs. One particular verse of interest describes Ibrahim as the "hanif", a believer in pure monotheism[24] and abstainer from "shirk" (polytheism) while commanding the Messenger, and to an extent all man, to follow this same path.

The Arabs were known to be extremely immersed in superstitious beliefs and activities, and these formed a large part of how society ran, namely: Tatayyur (belief in omens), Tanjeem (astrology), Tabarruk (seeking the blessing from objects) and Kahanah (soothsaying), were just a few, and were strongly rejected by Islam[25]. Moreover, a polytheistic altar was regularly joined in by new artifacts such as the al-Hamra cube (perhaps a pedestal), or the bull-god Apis, which resemble the reverent symbols of Egypt and Mesopotamia.

As many houses as many idols, that is to say, every community in Mecca had its own idol-guardian which was meant to protect the house. Al-Uzza was placed next to Arafat`s temple, where the pilgrims were coming to worship her. Quraysh, who venerated al-Uzza as their main

---

[22]   Cook, Michael. Muhammad, Oxford University Press, 1983, pp.37-39.

[23]   *Ibid*

[24]   Berkey, Jonathan. The Formation of Islam, Cambridge University Press, 2003, p. xii.

[25]   Wahhab, Mohamed. Kitab At-Tauhid, Dar-us-Salam Publications, 1996, pp. 49, 101, 106, 110.

---

deity, used to seek answers from her by placing divining arrows in front of her altar before taking any significant decisions. Another deity al-Khalsa found its place at the Mecca's valley. The Arabs used to adorn it, make sacrifices and hang the eggs of an ostrich over it. Its replicas, which, supposedly, brought good luck and assured protection from all evil, were a popular merchandise at the Mecca's market.

The Quraysh remained one of those tribes, which continued the monotheistic tradition of Ibrahim and Ismail. However, when Amr Luhay became the chief of Khuzaites, he brought the idols with him in Mecca and ordered people to worship them. One of his novelties was introduction of saiba. The main deity of the Nabatean culture in northern Arabia was Dushara[26]. Dushara was represented in the form of a stone cube or more generally in the form of cuboid architecture which can be seen throughout the remains of the Nabateans' principal city, Petra[27]. The history tells that once upon a time Amr Luhay was on his way from Mecca to Syria where he met the people worshipping idols. He could not wish for more, but to bring some idols with him to Mecca.The other version of this story says that it happened on his way to Syria, when he was passing through Betra (another spelling for Petraea and Petra). It is today's Transjordania. The city was inhabited by the Nabataeans, who were constructing their deities from the graven stone. Philip K. Hitti described the religion of Nabataean kingdoms as follows:

"At the head of the pantheon stood Dushara (dhu-al-Shara, Dusara), a sun deity worshiped under the form of an obelisk or an unknown four-cornered black stone.... Associated with Dushara was Al-Lat, chief goddess of Arabia. Other Nabataean goddesses cited in the inscriptions were Manat and al-Uzza, of Koranic fame, Hubal also figures in the inscriptions." For example, there is the extremely common type of inscription introduced by the formula "Remembered be..."*(dhykr)*[28].The inscriptions in question frequently suggest that the named person is to be commemorated in the presence of a particular god and they imply a religious attitude of dependence on particular deities[29].

The Dilmun civilization, which existed along the Gulf Coast and Bahrain until the 6th century BC, worshipped a pair of deities, Inzak

---

[26] Warwick Ball (4 January 2002). Rome in the East: The Transformation of an Empire. Routledge. pp. 67–68.

[27] *Ibid*

[28] Healey, John. The Religion of the Nabataeans: A Conspectus. Leiden: Brill. 2001, p. 8.

[29] *Ibid*

---

and Meskilak[30]. Beth Qatraye which translates "region of the Qataris" in Syriac was the Christian name used for the region encompassing north-eastern Arabia[31]. It included Bahrain, Tarout Island, Al-Khatt, Al-Hasa, and Qatar[32]. Oman and the United Arab Emirates comprised the diocese known as Beth Mazunaye.

The Arabian deities were of different categories. Some of them were responsible for jadd (luck), saad (fortunate, auspicious), rida (goodwill, favour), wadd (friendship, affection), and manaf (height, high place). Some deities bore the names of the places where they were venerated, e.g. Dhu al-Khalasah and Dhu al-Shara. For example, Dhul-Halasa was an oracular god in Yemen worshiped by the Bajila and Khatham tribes. He was venerated in the form of a whitestone. His sanctuary known by the same name was called the Kaaba of Yemen and rivaled the Kaaba of Mecca[33]. Other deities included:

- Talab, a god worshiped in southern Arabia, particularly in Saba and also a moon god. His oracle was consulted for advice.
- Wadd, a moon-god in Main.

Also, natural phenomena were represented in the "shirk" pantheon. Here belong: the sun (shams, feminine). The name Abd Shams, "Servant of the Sun", was considered to ensure protection to the owner of this name. The constellation of the Pleiades (al-Thurayya), which was believed to provide for rain, also appears as a deity in the name Abd al-Thurayya. The planet Venus was revered as a powerful goddess under the name of al-Uzza ("the Most Mighty"). It had a sanctuary at Nakhla near Mecca. The name Abd al-Uzza was widespread among the pre-Islamic Arabs. The Arabian adoration for the Venus became legendary, having become a symbol of carnal love. The planet Saturn was treated as phlegmatic and evil for its slow motion. The planet Mars with its fiery red light was believed to bring

---

30 Harriet E. W. Crawford (12 March 1998). Dilmun and Its Gulf Neighbours. Cambridge University Press. p. 79.
31 Hellyer, Peter. Nestorian Christianity in the Pre-Islamic UAE and Southeastern Arabia, Journal of Social Affairs, volume 18, number 72, winter 2011, p. 88.
32 Kozah, Mario; Abu-Husayn, Abdulrahim; Al-Murikhi, Saif Shaheen. The Syriac Writers of Qatar in the Seventh Century. Gorgias Press LLC, 2014, p. 24.
33 Robertson Smith, William. Kinship and Marriage in Early Arabia. Forgotten Books, 2010, p. 297.

havoc. Jupiter, with its magnificent golden light, was treated as lucky. Other deities were: al-Malik ("the King"); Ba1, "the Lord" etc.

Sacred stones, which embodied the gods, served as altars, where the blood of the victims was poured over. Then the Arabs sacrificed camels, sheep, goats, and, less often, kine. The flesh of the sacrificed animal was usually eaten by the worshippers, and the blood was left for the god. Originally, every food was believed to be a means to pacify the god. Hence the Arabic terms, qurba and qurban (derived from the root, q-r-b, to be near), which are used for a sacrifice. The names of the five false gods and the symbols under which they were represented are given in the Table 3.1.

Customs and Cults

Jahiliya was notorious for its barbaric practices, many of which were banned by Prophet Muhamed. One of such traditions stated that after the death of husband the woman, as a part of his

Table 3.1 Names of the Pre-Islamic Gods and Their Meanings

Pagan god	Shape	Quality represented
1. Wadd	Man	Manly Power
2. Suwa	Woman	Mutability, Beauty
3. Yaguth	Lion (or Bull)	Brute Strength
4. Yauq	Horse	Swiftness
5. Nasr	Eagle, or Vulture, or Falcon.	Sharp Sight, Insight

N.B. The classical work on Arabian idol-worship is Ibn al-Kalbi's "Kitab-ul-asnam".

"property", was inherited by his son who used to marry her and give birth to their children. Islam totally abolished this heinous custom (sura 4, ayat 22).

Nonetheless, not all pre-Islamic customs relinquished. There still exist pre-Islamic rites integrated, or slightly modified in the modern Islamic society.

Among the revised attitudes, the Hajj stands out. The Islamic era persisted with many Hajj's rites inherited from the jahiliya, i.e. the tawaf and the seasonal timing being preserved. In brief, the Hajj was one of the practices that survived into Islam in "revalorized form"[34], according to Jonathan Berkey. The reason can be found in the Quran: Hajj was a pilgrimage ordained by God to the House of God and is to be restored to its Abrahamic roots. On the other side, certain demeanours were rejected such as that of the method of prayer through "whistling and clapping"[35], the Tawaf around the sanctuary naked[36], and of course, the idolatry. As Muir explained it: "The rites of the Kaaba were retained, but stripped of all idolatrous tendencies" (this would also apply to other forms of worship such as the making of the Qasam (oath) or Nadhr (vow). Originally the above-mentioned rituals were made in the name of an idol.

Not only the holiness of the Kaaba perpetuated, but also the holy months survived with a minor adaptation. Fighting in these months was condemned in jahiliya, which the Quran supports: "Say: fighting therein is a great (transgression)..." However, in the context of a strategic military move by some Muslims that allegedly broke this tradition, the verse continues to introduce the new law: "...but a greater (transgression) with Allah is to prevent mankind from following the Way of Allah, to disbelieve in Him, to prevent access to Al-Masjid-al-Haram (in Mecca), and to drive out its inhabitants, and Al-Fitnah is worse than killing."

"We were a people of Jahiliyah worshipping idols, eating the flesh of dead animals, committing abominations, neglecting our relatives, doing evil to our neighbours and the strong among us would oppress the weak..." This was the ambassadorial speech of Jafar Ibn Abi Talib to the Negus of Abyssinia, describing the days of ignorance before Islam. From the above-mentioned we can affirm that Quran was reforming the original pre-Islamic way of the Arabs; the way of their ancestor Ibrahim (Abraham), by sending guidance through Prophet Muhamed.

Safi-ur Rahman Al-Mubarakpuri attributes the actions of the jahiliya people to the "imaginary fear of poverty and shame weighed heavily on them." This is attested to in the Quran: "And do not kill your children for fear of poverty. We provide for them and for you."

In what it concerns the practices of zina (adultery), it was largely widespread. According to Muhammad Ali, women were often viewed as "a mere chattel", while prostitution was a part of jahiliya's life. Quran rigidly reprimanded all forms of prostitution, including, forcing homemaids to

---

34 Berkey, Jonathan. The Formation of Islam, Cambridge University Press, 2003, p.42.

35 *Ibid, p.35.*

36 Banna, Hassan. The Seerah of the Final Prophet, Awakening Publications, 1999, p.32.

sell themselves out in order to provide income for their owners, as well as marrying close relatives. Notwithstanding, other elements of pre-Islamic Arabia were praised and fully supported by Islam, like Arab`s muruwa (chivalry), honour and hospitality amongst other traits.[37] They would often "kill their last sheep or goat to entertain their guests",[38] and this hospitality, demonstrated by Ibrahim as the angels visited him, is extolled in the Quran. Moreover, admiration for those characteristics was expressed by the Prophet who wished that those still in jahiliya carrying those qualities would enter Islam with them, as it became so with the likes of Hamza ibn Abdul Mutallib and Umar ibn Al Khattab[39].

In what it concerns other cults, such as the Berber`s cult of dead, it differed from that of other ancient peoples. Herodote remarked the same cult practiced by the Nasamons, who were dwelling around Syria and Augila: "That is their manner of making spells and exercise divination. They put a hand on the grave of those people, who among them have the justest reputation, and who are considered as good people, and swear by them. To make predictions, they go to the graves of their forefathers: they prey there and fall asleep afterwards. If during their sleep, they had a dream, they refer to it in their future." The ancient Egyptians were Berbers` neighbours, and their mythology has many traits in common. The ancient Oriental Berbers were venerating Isis and Seth, as the following paragraph of Herodote`s shows: "[The Libyans] do not eat cows, just like the Egyptians, they neither consume pork. The women of Cyrene do not allow themselves to eat the cow out of respect to the goddess Isis, who is adored in Egypt; they even fast and celebrate solemn feasts in her honour. The women of Barce do not just eat the cow, but also abstain from eating the pork`s flesh." Osiris, of Libyan origin, was also worshiped in Libya. All known sources show that it was originally a god from the north-eastern Africa, possibly Libya. For their part, the Egyptians knew the Libyan origin of Neith, who, according to mythology came from Libya to settle in the Nile Delta.The most remarkable common god was, perhaps, Amon. Honored by the Greeks of Cyrenaica, it was unified in Baal under the Libyan influence. The biggest Libyan temple of Amun is the Siwa Oasis.

---

[37]   Bashier, Zakaria. The Makkan Crucible, The Islamic Foundation, 1978, pp. 24-36.

[38]   Banna Hasan. The Seerah of the Final Prophet, Awakening Publications, 1999, p.31.

[39]   Bashier, Zakaria. The Makkan Crucible, The Islamic Foundation, 1978, p. 25.

There were undertaken numerous attempts to send guidance to the Arabian people. Notably, Arabia had been the birthplace of several Prophets of God long even before Muhamed's arrival. The Quran says: "And make mention (O Muhamed) of the brother of Aad when he warned his folk among the wind-curved sandhills—and verily warners came and went before and after him—saying: Serve none but Allah. Lo! I fear for you the doom of a tremendous Day." (sura 46, ayat 21)

Among the first prophets, there was Hud. He was sent to the Aad's people, who, according to historical sources, belonged to the Arab Baida. Those people lived in white and reddish sand dunes to the south-west of al-Rub al-Khali near Hadramaut. In ancient times there were bountiful cities, where a people of gigantic strength and stature dwelled. However, the whole area was covered up with the sand by Sahara's winds. Salih was another Messenger sent to the people called Thamud who lived in al-Hijr, which is between Tabuk and Hijaz. Prophet Ismail lived and died in Mecca. Another Prophet Shuaib was living in Midian near Maan. So, we can see that many messengers were coming and going while attempting to bring the God's word to the community. However, many of them became strangers in their own homeland or were obliged to seek new homes. For example, Ibrahim (Abraham) had to migrate to Mecca, whereas Moses had to flee to Midian.

Poetry

Why do we draw importance to the poetry here? Not just because poems were the greatest intellectual accomplishment of the pagan Arabs, but, also, because, they have always been the principal form of self-expression on this land. It was believed that God had bestowed the most distinguished talents of the head upon the Greeks (as a proof is their science and philosophy); of hand upon the Chinese (artisanship); and of the tongue upon the Arabs (eloquence). The significance of poetry can be found in the following testimony:

In nomad Arabia, the poets were part of the war equipment of the tribe; they defended their own, and damaged hostile tribes by the employment of a force which was supposed indeed to work mysteriously, but which in fact consisted in composing dexterous phrases of a sort that would attract notice, and would consequently be diffused and remembered widely[40]. Among the most eminent pre-Islamic poets here were Imru Al-Qays, Tarafa, Amr ibn Kulthum, and Antara ibn Shaddad. They initiated a poetic tradition

---

[40] Margoliouth D., Mohammed and the Rise of Islam, Cosimo Inc., 2010, p.53.

of artificial style, a stress on linguistic ingenuity, a predilection for allusive expression, the habit of emulating the work of famous predecessors, and of playing with strict literary conventions. The mastery of the poet consisted in his ability to deepen the metaphors and images to express the emotions. So, whenever an Arab is overwhelmed by grief, or, on the contrary, is in love, he usually expresses it through the verses. Therefore, in poetry, an Arab was finding a safe refuge for the emotional distress. For these means, poetry was found to be more convenient than the prose.

The poet was oftentimes referred to as "possessed" by jins (majnun). Suzanne Stetkevych has posited that the jahili poetry can be seen as resembling ritual in form and structure and, with reference to Freud, we can read these rituals as a cathartic mechanism for the Id impulses of the later Islamic community and thereby understand the textual ambiguity which emerged. Temptations should not release of which art permits, shall not be necessarily associated with Freud's Oedipal theory but, rather, with a desire to become homogenous with the natural forces found both in the world and the depths of the individual's mind. For example, we can see in the Suluk genre that the poet is able to enter the wilds and become associated with animals while increasing his own virtue: "I have folk [to keep me company] without you; swift wolf, sleek, spotted [panther]; and shaggy-maned, loping [hyena]."

The jahiliya poetry was of two forms: the qita and the qasida. It is widely believed that the qita was the original structural model of verses composing. Whilst the qasida rapidly became the most popular one for its fine style and structure, by means of which the poet would exalt oneself or the other distinguishing characters. The term qasida derives from Arabic word root (qa-sa-da) which means "to intend". Qasida points to the basic feature that, the author or the poet does not proceed straight on the subject of his poem but reaches his end in a rather complicated, roundabout way.[41] The verses or lines in the qasida are called "abyat" (literary means houses and its singular is bayt). Each bayt is laid out so as to emphasize the end-rhyme of each line; the gap that separates the two halves of the line indicates the point at which the metrical pattern is represented in accordance with the prosodic system of al-Khalil ibn Ahmed.[42]

Ibn Qutayba explained it as follows: "The composer often begins by describing the deserted habitation of his ancestors. He then weeps for a lost love (separation/nasib) before embarking or describing the trials and

---

[41]   Desomogyi J., A Short History of Classical Arabic Literature, Hildesheim, 1966, p.10.

[42]   Nicholson R., A Literary History of the Arabs, Kitab Bhavan, 1994, p.77.

pain of a desert journey with his camel (liminality/rahil). Very often there is a glorification or praise of the patron, tribe or of the poet's own deeds (aggregation/fakhr), "hija" or satire or lampooning the enemy or rival tribal or "hikam" or moral aphorisms.[43] Suzanne Stetkevych stated that the given consequence resembles a certain a ritual form. Within the verse's corpus, and especially in the fakhr sections we can find the examples of morality, the exaltation of good deeds.

An image in Arabic poetics is not simply a pictorial representation. It is the unification of disparate ideas and emotions into complex spatial instances of time, which aim to strike the reader's sensibility with a momentous impact. The concept of image in Arabic poetry is based on three fundamental principles, which are: direct treatment of the "thing"; unification of disparate ideas and emotions; and formation of new entities to fuse disparate experiences into an organic unity.

In what it concerns the symbolic implication of Arabic verses, it has dual connotations: "symbols may derive from the literal or figurative language which is represented, by virtue of some semblance, suggestion or association means something more or something else."[44] Furthermore, "Symbolism resembles figures of speech in having basic doublings in meaning between what is meant and what is said, but it differs in that what is said also what is meant."[45]

As an example here will be given interpretations of two representative pre-Islamic qasidas from "Seven Muallaqa" for the basic reason that they are considered to be the best poetic collections of the entire Arabic literature. The masterpieces were selected by some eminent experts and were written in golden letters and suspended on the Kaaba, and hence the title "Muallaqa", which can be translated as "suspended". Here is English translation (by Sir Charles Lyall, 1877) of an excerpt of The Muallaqa by Imru al-Qais:

O friend - see the lightning there! It flickered, and now is gone, as though flashed a pair of hands in the pillar of crowned cloud. Nay, was it its blaze, or the lamps of a hermit that dwells alone, and pours o'er the twisted wicks the oil from his slender cruse?

---

[43] Ibn Kutaiba, Kitabu'l' Shi'r wa-'l-Shu'ara,qouated from Nicholson, R. A Literary History of the Arabs, pp. 77-78.

[44] Friedman M., "Symbol" in The New Princeton Encyclopedia of Poetry and Poetics, eds. A. Preminger and T.V.F. Brogan, Princeton: Princeton University Press, 1993,p. 1252.

[45] *Ibid,p. 1253.*

[...]
At earliest dawn on the morrow the birds were chirping blithe,
as though they had drunken draughts of riot in fiery wine;
And at even the drowned beasts lay where the torrent had borne them, dead,
high up on the valley sides, like earth-stained roots of squills.

We can see that this Muallaqa is entirely self-centered, abundant in descriptions of nature's phenomena, such as the thunderstorm, dawn, draught. The Muallaqa depicts poems of the unhappy vagabond prince of Kanda faithfully reflecting the event of his adventurous life. In singing his wanderings, he had ample opportunities to display his talent for depicting natural phenomena and narrating his love in delicate tones.

The next qasida, the Muallaqa of Antara, begins with the description of the place where the poet's beloved had once dwelt, he yearned over it recollecting the memories when she was there and describing the scene of her departure. The nasib of his Muallaqa constitutes verse 1-9 below:

1.   Have the poets left a single spot for a patch to be sown?
Or did you recognize the abode after long meditation
2.   O abode of Abla at El-Jawa let me hear you speak;
I give you good morning, abode of Abla and greetings to you
3.   For there, I halted my she-camel, huge-bodied as a castle
That I might satisfy the hankering and lingerer
4.   While Abla lodged at El-Jawa and our folk dwelt
At El-Hazn and Es-Samman and El-Mutathallim
5.   All hail to you, ruins of a time long since gone by,
Empty and desolate since the day Umm el-Haytham parted
6.   She alight in the land of the bellows and it has become
Very hard for me to seek you out, daughter of Makhram
7.   Casually I fell in love with her as I slew her folk
By your father's life such a declaration is scarce opportune
8.   And you have occupied in my heart, make no doubt of it
That place of one dearly beloved and highly honored
9.   But how visit her, now her people are in spring quarters
At Unaizatan, while ours are dwelling in El Ghailam?
10.   Nothing disquieted me, but that her people burthen beats
Were champing khimklim- berries amid their habitation
11.   Two and forty milch-camel among them all black
As the inner wring feathers of the sable raven

The above nasib (verses 1-9) and a part of ghazal (verses 10-11) depict the way Antara laments the departure of the family of his beloved, who were forced to search for a new home, close to the water. The poet also depicts his beloved in a form of images of fragrance, water, and abundant vegetation. The following verses attest to that:

12.   She takes your hear with the flash edge of her smile,
Her mouth, sweet to the kiss, sweet to the taste
13.   As if a draft of must from a specimen's pouch
Announced the wet gleam of her inner teeth
14.   Or an untouched meadow bloom and grass,
Sheltered in rain, untrodden, dung free hidden
15.   Over it the white, first clouds of spring
Pour down, leaving small pools like silver dirhams.
16.   Pouring and bursting, evening on evening,
Gushing over it in an endless stream
17.   The fly has it all to himself, and is not about to leave,
Droning softly, like a wine drinker humming a tune,
18.   The buzzing, elbow on elbow like a one-armed man,
Kindling a fire, bent down over the flint

In portraying his beloved, Antara in verse 13 he centralizes an image of the wet mouth of Abla. Verse 14 is related to her inner teeth "awaridaha", thus evoking a strong image of her open, wet mouth. This image leads to other sensorial analogies. The garden scene compares between the taste of her wet mouth and the scent of musk. The language, which Antara uses to describe Abla changes from erotic into purifying. He views the garden as untouched "unuf" and the clouds that water it are virgin "bikr". This qasida, like many others, starts with the separation, and symbolizes the end of union of two lovers.

By and large, the pre-Islamic worldview is a foundation, on which the subsequent layers of a Muslim identity are posited. He lives it and finds satisfaction in it.

CHAPTER 4

ADVENT OF ISLAM

The rise of Islam was a turning point for the Arabs, as well as the beginning of new transformations, which affected the perception of their selves and the world. It favoured the restructuralization of the archaic elements, which were dominating the jahiliya psyche, into a cohesive and dynamic source of the Islamic being.

Muhamed himself did not recognize idols. Symbolically he put an end to shirk in Mecca by destructing 360 idols, which had been placed in the Kaaba. Then, after his own Tawaf (circumambulation) of the sanctuary, he noticed images of Ibrahim and Ismail throwing "divination arrows" and likewise ordered that all images be removed.[46] Therefore, the history of the Islamic civilization starts with the birth of Muhamed. The Table 4.1. provides the chronological timeline of its main events.

The history narrates that the Prophet Muhamed was born to the Quraysh family in Mecca around year 570. At his forties, Muhamed started receiving the messages from the angel Gibrael, which marks the beginning of Quran revelation. At first, Muhamed's mission was not widely supported by the Meccans. Moreover, it was severely opposed. In 618, after the death of his uncle Abu Talib, Muhamed was obliged to flee to the city of Yathrib (eventually named Medina) where he could establish the new Islamic society respecting all Quranic laws. In Yathrib, Muhamed was welcomed as a wise man and arbitrator. He was continuing receiving

---

[46] Mubarakpuri S., The Sealed Nectar, Darrussalam International Publications, 2002, p.348.

revelations, which were attesting to his place among the God`s prophets, but also differentiated the message of the Quran from Christianity and Judaism. During this time and until his death in 632, the most influential tribal chiefs of the Arabian peninsula were entering into agreements with him to acknowledge his prophethood and agree to follow Islam.

Revelation of Quran

The Arabic word for revelation is *wahi*. Linguistics defines the word wahi as "a quick indication", "to give or convey a message" or "gentle speech". Whilst Islamic tradition interprets wahi as Allah's message conveyed to the chosen persons. The Quran, accepted as the eternal word of God, contains the whole of God`s final revelation to man.[47]

As his mother Aminah, gazed at her first son, she heard a voice "The best of mankind has been born, so name him Mohamed."[48] Since the childhood, Muhamed was distinct from his peers. He was highly conscious and frank with the people around him, he used to listen more than talk. As a young man, Muhamad would be called "al-Sadiq" (the Truthful One) and "al-Amin" (the Trustworthy One)[49]. Since the situation in his society was gradually degrading, Muhamed could not help reflecting upon it. Until the time when he was nearly forty, he was intentionally isolating himself from the outside world and was spending hours in meditation over the concerns such as, social unrest, injustice, discrimination (particularly against women), fighting among tribes and abuse of tribal authorities prevalent in pre-Islamic Arabia.

Table 4.1 Timeline of the Arabo-Islamic Civilization

(All dates given in the table are those of the Christian calendar)

Year	Historical event
570	The Prophet Mohammad is born in Mecca
622	The Prophet and followers emigrate to Medina. The first year of Islamic calendar
632	Death of the Prophet
632	Muslim armies consolidate their power over Arabia

---

[47] Arberry A., Revelation and Reason in Islam, Routledge, 1957, p.11

[48] Storm M., Agent Storm: My Life Inside al-Qaeda, Grove Press, 2015, p.44.

[49] Storm M., Agent Storm: My Life Inside al-Qaeda, Grove Press, 2015, p.44.

634–644	Muslim forces advance through the Persian and Byzantine empires
636	Battle of Yarmuk. Byzantine emperor Heraclius is defeated by Muslim army in Syria
642	Arabs conquer Byzantine Egypt and expand into North Africa
656	Mohammad's son-in-law, Ali, succeeds to the leadership of Islam
661–750	Umayyads rule in Damascus
711	Tariq with a mixed force of Arabs and Berbers invades Spain
712	Muslims advance into Sind (modern-day Pakistan) and Central Asia
725	Muslims occupy Nimes in France
756–929	Umayyad emirs rule in Spain
762	Al-Mansur founds Baghdad
786	Haroun al-Rashid becomes caliph in Baghdad
792	The first papermaking factory in the Muslim Empire is built in Baghdad
813–823	Al-Mamun reigns in Baghdad. He founds the House of Wisdom
823	Beginning of Muslim conquest of Sicily
909–1171	Fatimids expand in North Africa
929–1031	Umayyad caliphate reigns in Spain
969	Fatimids conquer Egypt and transfer their capital to Cairo
973 976	Al-Azhar university is founded in Cairo
1058	Seljuks take Baghdad
1090	Cordoba is sacked by Almoravids
1096	First Crusade. Christians rule in Jerusalem in 1099
1145–1232	Almohads rule in Spain
1171	Saladin overthrows the Fatimids in Egypt
1171–1250	Ayyubid Dynasty rules in Egypt and Syria
1187	Saladin returns Jerusalem to Arab–Islamic rule
1206–1406	Mongol Empire
1492	Christian Reconquest of Spain
1453–1922	Ottoman Empire
1494–1566	Suleiman I guides the Ottoman Empire to its fullest extent, ranging from Morocco to the Caspian Sea and the Persian Gulf and into Europe through the Balkans to Hungary
1922	The end of the Ottoman Empire

Muhamed's first revelation opened the initial page in the history of Islam. That night Muhamed saw the archangel Gabriel who commanded Muhamed to read a verse (which are the first lines of the sura 96) from the Quran. The archangel said: "Read", to which he replied, "I am unable to read". Thereupon the angel held him and embraced heavily. It happened two more times and the angel commanded Muhamed to recite theses verses:

"Proclaim! In the name of thy Lord and Cherisher, Who created-
man, out of a clot of congealed blood:
Proclaim! And thy Lord is Most Bountiful,-
Who taught by the pen-
Taught man that which he knew not." (sura 96, ayats 1–5)

The event occurred in the cave called Hira, which is the "Jabal an-Nour" mountain, near Mecca. The revelation of the Quran was sent during the Laila al-qadr in Ramadan (one of the odd nights after the 21st till the end of Ramadan).

This is what the Quran tells about Muhamed's experience (sura 53, ayats 4-9):

"It is no less than inspiration sent down to him:
He was taught by one Mighty in Power,
Endued with Wisdom: for he appeared (in stately form);
While he was in the highest part of the horizon:
Then he approached and came closer,
And was at a distance of but two bow-lengths or (even) nearer."

Muhamed was ready to accept his mission even earlier the time when Gabriel came to visit him. Being well aware of the Gabriel's status among the other God's angels, Muhamed understood this as a signal to start. However, what really perplexed him was the inevitable opposition on the way to professing Islam.

Anxious and trembling after this experience, Muhamed headed home to confess to his wife Khadijah of what had happened. He said, "Cover me! Cover me!" She covered him till his fear was over and after that, he told her everything that had happened, "I fear that something may happen to me". Khadija replied, "Never! By Allah, Allah will never disgrace you. You keep good relations with your kith and kin, help the poor and the destitute, serve your guests generously and assist the deserving calamity-afflicted ones."[50] Having comforted him, they went to her Ebionite cousin

---

50   Akhtar M., Oracle of the Last and Final Message: History and the Philosophical Deductions of the Life of Prophet Muhammad, 2008, Xlibris, p.77.

Waraqa ibn Nawfal. Waraqa was knowledgeable about the Jewish and Christian traditions. Khadija said to Waraqa, "Listen to the story of your nephew, O my cousin!" Waraqa said, "O my nephew! What did you see?" When Muhamed told him what had happened to him, Waraqa replied, "This is Namus (meaning Gabriel) that Allah sent to Moses. I wish I were younger. I wish I could live up to the time when your people would turn you out." Muhamed asked, "Will they drive me out?" Waraqa answered affirmatively and added, "Anyone who came with something similar to what you have brought was treated with hostility; and if I should be alive until that day, then I would support you strongly." A few days later Waraqa died.

The following lines describe Ibn Ishaq narrating about Muhamed's first meeting with Gabriel: When it was the night on which God honoured him with his mission and showed mercy on His servants thereby, Gabriel brought him the command of God[51]. "He came to me", said the apostle of God, "while I was asleep, with a coverlet of brocade whereon was some writing, and said, "Read!" I said" "What shall I read?" He pressed me with it so tightly that I thought it was death; then he let me go and said, "Read!" I said, "What shall I read?" He pressed me with it again so that I thought it was death; then he let me go and said, "Read!" I said, "What shall I read?" He pressed me with it the third time so that I thought it was death and said, "Read!" I said, "What then shall I read?"—and this I said only to deliver myself from him, lest he should do the same to me again. He said, "Read in the name of thy Lord who created, Who created man of blood coagulated. Read! Thy Lord is the most beneficent, Who taught by the pen, Taught that which they knew not unto men." So I read it, and he departed from me. And I awoke from my sleep, and it was as though these words were written on my heart. Now none of God's creatures was more hateful to me than an (ecstatic) poet or a man possessed: I could not even look at them[52]. I thought, Woe is me poet or possessed—Never shall Quraysh say this of me! I will go to the top of the mountain and throw myself down that I may kill myself and gain rest. So I went forth to do so and then when I was midway on the mountain, I heard a voice from heaven saying, "O Muhammad! thou art the apostle of God and I am Gabriel."[53]

[51]   Peters F., Muhammad and the Origins of Islam, State University of New York Press, 1994, p.148.

[52]   Gabriel R., Muhammad: Islam's First Great General, University of Oklahoma Press: Norman, 2007, p.65.

[53]   Ibn Ishaq, Sirat Rasul Allah, Oxford University Press, 1955, p. 106.

According to Tabari and Ibn Ishaq, Muhammad told Zubayr[54]:"When I was midway on the mountain, I heard a voice from heaven saying "O Muhamed! you are the apostle of Allah and I am Gabriel." I raised my head towards heaven to see who was speaking, and Gabriel in the form of a man with feet astride the horizon, saying, "O Muhamed! you are the apostle of Allah and I am Gabriel." I stood gazing at him moving neither forward nor backward, then I began to turn my face away from him, but towards whatever region of the sky I looked, I saw him as before."

The cessation period between the first revelation and the next one (called fatra) lasted for three years (in accordance to Ibn Ishaq). It resumed with the first verses of chapter 74 when Muhamad heard a voice from the sky and saw the same angel "sitting between the sky and the earth"[55].

Narrated Jabir bin Abdullah Al-Ansari while talking about the period of pause in revelation reporting the speech of the Prophet, "While I was walking, all of a sudden I heard a voice from the heaven. I looked up and saw the same angel who had visited me at the Cave of Hira sitting on a chair between the sky and the earth. I got afraid of him and came back home and said "Wrap me (in blankets)" and then Allah revealed the following holy verses (of the Quran): O you covered in your cloak, arise and warn (the people against Allah's punishment) ... up to "and all pollution shun."[56]

After this revelations were coming regularly. Bukhari considers the sura 74 as the second revelation, even though, the sura 68 has strong claims to be the second revelation. However, many experts maintain that sura Al-Muzzammil (73) was the next revelation. According to others, sura Al-Fatiha (1) was the third sura to be revealed[57]. Among other early revelations, which the Prophet declared in Mecca, are, according to some sources, sura 111, sura 81, sura 87, sura 92, sura 89, etc. Then revelation continued, "mentioning Paradise and Hell, and until mankind turned to Islam, then came revelation about halal and haram ... "[58]

---

[54] Rosenwein B., Reading the Middle Ages, Volume I: Sources from Europe, Byzantium, and the Islamic World, c.300 to c.1150, University of Toronto Press, 2013, p.116.

[55] Mahmoud O., Muhammad: an evolution of God, AuthorHouse, 2008, p.31.

[56] Von Denffer A., Ulum al Qur'an: An Introduction to the Sciences of the Qur'an, The Islamic Foundation, 1994, p.14.

[57] Von Denffer A., Ulum al Qur'an: An Introduction to the Sciences of the Qur'an, The Islamic Foundation, 1994, p.15.

[58] *Ibid*

Many Muslim scholars agree that the last revelation was sura 2, verse 281:[59] "And fear the day when ye shall be brought back to God. Then shall every soul be paid what it earned and none shall be dealt with unjustly." Some also say that it was 2:282 or 2:278[60]. There was also an assumption that all three verses were revealed on one occasion. The Prophet died nine nights after the last revelation.[61] Others hold that sura 5:4 was the last to be revealed:[62] "This day I have perfected your religion for you, completed My favour upon you and have chosen for you Islam as your religion." In conformity with the hadith from Umar, this verse cannot be the last revelation, since it was sent during the final pilgrimage of the Prophet. Suyuti explains concerning the verse in sura 5 that after it nothing concerning ahkam and halal and haram was revealed, and in this sense it is the "completion" of religion.[63]

The revelations were being conveyed to the Prophet throughout his lifetime, both in Mecca and Madina, i.e. over a period of approximately 23 years,[64] until shortly before his death in the year 10 after Hijra (632). There were chosen different manners to transmit the God`s message to Muhamed, in particular in a form of:

1.   Dreams:

Prophet Muhamed used to receive clear revelations of the Holy Quran in the form of dreams.[65] Ayesha narrates that the beginning of wahi began in the form of true dreams. The next morning after dreaming, the Prophet`s dream would become clear (Bukhari).

2.   Directly into the heart:

The Prophet also used to have deep insights. Imaam Hakim narrates that the Prophet stated: "Angel Gibraeel conveyed a message into my heart.

---

[59]   *Ibid*

[60]   Kamal A., Adil: 'ulum al-Qur'an, 1974, p.18, consulted on 01.05.2016

[61]   http://www.irfi.org/articles3/articles_4601_4700/revelation%20and%20 how%20it%20came%20to%20prophet%20muhammadhtml.htm, consulted on 01.07.2016

[62]   Journal of Global Religious Vision, International Centre for Religious Studies, 2001, vol. 2, p.133.

[63]   Von Denffer A., Ulum al Qur'an: An Introduction to the Sciences of the Qur'an, The Islamic Foundation, 1994, p.16.

[64]   Al-Azri K., Social and Gender Inequality in Oman. The Power of Religious and Political Tradition, Routledge, 2013, p.22.

[65]   http://www.sacred-texts.com/isl/hadith/had04.htm,   consulted   on 01.07.2016

That no man can die until his "rizk" or resources have been completed. So Man should fear God and try all means to achieve his resources. If there is a delay in receiving your due then do not go astray to achieve it for whatever you will receive will be through Allah and what he has already ordained."*

3. Revelations, which followed the sound of a bell:

Another way of revelation came down after the sound of a bell. The Prophet would hear the ringing of a bell or a musical instrument, which would be immediately followed by divine revelation. According to Ayesha once the divine revelation began, Angel Gibraeel would come at various times with different ayats of the Quran. According to her, the Prophet himself stated that "Sometimes wahi comes to me after a bell rings and that is a heavy time for me." This way of revelation happened to be the most challenging for the Prophet. If he was mounted on a camel and received revelation after the ringing of a bell, the camel would be unable to bear its weight and be forced to come down upon its knees[66]. On another occasion it is narrated by Hadrat Zaid bin Thabit that the Prophet's thigh was resting on his thigh at the time of receiving wahi. The force of the revelation was so strong that it felt as if his own thigh was breaking. Ayesha also reports that during these occasions the Prophet's brow would sweat or that his face would become very red.[67]

4. Revelation in the form of a Man:

The most common way of receiving revelation was through Angel Gibraeel. The Quran states:

"Say: Whoever is an enemy to Gibraeel – for he brings down the (revelation)to thy heart by Allah's will, a confirmation of what went before, and guidance and glad tidings for those who believe, - Whoever is an enemy to Allah and His angels and apostles, to Gibraeel and Michale, - Lo! Allah is an enemy to those who reject faith." (sura 2, ayats 97-98)

Angel Gibrail would sometimes come to the Prophet in the form of a man[68]. Ummi Salma reports that, "once I saw Dhaya Qalbi in front of the Prophet talking to him. The Prophet then asked me, "Do you know who this man is?" I replied, "That was Dhaya Qalbi" By God I thought

---

[66] *According to hadiths of Al-Mustadarak lil-Hakim
**According to Imam Muslim"Bab-ul-Miraj"
http://hadithway.com/Mecca08.html, consulted on 30.04.2016

[67] http://hadithcollection.com/sahihbukhari.html, consulted on 01.05.2016

[68] As-Sallaabee A., The Noble Life of the Prophet, Darussalam, vol. 1, 2005, p.141.

it was him but the Prophet of God later announced in his Kutbah it was the Angle Gibraeel"[69]

5.   Revelation through an Angel in his true form:

Angel Gibrail also came to the Prophet in his actual angelic form. Abdullah ibn Masood narrates that Prophet Muhamad said, "When I saw Angel Gibraeel he had 600 wings"**

6.   Revelation directly from God:

God has directly communicated with some of His Prophets as with Prophet Musa on Mount Toor.[70] Allah talked directly about the obligation of five daily prayers to Muhamad during his ascent into the heavens (the Miraj Night). Here we observe a peculiar system of communication between Allah and His Chosen people. Initially, Allah contacts His Prophet through dreams. Then the revelation reaches his heart. Afterwards, the Angel Gibrail is sent down with the revelation in the form of a man. As the contact between Prophet and Allah strengthens, Angel Gibrail descends on the earth and appears himself in front of the Prophet's eyes. Finally, Allah calls His Prophet to the heavens and talks to him, which is known as Miraj-an-Nabi.

Besides the Quran, Muslims draw information on day-to-day Islamic practices from another prime source, which is the hadith (literally means "speech"). These are the recorded sayings of Muhamad certified by isnad; which with Sirah Rasul Allah form the suna and Islamic law sharia. As Aisha confirms, the life of Muhamed was the practical implementation of Quran.

The Quranic verses were preserved till nowadays through memorization. Muhamed was making sure that he retained well the revealed passages, for these means he would be revising them numerous times. This practice is known as hifz: "...an apostle from God, rehearsing scriptures, kept pure and holy...(sura 98, ayat 2). He would recite them to his allies and followers. The Arabs, although being illiterate, cherished poetry more than anything else. So, it was fun for them to memorize ayats in order to communicate them to others, which was encouraged by the Prophet. Hadrat Uthman bin Affan narrates the Prophet as saying the most superior amongst the Companions were those who learn the Quran and then taught it to others[71]. The ayats were daily recited in five prayers, so, as it

---

[69]   http://hadithcollection.com/sahihbukhari.html, consulted on 01.05.2016

[70]   http://hubpages.com/religion-philosophy/Does-Allah-God-Speak-To-Us, consulted on 01.07.2016

[71]   *According to Zaid bin Thabbit

Bukhari S., book 61: Virtues of the Quran

---

seems, there was no difficulty with memorization of Quran. The Prophet delighted in listening to his Companions reciting Quran. Hadrat Ibn Masud affirms that once Prophet shed tears after listening to his recitation of sura Nisa.

During the lifetime of the Prophet, Quran began to be inscribed on different materials. These varied from pieces of parchment to leather and leaves*. Once a passage engraved, the Prophet personally checked its correctness and order. Hadrat ibn Abbas[72] reports that Hadrat Othman bin Affan stated that when the Prophet received revelation he would call a companion to write it down and then tell them where to place the ayat in the Quran. Imam Ahmad bin Hanbal reports the narration of Hadrat Othman bin abi-ul-Aas as follows, "I was once sitting with the Prophet when he received revelation. Then he lowered his eyes and the Prophet stated that "Angel Gibrail has come to me and ordered that I should place this ayat with this sura. Quran, as the greatest book of Muslims, has its precise structural organization. Regarding the order of sura's appearance in Quran, it is believed to be established by Allah. It has been recorded that the Prophet reviewed the Quran with the archangel Gabriel 24 times all within his life[73]. Muhamed was reviewing it during Ramadan with Gabriel. And Gabriel revised the Quran twice with the Prophet during the last Ramadan of his life. So, the Prophet followed this order of Quran, which is preserved till nowadays (see Table 4.2).

Table 4.2 Revelation Order of the Quran

Revelation Order	Sura Number	Sura Name
1	96	Alaq
2	68	Qalam
3	73	Muzammil
4	74	Mudathir
5	1	Fatehah
6	111	Lahab
7	81	Takwir
8	87	Ala

[72] Al Hindi Ali, Kanz al umal,Beyt Al Afkar, 2005, p.79.

[73] http://www.missionislam.com/quran/revealationorder.htm, consulted on 01.07.2016

9	92	Leyl
10	89	Fajr
11	93	Duha
12	94	Inshira
13	103	Asr
14	100	Aadiyat
15	108	Kauthar
16	102	Takatur
17	107	Alma'un
18	109	Kafirun
19	105	Fil
20	113	Falaq
21	114	Nas
22	112	Iklas
23	53	Najm
24	80	Abasa
25	97	Qadr
26	91	Shams
27	85	Buruj
28	95	Tin
29	106	Qureysh
30	101	Qariah
31	75	Qiyamah
32	104	Humazah
33	77	Mursalat
34	50	Qaf
35	90	Balad
36	86	Tariq
37	54	Qamr
38	38	Sad
39	7	Araf
40	72	Jinn
41	36	Yasin
42	25	Furqan
43	35	Fatir
44	19	Maryam

45	20	Ta Ha
46	56	Waqiah
47	26	Shuara
48	27	Naml
49	28	Qasas
50	17	Bani Israil
51	10	Yunus
52	11	Hud
53	12	Yousuf
54	15	Hijr
55	6	Anam
56	37	Saffat
57	31	Luqman
58	34	Saba
59	39	Zumar
60	40	Mumin
61	41	Hamim Sajdah
62	42	Shura
63	43	Zukhruf
64	44	Dukhan
65	45	Jathiyah
66	46	Ahqaf
67	51	Dhariyat
68	88	Ghashiya
69	18	Kahf
70	16	Nahl
71	71	Noah
72	14	Ibrahim
73	21	Anbiya
74	23	Muminun
75	32	Sajdah
76	52	Tur
77	67	Mulk
78	69	Haqqah
79	70	Maarij
80	78	Naba

81	79	Naziat
82	82	Infitar
83	84	Inshiqaq
84	30	Rum
85	29	Ankabut
86	83	Tatfif
87	2	Baqarah
88	8	Anfal
89	3	Aal-e-Imran
90	33	Ahzab
91	60	Mumtahana
92	4	Nisa
93	99	Zilzal
94	57	Hadid
95	47	Muhammad
96	13	Rad
97	55	Rahman
98	76	Dahr
99	65	Talaq
100	98	Beyinnah
101	59	Hashr
102	24	Nur
103	22	Hajj
104	63	Munafiqun
105	58	Mujadila
106	49	Hujurat
107	66	Tahrim
108	64	Taghabun
109	61	Saff
110	62	Jumah
111	48	Fath
112	5	Maidah
113	9	Taubah
114	110	Nasr

On balance, it took over twenty-three years for the Quran to be revealed and structured, which did not happen in one single act, but in continuous stages. And there are a number of reasons for that:

- To show continuous guidance and true support to the Prophet as different life circumstances arose;
- To implement the laws of God steadily;
- To give more time for the Muslims to perceive, realize and memorize the revelation;
- Out of consideration for the Prophet, for who revelation was, truly, challenging experience.

Hijra

Muhamed`s prophecy did not receive acceptance from all of his people, moreover, he fell under persecution in his native town. To survive, he was obliged to flee from Mecca, which nominated the beginning of Hijra ("Emigration"). Hijra is the Prophet Muhamad's dislocation (622) from Mecca to Medina in order to escape persecution.[74]

The ill-wishers of Muhamed were deciding on the most effective way to eliminate the peril that Muhamed had brought in with the monotheistic faith. So, they agreed to kill Muhamed himself. The consensus was reached that one warrior from each clan in Mecca and its suburbs, would attack the house of Muhamed at once, and kill him before dawn. However, the Prophet was well aware of this conspiration plan owing to one convert, who had warned Mohamed in advance. Ali ibn Abi Talib suggested his own plan to circumvent the Quraysh. He advised to put Ali in the Prophet`s bed, and then flee the house when an opportunity presents itself.

The Quraysh, seeing Ali covered in a mantle, would imagine that Muhamad was sleeping, he explained[75]. He also asked Ali to restore all the deposits of the pagans to their owners, and then to leave Mecca and to meet him in Yathrib[76].

Muhamed Husayn Haykal was the young men whom the Quraysh had prepared for performing Muhamed's assassination had blockaded his house during the night lest he ran away. On the night of the Hijrah, Muhamed confided his plan to Ali ibn Abi Talib and asked him to cover himself with

---

[74] http://www.britannica.com/event/Hijrah-Islam, consulted on 31.04.2016

[75] Razwy A., A Restatement of the History of Islam and Muslims, World Federation of Khoja ShiaIthna-Asheri Muslim, 2001, p.87.

[76] *Ibid*

the Prophet's green mantle, and to sleep in the Prophet's bed.[77] Muhamed also asked to return all deposits, stored at Muhamed`s, to their owners, and only then come to join them in Yathrib. That said, he gave his cloak to Ali, bidding him lie down on the bed so that anyone looking in might think Muhamad lay there.[78]

When the night fell down, the instigators encircled Muhamed`s house. They approached it closer to make sure that the figure covered in a blanket was sleeping. The Prophet managed to escape the ambush after the inflamers had dozed off. He silently walked through them and out of the precincts of his house[79]. Muhamed left Mecca unnoticed.

Ali kept sleeping in the Prophet`s bed until the dawn, that is when the pagans woke up and intended to kill him. However, they discovered that there was Ali, instead of Muhamed. They were more than overwhelmed and decided not to kill him, but to find out where Muhamed was. Not having received the information, and only wasted time, they let Ali go. In remembrance of this event and appreciation of Ali`s readiness to self-sacrifice, the following Quranic verse was revealed:

"And among men, there is one who sells his life to win the pleasure of Allah. Allah is very kind to His devotees." (sura 2, ayat 207)

When Muhamed`s house was far behind, he went to Abu Bakr, and told him that Allah had ordered him to leave Mecca as well. So, together they advanced to the city and hid in a cave called Thaur (in the south of Mecca) while it was still dark.

According to tradition, a spider had spun its web across the entrance to the cave, and a bird had laid an egg at it.[80] The Quraysh, who were already searching for Muhamed, were persuaded that nobody could have entered the cave during the last night. And if anyone had entered it, the web and the egg would have been broken, but since both were intact, no one had been in there. Thus they returned to Mecca. While the Quraysh were debating outside, Abu Bakr addressed to Muhamed, "We are only two and our enemies are so many. What chance we have of saving our lives if they

---

[77] Haykal M., The Life of Muhammad, American Trust Publications, 1935, p. 157.

[78] Razwy A., A Restatement of the History of Islam and Muslims, World Federation of Khoja ShiaIthna-Asheri Muslim, 2001, p.87.

[79] *Ibid, p.88.*

[80] Storm M., Agent Storm: My Life Inside al-Qaeda, Grove Press, 2015, p.44.

enter the cave?"[81] The latter said, "No. We are not two. There is a Third One with us, and He is Allah." This occurrence is present in Al-Quran al-Majid as follows:

"And God helped His Apostle when the unbelievers banished him. And when they were in the cave, he said to the second of the two: "do not be grief-stricken. God is with us." And God bestowed His peace upon him (upon His Apostle)." (sura 9, ayat 40)

They had to spend three days hiding in the cave.[82] The Meccans were no longer searching for the fugitives. On the fourth day, Abdullah, the son of Abu Bakr, appeared with two camels and offered them. But the Apostle refused to ride an animal which was not his own, and when Abu Bakr wanted to give him it, he demanded to know what he had paid for it and bought it from him.[83] By riding camels they reached Quba on the tenth day, a place, which is in the south of Yathrib, where they were accommodated by Kulthum bin Hind. The Apostle preferred to enter Yathrib together with Ali, so he accepted the Kulthum`s hospitality and waited at his house for Ali`s return. While waiting, he proceeded with the arrangement of the first mosque ever, which happened to be in Quba. The Prophet was engaged with construction process during fourteen days.

When the Prophet entered Yathrib, he was welcomed by his supporters, which later came to be known as the anṣar ("helpers"). They were Medinese who aided Muhamad and other muhajirun (immigrants) to settle down. The anṣar belonged to two major Medinese tribes, which are al-Khazraj and al-Aws. They came to be his devoted supporters.

The significance of hijra is not limited exclusively to Islamic history or to Muslims only. The hijra not only reshaped – socially and politically – the Arab Peninsula but also had its impact on worldwide civilizations.[84]

Hijra marked a transitional period between the era of Mecca and the era of Madina, which, essentially, means the transition to a new Islamic way of life, which combined politics, economy, social and marital relations. Islam positioned itself as a complete religion in form of:

---

[81]   Razwy A., A Restatement of the History of Islam and Muslims, World Federation of Khoja ShiaIthna-Asheri Muslim, 2001, p.88.

[82]   Lipovsky I., The Socialist Movement in Turkey: 1960-1980, Brill, 1996, p.222.

[83]   Haykal M., The Life of Muhammad, American Trust Publications, 1935, p.158.

[84]   http://www.irfi.org, consulted on 01.07.2016

- Shift in the perception of Muslims from a tribal structure to a regional power;
- Transformation into a strong Islamic nation (umma), and, a state, consequently;
- Passing on to the world level alongside with Islam`s expansion reaching out Persia, Egypt, the Byzantine Empire etc.

The date the Prophet left Mecca embodies the beginning of the Muslim calendar and the start of the Islamic era. It was Umar I, the second caliph, who in the year 639 introduced the Hijra era (now recognized by its initials ah or anno Hegirae, "in the year of Hijra"). Umar started the first year *ah* with the first day of the lunar month of Muḥarram, which corresponds to July 16, 622, on the Julian calendar. The calendar has twelve lunar months, the beginnings and endings of which are determined by the appearance of the crescent moon.

Islamic months begin at sunset of the first day, the day when the lunar crescent is visible with naked eye. The lunar year lasts around 354 days, so the months rotate backward through the seasons and are not fixed to the Gregorian calendar.[85]

The months of the Islamic year are named in this way:

1. Muharram ("Forbidden" –during this month it is forbidden to wage war or fight)
2. Safar ("Empty" or "Yellow")
3. Rabi' Awal ("First spring")
4. Rabi' Thani ("Second spring")
5. Jumada Awal ("First freeze")
6. Jumada Thani ("Second freeze")
7. Rajab ("To respect" – this is another holy month when fighting is prohibited)
8. Shaaban ("To spread and distribute")
9. Ramadan ("Parched thirst" – this is the month of daytime fasting)
10. Shawwal ("To be light and vigorous")
11. Dhul-Qidah ("The month of rest" – another month when warfare is not allowed)
12. Dhul-Hijja ("The month of Hajj" – this is the month of pilgrimage to Mecca, again when fighting is prohibited).

---

[85] http://www.irfi.org/articles/articles_451_500/significance_of_the_hijrah.htm, consulted on 01.07.2016

In any event, hijra personifies changing to a better situation with assured support coming from above. It does not mean to rest on one's laurels once the destination is reached. Rather, to finally find one's own (aspired and promised) place so that to deepen the belief in one's own mission and to proceed further even stronger and better. That is exactly what the Prophet did, having reached Medina. He laid the first stone of creation of a God-fearful and powerful Islamic society.

The Death of Prophet

Muhamed was expecting his death after he received such prediction in sura "Nasr": "When comes the help of God, and victory, And thou dost see the people enter God's religion in crowds, Celebrate the praises of thy Lord, And pray for His Forgiveness: For He is oft-Returning (in grace and mercy)."

Imam Bukhari reports that when this chapter was revealed, Umar bin al-Khattab asked Abdullah ibn Abbas if he could enlighten him on its meaning. Ibn Abbas said: "These verses mean that the time for the Messenger of God to part company with us is approaching."[86]

Nothing was ever so blissful to him in his last days as prayers and expressions of deepest devotion to Allah, who he was preparing to meet after his decease.

The Prophet was alluding to his imminent decease when:

1. In his address of the Farewell Pilgrimage in Arafat on Friday, the 9th of Dhil-Hajj, 10 A..H., he said: "Perhaps, this is my last Hajj."[87]

In concluding his speech, he posed a question to the pilgrims, "When you are questioned by your Lord about my work, what will be your answer?" The pilgrims shouted with one voice: "You delivered the message of God to us, and you performed your duty." When he heard this answer, he lifted his gaze toward Heaven, and said, "O God! Be Thou a Witness that I have done my duty"[88]

At the "coronation" of Ali ibn Abi Talib at Ghadeer-Khumm, on 18th of Dhil-Hajj, 10 A.H., Muhammad stated, "I am also a mortal, and I may be summoned into the presence of my Lord any moment".[89] Thousands of Muslims understood that the time for the Prophet to leave

---

[86] Razwy A., A Restatement of the History of Islam and Muslims, World Federation of Khoja ShiaIthna-Asheri Muslim, 2001, p.198.

[87] *Ibid, p.197.*

[88] *Ibid, p.196.*

[89] *Ibid, p.200.*

was approaching. Muhamed had accomplished his mission, and nothing else could have impeded him from meeting his Lord. The Prophet kept going with his life, as usual. He spent his nights with his various wives by turns. On the 19th of Safar of 11 A.H., he was supposed to sleep in the Ayesha`s room. Before visiting her, Muhamed stopped by the cemetery of Al-Baqi accompanied by his servant, Abu Muwayhiba, who later narrated that "The Apostle stood between the graves and addressed them in the following words: "Peace be upon you who are in these graves. Blessed are you in your present state to which you have emerged from the state in which the people live on earth. Subversive attacks are falling one after another like waves of darkness, each worse than the previous ones"[90].

Muhamad Husayn Haykal said that the Prophet had fallen terribly sick in the morning after the night`s avowal at the cemetery, i.e. on 20th of Safar. He further added, "It was then that the people became concerned and the army of Usama did not move. True, the report of Abu Muwayhiba is doubted by many historians who believe that Muhamed's sickness could not have been the only reason that prevented the army from marching to Al-Sham, that another cause was the disappointment of many, including a number of senior Muhajireen and Ansar, in regard to the leadership of the army."[91]

The following incident appears to have taken place on the morning of the 20th of Safar: One night the Prophet walked to the burial ground in the outskirts of the city. There he waited long absorbed in meditation and praying for the dead. In the morning, passing by the door of Ayesha, who was suffering from a severe headache, he heard her moaning: my head! oh, my head! He entered and said: "Nay, Ayesha, it is rather I that have to cry my head, my head!"[92] Then in a tender strain: "But wouldst thou not desire to be taken whilst I am yet alive; so that I might pray over thee, and wrapping thee, Ayesha, in thy winding sheet, thus commit thee to the grave?"

"That happen to another," exclaimed Ayesha, "and not to me!" archly adding: "Ah, that is what thou art desirous of! Truly, I can fancy thee, after having done all this and buried me, return straightway to my house, and spend that very evening in sporting in my place with another wife!". The

---

[90] Haykal M., The Life of Muhammad, American Trust Publications, 1935, p. 477.

[91] *Ibid, p.478.*

[92] Razwy A., A Restatement of the History of Islam and Muslims, World Federation of Khoja ShiaIthna-Asheri Muslim, 2001, p.232.

Prophet smiled at Ayesha's raillery, but his sickness pressed on him too heavily to admit of a rejoinder in the same strain.[93]

The pain was coming and going as he was visiting his other wives, like always. On the 24th of Safar he paid the visit to his wife Maymuna. At that time a sudden severe headache struck him and the body temperature increased. Then he called upon all his wives and asked them to gather in the chamber of Ayesha. So, they obeyed. Ali and Abbas stood by his sides, as he was too weak to walk alone, and helped him to move to the apartment of Ayesha, where he would meet his death in the end. No matter how weak the Prophet felt himself, he was not missing the prayers at the mosque and was leading the Muslims in prayer. On the 26th of Safar, supported by Ali and Abbas, Muhamed was resolve to lead the zuhr (midday) prayer. At the end of the prayer, he addressed the umma, adding the following: "With Allah, the months are twelve; four of them are holy; three of these are successive and one occurs singly between the months of Jumada and Shaban." (Al Bukhari)

Abu Bakr who was present during his speech understood that the Prophet's days are counted and he could not help crying. To which the Prophet responded, "I am more grateful to Abu Bakr than to anyone else for his material and moral support, and for his companionship. If in this umma, I were ever to choose any man for a friend, I would have chosen him. But it is not necessary because the Islamic brotherhood is a stronger bond than any other, and it is enough for all of us. And remember that all doors which open into the mosque, should be closed except the door of the chamber of Abu Bakr."[94]

The Prophet warned the Muslims not to relapse into idolatry, and to remember that they were monotheists, and he added, "One thing you must never do, is to worship my grave. Those nations of the past which worshiped the graves of their prophets, earned the wrath of the Lord, and were destroyed. Beware, lest you imitate them."[95]

This was the last time the Prophet appeared in public. The Islamic tradition assumes that during the mosque's speech Muhamed confirmed that he did not intend to make Abu Bakr his successor. Therefore, his statement reads: "If I were to choose a friend, I would choose Abu Bakr. But

---

[93] http://www.alseraj.net/maktaba/kotob/english/historyofislam/ARestatement/html/eng/books/restatment/43.htm, consulted on 31.04.2016

[94] Razwy A., A Restatement of the History of Islam and Muslims, World Federation of Khoja ShiaIthna-Asheri Muslim, 2001, p.234.

[95] Razwy A., A Restatement of the History of Islam and Muslims, World Federation of Khoja ShiaIthna-Asheri Muslim, 2001, p.233.

I am not choosing him. All of us are members of the universal brotherhood of Islam, and that's enough for all of us"[96]. Starting from the next day, Abu Bakr was leading the prayers at the mosque, as the Prophet instructed him. Muhamed himself remained seated during the prayers.

Bukhari claims the following in his hadith:"On the 28th of Safar, Abbas ibn Abdul Muttalib came to see Ali, and said, "By God, Muhamed is soon going to die. I can tell from the expression on the faces of the children of Abdul Muttalib when they are going to die. I, therefore, suggest that you talk to him and ask him about the matter of his succession". But Ali said, "No. Not in the state in which he is now. I do not wish to bring up the subject"[97].

However, the Shias disregard these sayings and believe that the Prophet had announced many times that Ali was to be chosen his successor. In the afternoon, Muhamed Mustafa confessed to Ali, "For me, it is the journey's end. When I die, you wash my body, cover it in a shroud, and lower it into the grave. I owe money to such and such people, among them a Jew who gave me a loan to equip the expedition of Usama. Pay these debts to all of them including the Jew."[98] Muhamed granted his ring, sword, spear, armor, and other weapons to Ali.

Monday, Rabi al-Awwal 1 of 11 Hijri was the last day of Muhamed ibn Abdullah, the Messenger of God, on this earth. Ayesha, his wife, reports the following: "As the day crept up toward noon, Fatima Zahra, the daughter of the Messenger of God, came to see him. He welcomed her and asked her to sit beside him. Then he said something to her which I could not hear but she began to weep. Noticing the tears of his daughter, he said something else to her which again I could not hear but she began to smile. She was so much like her father in temperament, character, and appearance."[99]

Later Ayesha asked Fatima what father`s words said made her cry and smile. Fatima replied: "First my father told me that he was going to die. When I heard this, I began to cry. Then he informed me that I would be

---

[96]   *Ibid, p.234.*

[97]   *Ibid*

[98]   http://www.al-ijtihad.com/library/history%20of%20islam/History%20 Of%20Islam_book.pdf, consulted on 31.04.2016

[99]   http://www.sunnah.org/history/Life-of-Prophet/Life_Story_of_Fatima_ bint_Muhammad.htm, consulted on 01.07.2016

the very first to meet him in heaven, and that too, very soon. When I heard this, I was very happy, and I smiled."[100]

The Western historians reached the conclusion that the Prophet died on June 8, 632, which is the same day (8th July) of his birth.On Tuesday Osama was pouring water on the Prophet`s body and Ali washed it. When finished, Ali wrapped it in a shroud and prayed over it. He then went out and asked the Muslims, who were in the mosque, to go into the chamber and say the funeral prayers. Banu Hashim were the first to offer prayers, and then the Muhajireen and the Ansar carried out this duty.[101] And in the presence of six men, Muhamed was buried. The men, who attended the funerals were Ali ibn Abi Talib, Abbas ibn Abdul Muttalib, Fadl ibn Abbas, Qathm ibn Abbas, Usama bin Zayd bin Haritha, Aws bin Khuli Ansari. The earth was strewn over the grave, and water showered over it.

The farewell procession was carried out in a modest way in the presence of Muhamed`s closest people. However, not all from those, who claimed to be his friends, attended the funerals. Ibn Saad says in his Tabqaat that Ali ibn Abi Talib paid all the debts of Muhammad, the Prophet of Islam[102]. Ali declared that he would pay all Muhamed`s debts. So, anyone, who was coming to him with claims, was receiving compensation. And Ali was not asking for any proof.

Obviously, during the Muhamed`s lifetime, one big epoch in the Arab history closed, and yet another opened. A Man, who stressed on his primary function of passing "the divine" to "the human", symbolized himself the transition from the archaic to the Islamic. He filled in space between the two. He signaled the initiation and led the passage, which marked the incorporation of a Bedouin and his introduction into a new, Islamic setting.

---

[100] Razwy A., A Restatement of the History of Islam and Muslims, World Federation of Khoja ShiaIthna-Asheri Muslim, 2001, p.236.

[101] Razwy A., A Restatement of the History of Islam and Muslims, World Federation of Khoja ShiaIthna-Asheri Muslim, 2001, p.237.

[102] *Ibid, p.238.*

CHAPTER 5

PRE-COLONIAL PERIOD

Carl Jung claims that "Instead of learning spiritual techniques of the Orient by heart and imitate them [...], it would be much more important to discover, if there exists in unconscious the introvert tendency analogous to the spiritual principle dominant in the Orient. We will even construct on our land and with our methods[...] It is from the interior, and not from the exterior that we should approach our Oriental values; it is inside ourselves, in the unconscious, where we should look for them."[103]

The Arab Medicine and Philosophy

Islamic philosophy and medicine have world glorious history, whose first achievements date back to as early as the 2nd century AH of the Islamic calendar (early 9th century CE). The period, which is known as the Islamic Golden Age, lasted until the 6th century AH (late 12th century CE).

---

[103] Jung C., Psychologie et orientalisme, Albin Michel, 1985, p. 138.

The history of Islamic medicine shows four stages[104]. Each of them is renowned for the specific methods, which were mastered. The first stage followed soon after the death of the Prophet, and was, consequently, called the Prophetic medicine. This period venerated the sayings of the Prophet, so, mainly Muslims were searching for relief in Quranic verses and Prophetic suna. It lasted for the first two centuries of Hijra calendar until the translation of Greek medical scripts became available to the Arabs. Then the second stage, which is the Experimental medicine, followed. It was dominated by an Arab philosophical thought and new inventions. Its beginning is marked by works of Al-Kindi (died in 252H) and its termination by the end of Averroes`s life (died in 595 H). As soon as the third period, the Spiritual medicine, neared, the Arabic mind was dominated by mysticism during six centuries (7th till 12th century). The description of psychiatric symptoms such as delusion, hallucination and affective conditions by Sayyed Esmaeil Jorjani, an Iranian scientist, who was also writing in Arabic, is still valid. His most famous and important book is Zakhireh Khwarazmshahi or The Treasure of King Khwarazm, which is really a complete and valuable medical encyclopedia in Persian language.[105] Later it was translated into Arabic and made up a basis of a common heritage of the Islamic medicine.

In summary, the fourth period, the Phenomenological medicine, included the accomplishments of all previous stages

Prophetic Medicine

Early Muslims were collecting plants mentioned in the Holy Quran and in the Hadith of the Prophet in order to stay healthy. Among the products, which formed the basis for the Prophet's medicine (Al-Tibb al-Nabawi) there are dates, black seeds, olive leaf and olive oil, honey, and camel milk. The Prophet`s medicine included medical treatments, prescriptions of diseases, prevention, health promotion. The book of medicine (Kitab

---

[104] Hanafi H.,Islam in the modern world. Religion, Ideology and Develoment,Dar Kebaa Bookshop, Heliopolis, vol. I, p.469.

*The three collections of Bukhari, Ibn Daoud and Ibn Maja contain a separate chapter on medicine, while collection of Muslim does not. Muslim refers to the sayings containing the prophetic medicine in the book of peace Kiatab-al-Salam.

**For example, Al-Razi critique of Hippocrates and Galen

[105] http://www.ncbi.nlm.nih.gov/pmc/articles/PMC3929806, consulted on 31.04.2016

al-Tibb) of Sahih al-Bukhari by Imam Bukhari is recognized by the majority of the Muslim scholars to be one of the most authentic collections of what had been said and practiced by the Prophet. The scope of the Prophetic medicine has been explained in the very well known commentaries of Sahih al-Bukhari by Ibn Hajar al-Asqalani and Abu Mohammad al-Ayni. Certain imams were known for their wise guidance provided to Muslims at the time when the Prophet was dead. Their expressions make up the heritage of Islamic spiritual tradition, and until nowadays are observed by millions of Muslims. Here are some of them:

"I would rather eat quickly while thinking about the prayer than pray quickly while thinking about the food" (Abu Hanifa). Abu Hanifa also reported that the Prophet said:

"The best among you is the one who does not harm others with his tongue and hands."

"Do not let your difficulties fill you with anxiety. It is only the darkest nights that the stars shine more brilliantly." (Hazrat Ali)

"Body is purified by water, self (nafs) is purified by tears, intellect is purified by knowledge, and the soul is purified with love." (Imam Ali)

"This world is a bridge and a bridge should not be taken as home." (Ibn Al-Jawzi)

"Where your mind is going during a prayer it is where your heart is. Take it back to your Lord." (Abdulbary Yahya)

"Sometimes your prayers are turned down, because you often, unknowingly, ask for things that are really harmful to you." (Imam Ali)

Abu Bakr was saying, "Taking pains to remove the pains of others is the true essence of generosity." The principal and unique source of the Prophetic medicine can be found in the early collection of the Hadith, except Al-Tirmithi. The book of medicine Kitab Al-Tibb begins with the book of drinks (Kitab Al-Ashribah) and the book of food (Kitab Al Atimah). The book of medicine provides the description of certain diseases, symptoms, therapies as well as the general medical overview of possible treatment. The alimentative rules and healthy habits in drinking and eating are provided there as well. However, this source cannot be considered as authentic, since many sayings there remain unverified. Moreover, the multilateral transmission (tawatur) might only confirm the common sense, and not essentially attest to what happened during the Prophet's time. The other point evokes doubts regarding their religious character. It is quite possible that these are the expressions of true taste and preferences of the Prophet in food, drinks, smells, etc. So, the line between the science and religion is practically invisible.

Experimental Medicine

Experimental medicine appeared as a response to the Scriptural (Prophetic) medicine. It was looking for the logical explanation of natural phenomena without recurring to the scriptures. The Arabs at the epoch were eagerly exploring the limits of human potential and the rules, which were governing the universe. The Quran supports the search for knowledge. At that time the Greek medicine became available in Arabic language, the Muslims absorbed it, criticized some of its theories and verified the rest in their own experience**. And the Islamic scientific medicine was worked on by philosophers and translated into Hebrew and Latin to the West. In such a way, advanced Islamic medicine became the essential source of modern Western science. Islamic medicine was progressing steadily both in theoretic and practical dimensions. The Islamic medicine at this stage was deriving from the knowledge on body`s organic functions, i.e. humour, temper, mazaj. Arabs were constantly looking for causes and effects, trying to reach the deepest understanding of the symptoms and their treatment.

Experimental medicine marked a shift in Arab mind from total submissiveness to fatalism to the discovery of limitless human potential. Thus, both reason and senses became indispensable tools in the exploration of the laws of human existence. Mysticism, which grew popular at the epoch, was acknowledged as a deeply spiritual and gnostic practice on a path to Allah. The mystical experience was considered just another way of receiving knowledge. In no way, experimental medicine was a replica of the Greek`s science. On the contrary, the Western world was following the attainments of the Arabs and was consequently adapting them into their own system. It was not a reaction to theory or to a priories, as in the West, but a continuation and an extension of the theory[106].

Spiritual Medicine

Spiritual medicine did not add much new to the scientific progress in Islam world. It was a mere continuation of the previous stage during the 8th and the 14th centuries. The Arabs call it the stagnation period. Culture and science are the mere reflections of the societal and political state of affairs, which were not living their best times then. So, the experimental medicine was continued, as a craft by amateurs, and not by physicians; by imams, and not by philosophers. The mosques regained their value as scientific

---

[106] Hanafi H.,Islam in the modern world. Religion, Ideology and Develoment, Dar Kebaa Bookshop, Heliopolis, vol. I, p.476.

centers, which, was bringing the scientific achievements back to the earliest stage, the prophetic medicine. The scriptural medicine came back, and the experimental medicine was rarely practiced. Muslims were referring to the prophetic sayings again and again in search of consolation. However, this time, spiritual comfort was found also in poems, magic, myths, as there was no distinction between the prophets, the poets, the magicians and the heroes. Subsequently, such state of affairs led to the predominant use of magic and superstitions. The talismans and other protecting stones became the saviours in eyes of many Arabs. The Talsams became the only treatments given to the patients and prescribed by the imams and the sheikhs in the mosques. This all became contrary to both prophetic and experimental medicine. A simple Quranic verse, written on a small piece of paper, folded several times, put in the pocket, or hung on the door, or put secretly between two stones, was supposed to cure the plague.

Phenomenological Medicine

It is believed that the time of the phenomenological medicine has not come yet. The Arab society is still preceding on the stage of the spiritual medicine. Phenomenological medicine is a middle road between the analysis of the body and the salvation of the soul, with no fear of falling, not in the biology nor in magic.[107]

In the long run, the Arab culture has developed complex medical and philosophical beliefs during the Islamic era. It also inherited the knowledge, which existed long before, e.g. in the Babylonian Empire. From these perspectives, they believed that 1. the heart is the seat of the mind, 2. the liver is the seat of emotion, 3. the stomach is the seat of courage, and 4. the uterus is the seat of kindness. And these beliefs survived for several millennia until the civilizational progress permitted more scientific explanations.

Traditional Therapies

Traditional therapies have never, actually, lost their popularity since the time they appeared. The reason is that they have been the most available and accessible type of care. A traditional healer could find the indicative signs in any life occurrence and seek the cure from the herbal potion, which fitted well into the outlook of an ancient Arab.

---

[107] *Ibid, p.479.*

Ibn Arabi maintained that natural insights based on intellectual operations such as associations, theories, past experience, and logic were "but veils which can only be lifted by true spiritual insight". Shaikh or Guru was actually a sort of counselor or psychotherapist of his time, Jailani says, "The sheikh should treat his disciple with mercy and love. If the disciple finds difficulty in changing his bad habits and does what the guru wants, he must be gentle and gradually help him in the way that a mother or a loving father treats their child"[108]. Similarly, Abu Hamid Al-Ghazali describes the duties of the Shaikh and his treatment to his disciples as follows: "The first duty and attribute of a good sheikh is to be humble and gentle with those he is dealing with. He should not stress on giving knowledge or advising but rather choose the route of mild and tender gradualism. A good sheikh should also be ascetic and should not look at his disciple's money with greed. Another good quality of the guru is that if he comes to see or to know that one of his disciples committed some offense, he should not tell him directly about it. He must be indirect and rather meandering about helping him to see the wrong he had done. He can, for example, advise a whole group of disciples about the bad effects of what the person had done without making him feel that he is the one meant for the advice. This would be good to the whole group. And finally, the guru should keep the secrets of his disciples and his clients. These people trust him with personal experiences some of which may be embarrassing. The sheikh should put down a heavy lid over his heart and tongue in keeping these secrets in the dark." (AlIhya, vol.5, pp.206-28). The sheikh will always find something in the Quranic ayat to relieve the wounds of soul.[109]

Among other traditional healers, who have been incredibly popular in subharian Africa, are the marabouts. They are kind of shamans, to who multiple powers are attributed. They restore health or social order by means of talisman. In Maghreb, the marabouts are oftentimes the Muslims. Their techniques are based on the esoteric reading of Quran, numerological system and blessings (fatiha). The term "marabout" in Arabic Maghrib does not designate a magician since he does not practice any sacrificial or animistic rituals in a name of spirits.

The Arabic term "marabout" in North Africa corresponds in reality to a saint sufi mystic, who belongs to (mura-bet in Arabic, plural al-murabitin) to a chain (chain of transmission of spiritual mastery called hikma) and who follows an esoteric way (tariqa) of Islam (sufism). The first

---

[108]   http://www.zeriislam.com/artikulli.php?id=987, consulted on 31.04.206

[109]   http://next.liberation.fr/culture/2001/06/25/le-liban-hesite-devant-le-divan_369203, consulted on 01.05.2016

known reference to a word "marabout" dates back to 1600.[110] Marabouts are believed to possess qualities such as spiritual power, strength, and charisma. Marabouts are viewed as being closer to God than an ordinary human being. A marabout is supposed to have extensive knowledge of Quran. A marabout usually exercises dream interpretation, clairvoyance, divination, and meditation. They are also looked upon as visionaries, who can diagnose merely from seeing or feeling a person. The varieties of marabouts include: seetkat (a clairvoyant), guerisseur, feticheur, tradipractien, and the Wolof faikat: someone who uses medicine.[111] Seetkat offer mostly cowry shell divination, techniques involving knots in string, incantations, and healing.[112] They also offer services such as witch finding, jinn fighting, protection, spells, and removal of bad spells.[113] And the most applied methods for healing in traditional therapy is ruqiya. At the epoch the mental illnesses were considered as possessions, known in two forms: total possession and waswas. Allah said, "Those who fear Allah, when they are tempted by Shaitan, they have but to remember Allah and they shall see the light (right course of action)!" (sura 7,ayat 201).

It is too simplistic to claim that the traditional practices operate by persuasion or suggestion.They invite a patient to a word, a ritual, a trance, or all this at once. And healing is only one element of a global symbolic. Saints are the representatives of venerable institutions, the marabouts, who proved with their actions that they are disinterested in pursuit of any gain and that their lives were entirely devoted to an overall well-being - therapeutic, religious, social and even political of the population. Other social actors, motivated rather by greed, are real magicians or quacks who could take advantage of the symptoms to accede to considerable gains at the expense of human suffering.

Total Possession

As an example we can refer to the following story: according to Outhman Ibn Abi Al As, who told that as soon as the Prophet appointed him as the head of the city Taef as a local responsible, a strange occurrence happened to him during the prayer to the point that he did not know what

---

[110] http://www.merriam-webster.com/dictionary/marabout, consulted on 01.05.2016

[111] Gemmeke A., Marabout Women in Dakar: Creating Trust in a Rural Urban, Transaction Publishers, 2008, p.11.

[112] *Ibid*

[113] *Ibid*

to do in a prayer (that is to say there was confusion in a prayer, he was mixing up everything). He was not able to tolerate it any further and he went to see a prophet in Medina and narrated his story.The Prophet said that it was the demon and asked him to come closer. The Prophet hit his chest with his hand and inhaled in his mouth, then said, "Get out Allah`s enemy". He did it three times. Then the Prophet told Al As to return to his work. Outhman Ibn Al As said that since that day he has not felt anything (also authenticated by Sheikh Albani).

According to Kharija Ibn Soulte, who related from her uncle`s words, who said that when they had been returning from the Prophet`s, his friends and he had been passing by one Arabic tribe. The members of the tribe told them: It was told to us that you are returning from that man, who`s well told about. Do you happen to have cure or ruqiya for one ill person? We have one man with us, who has gone mad, and who we were obliged to tie up. He says: They have brought an ill man, who was tied up, and I started to read sourat Al Fatiha during three days. In three days he has woken up from his state of craziness. They gave me a pasture-raised animal and I said that I would not touch it before seeing the prophet. The Prophet told me to take it. So that I do not take it for illegal ruqiya, but for a legal ruqiya." (Narrated by Imam Ahmed, Abou Daoud, Nassai, Al Hakim).

Obviously, one should be careful in the relationship between man and woman when enacting a ruqiya ritual. This is not a man who will give slaps on the chest of a woman and vice versa. If a woman cannot find a woman raqui, a man can blow and read raqui Mouawidhates to a sick arm of a woman while she is covered.

Waswas

Clinically speaking, waswas is an obsession, which is manifested in a form of obsessive thoughts, compulsive acts, and accomplishment of certain unwanted rituals. Constant struggle against one`s thoughts only increases the appearance of undesirable symptoms. This waswas may occur during ablution, prayer, or any other daily activity. A person starts feeling spiritless since no method brings relief. And at this point, many sufferers address to traditional healers. As the first step to improvement, Arabic tradition prescribes strengthening of faith by reading Quran, constant evocations, and duas. Quran mentions: "And if there comes to you from Satan an evil suggestion, then seek refuge in Allah. Indeed, He is the Hearing, the Knowing" (sura 41, ayat 36). The thorough fulfillment of the above-mentioned makes a human more aware that these thoughts come from Iblis. Sheikh Al Islam Ibn Taymiya affirmed that the ayat "Throne" is the most efficient in this regard. Those who were reading the ayat from the Throne were released from waswas influence. For the same means there might be useful perfumes, colours, texts of the wise Islamic medicine, fabrication of the objects of protection. In addition to this, reputable Arabic texts recommended to use olive oil or Habba Saouda for massage, then read Mouawidhates on the hands and pass them through the body, etc.

The most vivid character of the Arabic folklore that settles in a human, is Ghoul, fem. Ghoula (from Arabic –ogre). This monster appeared in the stories of One Thousand and One Night. They constitute a class of Jinns, as the Efrits, for example, and therefore, coming from the devil. Ghouls change shape, taking on the appearance of a hyena or that of a woman, but they are recognized by their cloven hoofs, the only constant element of their appearance. The Ghoula, feminization of the Arabic word, is the equivalent of Persian Lilith (Lamia).

Al-firasa

Al-firasa is well-known medieval Arab scientific art of studying people by their physical appearance, i.e. colour, shape, body parts etc. An Arabic physiognomist Abul-Faraj (1226-1286) provided an accurate description of the physical traits and their connection with the character in his Book of Entertaining Stories. He came to the conclusion that a strong, brave man has a little long face, deep-set eyes, high forehead, "aquiline" nose, coarse hair, thick eyebrows, thin lips, while a wise man has a beautiful face, thin lips, and his eyes glow with force. A slow man has the thick tip of the nose and big ears. Yusuf Murad`s thesis on Fakhr al-Din al-Razi (died in 1209), an annotated translation of Kitab al-Firasa (The Book on Physiognomy), was intended to be of interest not only to orientalists but also to historians of science as part of a larger series of translated Arabic medico-psychological texts.[114]

Murad worked on translation of psychological terminology of Al-Razi`s works. Bringing knowledge of Arabic physiognomy to the outside world enabled him to trace the Arab influence in the Western scientific tradition. At this time the significance of al-firasa in the Arab world was rising in parallel with the inception of psychological science in the West. Al-firasa, or the art of seeing the hidden meaning through the external forms, was transmitted through the pseudo-Aristotelian text the Secretum Secretorum or Kitab Sirr al-Asrar. The text was regarded as

---

[114]   Al Shakry O., The Arabic Freud: the Unconscious and the modern subject", Modern Intellectual History, Volume 11, Issue 01, April 2014, p.110.

an epistolary book of useful advice to Alexander. This text brought even more significance to the Greek philosophical thought in the Arabic world. Its first printed edition by Abd al-Rahman Badawi appeared in 1954, a philosopher who was a student of Alexandre Koyre at Fuad I University and one of the main transmitters of the existential tradition into Arabic, most notably through Heidegger. Al-Ghazali considered al-firasa as a natural science while Ibn Rushd (Averroes) thought of it as occult sciences. Physiognomy was extremely popular in the Middle Ages up to the point that Hanbalis and al-Shafii were applying it juridically to determine culpability. Ibn Arabi, the medieval Sufi, was not only the transmitter of al-firasa knowledge but its translator. Ibn Arabi's contribution to the practice of physiognomy is considered to be extremely rich and productive. Ibn Arabi distinguished two forms of firasa: natural firasa and divine firasa. The former derived from the basic knowledge of human nature, whilst the latter could be granted only by God as a divinatory power, which is called mystical firasa (al-firasa al-dhawqiyya). Physiognomists judged the character based on physical appearance, while the mystics were reading spiritual essence. One chart could also determine whether a person will live or die based on the numerical value of the patient's name (Kitab Sirr al-asrar, 12: Rajab 1264 = 3 June-2 July 1848). According to Al-Qushayri (died in 1072) spiritual insights in al-firasa can come suddenly, and that the human heart cannot oppose the flashes of insight that strike it no matter how hard it tries. In the words of Ibn Arabi: "Know that insight is a light shed by the divine light, with which the faithful find their way to reach salvation. That light also makes visible all that there is to see in the material world. Firasa was therefore not a pure act of the intellect but a combination of feeling, sentiment, and Knowledge."[115]

Ilm al-Nafs

Ilm al-nafs became a separate domain of medicine in the Islamic world during the Middle Ages. In medieval Islamic medicine in particular, the study of mental illness was a speciality of its own,[116] and was variously known as al-ilaj al-nafs (approximately "curing/treatment" of the"ideas/

---

[115] Al Shakry O., The Arabic Freud: the Unconscious and the modern subject", Modern Intellectual History, Volume 11, Issue 01, April 2014, p.111.

[116] Youssef, Hanafy A.; Youssef, Fatma A.; Dening, T. R.,Evidence for the existence of schizophrenia in medieval Islamic society, History of Psychiatry 7 (25), 1996, p.58.

soul/vegetative mind"),[117] al-tibb al-ruhani ("the healing of the spirit", or "spiritual health") and tibb al-qalb ("healing of the heart/self", or "mental medicine").[118]Therefore, Islamic psychology, or Ilm-al Nafsiat (psychological sciences), refers to the study of Nafs (self or psyche) and is related to psychology, psychiatry and neurosciences.[119] Al-ilaj al-nafsy (psychological therapy) in Islamic medicine is simply defined as the study of mental illness and is equal to psychotherapy, as it deals with curing/ treatment of ideas, soul and vegetative mind. The psychiatric physician was referred to as al-tabib al-ruhani or tabib al-qalb (spiritual physician).[120] The most characteristic features of medieval Muslim psychotherapy were the use of clinical observations of mentally ill patients, which resulted in the provision of ground-breaking applications of moral treatment, baths, drug medication, music therapy and occupational therapy.

Mentally ill people were considered as disabled, and, in accordance to sharia, were to be protected on a state level. In this regard, Quran states, "Do not give your property which God assigned you to manage to the insane: but feed and clothe the insane with this property and tell splendid words to them." It was originally thought that mentally ill individuals could not differentiate between the real and the unreal, therefore, mentally ill was defined by Avicenna as "one who suffers from a condition in which reality is replaced with fantasy."[121]

At the epoch there was no clear distinction between self (nafs), intellect (aql), heart (qalb), spirit (ruh), will (irada), especially when it referred to the non-physical illness, since all of them designated a personality. If we refer to more ancient concepts of psychology we will find some at scripts of the Pharaonic epoch. Medical knowledge from the Ancient Egyptian time period is drawn from multiple sources:[122]

---

[117] Haque A., Psychology from Islamic Perspective: Contributions of Early Muslim Scholars and Challenges to Contemporary Muslim Psychologists, Journal of Religion and Health 43 (4), 2004, p.378.

[118] Deuraseh N., Abu Talib M. Mental health in Islamic medical tradition, The International MedicalJournal, 2005, 4, pp.76-79.

[119] *Ibid*

[120] *Ibid*

[121] http://www.ummah.com/forum/showthread.php?414109-Understanding-human-psychology-through-Islam, consulted on 01.07.2016

[122] http://mentalillness.umwblogs.org/ancient-egypt/, consulted on 31.04.2016

1. Kahun Papyrus (1900 BC): addresses morbid states attributed to the displacement of the uterus.
2. Ebers' Papyrus (1600 BC): the world's oldest medical document.
3. Edwin Smith Papyrus (1600 BC): narrates mainly about surgeries.
4. Hearst Papyrus: similar to Ebers' Papyrus.
5. Berlin Medical Papyrus (1250 BC): prescriptions are preserved in an unsystematic arrangement.
6. London Medical Papyrus (1350 BC): contains enchantments or incantations for diseases.[123]

The oldest of these documents is dedicated specifically to hysteria. This document is known as the Kahun Papyrus, after the ancient Egyptian city in the ruins of which it was found, and dates back to about 1900 BCE.[124] The Kahun Papyrus confirms an assumption that in ancient Egypt the hysteria was known even before Hippocrates, and it was treated in physical rather than esoteric way. The same can be stated about depression, which was described as follows: "He huddled up his clothes and lay, not knowing where he was. His wife inserted her hand under his clothing. She said, "my brother, no fever in your chest and limbs, but sadness of the heart in this dismal ode: "Now death is to me like health to the sick, like the smell of a lotus, like the wish of a man to see this house after years of captivity.""[125]

The psychotherapy of ancient Egypt was successfully practicing a method of sleep therapy, which was known as the "Temple sleep". It is believed that Imhotep, the earliest known physician in history, initiated this type of cure. I.em.ho.tep., "he who comes in peace," was the physician vizier of the king Djoser. Imhotep built the first pyramid, the Steppyramid at Saqqara after 2611 BCE. And a temple dedicated to him was built on the island of Philae. It became a popular center for sleep treatment. The treatment prescription depended greatly on the manifestations and contents of dreams, which were, of course, highly affected by the psycho-religious climate of the temple, or the confidence in the supernatural powers of the deity, and on the suggestive procedures carried out by divine

---

[123] Okasha A.,Mental disorders in Pharaonic Egypt. Egyptian Journal ofPsychiatry, 1978, pp.1-12.

[124] https://www.researchgate.net/publication/7426670_Mental_health_in_Egypt, consulted on 31.04.2016

[125] *Ibid*

healers[126]. The Egyptians were among the first ancient nations to have conducted the psychological, which occurred in the 7th century B.C.[127] The experiment hypothesized that, if Egyptian children were isolated during infancy without any means of language communication, they would spontaneously speak the original language of civilization: Egyptian.[128] This experiment underscored the interdependence between the language and the mind.

Therefore, Ilm al-nafs, the science of the nafs ("self" or "psyche")[129] encompasses a wide range of medical and philosophical studies of the psyche, such as psychology, neuroscience, philosophy, psychiatry and psychosomatic medicine from an Islamic standpoint.

"Bimaristan", the First Mental Hospital

In ancient Egypt three thousand years ago, Imhoteb, minister of King Zoser, the builder of the Sakkara pyramid, was a well known physician who treated mental patients in general hospitals.[130]This fact became known after discovery of the "Sleeping Temple" in Sakkara, south of Cairo.[131] In what it concerns the next major step in the evolution of psychology, the Golden Age of Islam, it was unique in the sense that the treatment of mental disorders was institutionalized at the hospitals. Psychiatric hospitals were constructed in Baghdad (Azudi hospital) in 705 and Cairo in 805, and there is evidence to suggest that there was also one such facility in

---

[126] https://www.researchgate.net/publication/7426670_Mental_health_in_ Egypt, consulted on 31.04.2016

[127] Hunt M., The story of psychology, Doubleday, 1993, p.1.

[128] http://www.apa.org/international/pi/2012/03/egypt.aspx, consulted on 01.05.2016

[129] Deuraseh N., Abu Talib M., Mental health in Islamic medical tradition. The International Medical Journal, 2005, 4, pp.76-79.

[130] http://scholarworks.wmich.edu/cgi/viewcontent.cgi?article=1980& context=jssw, consulted on 01.05.2016

[131] Ghaliongui P.,Magic and medical science in ancient Egypt, Hodder andStoghton, 1963, p.56.

---

operation Fez during the 8[132] century, and Marrakesh in 1190.[133] Another psychiatric hospital functioned in Aleppo since 1270.

The first biggest maristan in the North Africa was constructed by Sultan Yakoub al Mansour in the XIIth century, where the great Muslim scholars such as Ibn Rushd and Ibn Tufail were practicing medicine. The hospital was the centre of medical progress and the greatest achievement of Arab–Islamic civilization. It was called a Bimaristan, a derivate from the Persian words Bimar, "ill person" and stan "place". It shall be stressed out that the Prophet Muhamed initiated the construction of small mobile military Bimaristan. However, only Al-Waleed bin Abdel Malek (ruled from 705 to 715) realized practically this idea in Damascus with the founding of a leprosarium. The earliest hospital of Islamic epoch, the information of which was preserved was built in the 9th century in Baghdad, most likely by the Vizier to the Caliph Harun al-Rashid. In Egypt, the first hospital was built in the southwestern quarter of present-day Cairo in 872 by Ahmad ibn Tulun, the Abbasid ruler. Some time later, two other hospitals were constructed in Old Cairo (Fustat). In the 12th century the Nasiri hospital was raised in Cairo by Saladin and in 1248 the Mansuri hospital. The Mansuri hospital (with 8000 beds) was the top primary medical center in Cairo all long the 15th century. In Damascus, the Nuri hospital took a place of the major hospital until the 15th century. By that time the city had five new hospitals. Besides those in Baghdad, Damascus, and Cairo, hospitals were erected in other Islamic states. For example, in Al-Qayrawan (Tunisia), there existed hospital at the beginning of the 9th century, while in Mecca and Medina even earlier. The environment and location of the hospitals were thoroughly chosen. We can find the paintings of some ancient hospitals, which were presumably built over the hills or next to the water. The history tells when Harun al-Rashid asked Rhazes to build the first general hospital, so Rhazes selected the place after putting a few pieces of meat in different places in Baghdad to check which spoiled the least, thus identifying the place with the freshest air. A typical Islamic hospital was constructed on a cruciform plan with four central vaulted halls, with many adjacent rooms, such as kitchen, storage areas, a pharmacy, space for the medical staff were installed afterwards. Each Iwan had its own fountain, which served as a source of clean water. The hospital was divided into different departments, specialized in treatment of specific

---

[132] Wael M., Arab and Muslim Contributions to Modern Neuroscience, International Brain Research Organization History of Neuroscience, 2012

[133] https://www.cairn.info/revue-l-information-psychiatrique-2009-7-page-605.htm, consulted on 01.07.2016

diseases. There was a separate department for the mentally ill. The staff was made up of doctors, pharmacists and physicians who were serving shifts and prescribing medications. There were also doctors` assistants, who could take care of the basic needs of the patient. Such hospitals were well funded. By the way, the budget of the Mansuri hospital was the largest of any public institution. Medieval Arab–Muslim physicians relied mostly on clinical psychiatry and clinical observations on mentally ill patients. Islamic hospitals were the first to offer psychotherapeutic treatment for those, who were diagnosed with mental illnesses, in addition to baths, drug medication, music therapy, and aromatherapy. The following points summarize the main characteristics of Arab–Islamic hospitals:

Secular: Hospitals were owned by a state, and open to all people despite their ethnicity or religion. Physicians from all around the world collaborated for one common aim: the well-being of patients.

Separate wards: Male and female patients were placed in the different wards. Moreover, each disease, especially infectious one, was treated at different department. Male nurses were responsible for male patients, and female nurses took care of the females.

Proper records of patients: For the first time in history, hospitals recorded the patients` names, date of arrival and discharge, diagnosis and prescribed treatment.

Hygiene: Hospitals had a separate room for prayers, as well as a room for ablution.

Qualifications of physicians: The qualified physicians were subject to the procedure of examinations with the subsequent attainment of license. In 931 by the order of Caliph Al-Mugtadir from the Abbasid dynasty, the Chief Court Physician Sinan ibn Thabit checked over 860 physicians of Baghdad, and the medical license was accorded only to those who passed it successfully. In order to become a practitioner, students had to specialize in Islamic studies, philosophy, astronomy, art, chemistry, and other subjects even before beginning the medical studies. So, only a wise and intellectual person could have practiced medicine. To mention, the Arabic translation of a physician is hakim, which means sage.

Medical schools: But for treating patients, the hospital was managing numerous roles at once. It was also a centre for medical studies, exchange of professional knowledge, application of new therapeutic methods, and medicine development. An Islamic hospital had an extensive library, lecturing rooms, living space for students and technical staff.

Ethics and regulation: The law was very rigorous about the medical practice, and this profession, more than any other, conformed to the ethical regulations and conduct norms. First of all, they intended to control the relation between a doctor and a patient, its confidentiality and reliability.

Building hospitals: The Caliphs of the Arab–Islamic Empire tended to sponsor generously the construction of hospitals, for the main reason that, in accordance with Islam, charity is a good investment for Judgment Day. So, the medical field was well supported, and it kept on flourishing.

Funds of the hospitals: The hospitals were receiving funding from several different sources. The first, and, probably, the most substantial was the Caliphs' contributions. Another part of funds was obtained through Al-Waqf system, which was formed on the basis of citizens' donations. The donation was administered and distributed by the state. And the other source was coming from Al-Zakat charity (2.5% of property value).

In the 14th century mental disorders was one of the four departments in Cairo's Kalawoon Hospital, a precursor of the place of psychiatry in general hospitals that was accepted in Europe six centuries later.[134]

It is interesting to give a brief account of the 14th century Kalawoun Hospital in Cairo. It had separate sections for surgery, ophthalmology, and medical and mental illnesses. Generous contributions by the wealthy of Cairo allowed a high standard of medical care and provided for patients during convalescence until they were gainfully occupied. Two features are striking: the care of mental patients in a general hospital and the involvement of the community in the welfare of the patients, foreshadowed modern trends by six centuries.[135]

Muslim Scholars of Khalifat Period and Their Main Ideas in the Field of Psychology

The Islamic scientists became renowned for their fundamental contributions to the understanding of human nature, and, consequently, the evolution of the world civilization. It must be made clear that medieval Islamic psychology does not deal with the mind only[136]. The Arabic physicians gave a broad reference to the qualities and effects of the narcotics such as opium, hyoscyamus and hashish. The names of the Islamic scholars, which are mentioned in the Table 5.1, constitute the foundation of the modern human sciences.

---

[134] http://www.ncbi.nlm.nih.gov/pubmed/16342608, consulted on 01.07.2016

[135] http://scholarworks.wmich.edu/cgi/viewcontent.cgi?article=1980&context=jssw, consulted on 31.04.2016

[136] Ashy M., Health and illness from an Islamic perspective. Journal of Religion and Health, 38, 1999, pp.241-257.

Table 5.1 Muslim Scholars and Their Specialization

Name	Dates of life	Specialization
Ibn Sina Avicenna	980–1037	Medicine, philosophy, mathematics
Al-Razi Rhazes	864–930	Medicine, ophthalmology, smallpox, chemistry, astronomy
Al-Zahrawi Albucasis	936–1013	Surgery, medicine (father of modern surgery)
Al-Biruni Al-Biruni	973–1050	Physic, anthropology astronomy, chemistry, pharmacy
Ibn Zuhr Avenzoar	1091–1161	Surgery, medicine
Al-Antaki Al-Antaki	Died 1599	Pharmacy, natural product-based drugs
Al-Kindi	800–873	Philosophy, physics, optics, medicine, mathematics, metallurgy
Ibn Khaldun Ibn Khaldun	1332–1406	Sociology, philosophy, political science
Ibn Jazzar Ibn Jazzar	898–980	Medicine
Ibn Wahshiyyah	ca. 900	Alchemy and toxicology
Ibn Hayan Geber	Died 803	Chemistry (father of chemistry)
Ibn al-Haitham Alhacen	960–1040	Physics, optics, mathematics
Ibn Rushd Averroes	1128–1198	Philosophy, medicine, astronomy, theology
Ibn al-Nafis Ibn al-Nafis	1213–1288	Anatomy

Al Kindi (801–873 AD)

Al Kindi was the first of the Muslim peripatetic philosophers, who is unanimously hailed as the "father of Islamic or Arabic philosophy"[137]. He was responsible for supervision of Greek scientific and philosophical texts translation into Arabic at the palaces of the Abbasid Caliphs. Al Kindi`s

---

[137] Nasr S., Islamic philosophy from its origin to the present: philosophy in the land of prophecy. State Univ. of New York Press, 2006, pp. 137–138.

knowledge of ancient philosophy evoked his interest in exploration of other related disciplines, which ranged from metaphysics, ethics, logic and psychology, to medicine, pharmacology, mathematics, astronomy, astrology and optics, and many others.[138] His writings, arranged in a form of short treatises, are classified into seventeen groups: Philosophy, Logic, Arithmetics, Globe, Music, Astronomy, Geometry, Sphere, Medicine, Astrology, Dialectic, Psychology, Politics, Meteorology, Dimensions, First things and Metals and Chemicals. We have two works by al-Kindi devoted to the ontology of the human soul: That There are Incorporeal Substances and Discourse on the Soul.[139]The work That There are Incorporeal Substances elaborated the ideas from Aristotle's Categories regarding the issue of immaterialism of the human soul. He maintained that since the soul is the core of any living being, and a living being is a substance, therefore, a soul is a substance. A treatise Discourse on the Soul is a comprehensive compendium of quotes from Greek scholars, such as Plato, Pythagoras, and Aristotle regarding the soul.

Al-Kindi was also the first to introduce the experiment method in psychology. As a result of his experiments, the scholar found out that sensation is proportionate to the stimulus. He was also a pioneer in discovering the healing effects of music therapy. Among the other Al-Kindi`s psychology-related works are: On Sleep and Dreams, First Philosophy, and Eradication of Sorrow. He believed that a spiritual (nafsani) grief is provoked by a loss, so he said, "If causes of pain are discernible, the cures can be found." He recommended that "if we do not tolerate losing or dislike being deprived of what is dear to us, then we should seek after riches in the world of the intellect. In it we should treasure our precious and cherished gains where they can never be dispossessed...for that which is owned by our senses could easily be taken away from us."[140] He also stated that "sorrow is not within us we bring it upon ourselves." Al-Kindi`s interest also expanded to human cognition sphere and treatment of depression. Today, one of the biggest medical centres, Al-Kindi General Hospital is located in Baghdad.

---

[138] Corbin H., History of Islamic philosophy, Kegan Paul International, 1993, p. 155.

[139] http://plato.stanford.edu/entries/al-kindi/#Psy, consulted on 01.05.2016

[140] http://www.jstor.org/stable/27512819, consulted on 31.04.2016

Al-Farabi (870-950)

Al-Farabi or Alpharabius, was a renowned philosopher who contributed to the fields of political philosophy, law, metaphysics, ethics, logic, psychology and others. His birthplace is considered to be Farab on the Jaxartes (Syr Darya) in modern Kazakhstan. He was studying the behavior of people in communities, and his works are mainly focused on social psychology. One of his most famous citations reads: "an isolated individual could not achieve all the perfections by himself, without the aid of other individuals";[141] and "innate disposition of every man to join another human being or other men in the labor he ought to perform";[142] or "achieve what he can of that perfection, every man needs to stay in the neighborhood of others and associate with them."[143] He was writing excessively in the field of psychology, in particular, The Treatise on the Intellect (Risalah fil-aql) deals with the function of intellect. The Principles of Existing Things, also known as The Political Regime (Kitab al-siyasa al-madaniyya), and The Principles and Opinions of the People of the Virtuous City (Mabadi ara ahl al-madinah al-fadilah), are some of Al-Farabi's major works where he deals with psychological topics such as the nature of the soul, its cognitive capacities, and the doctrine of the intellect.[144] Both The Political Regime and The Virtuous City are essential resources for understanding the Al-Farabi's cosmology which consists of six hierarchical principles: (1) the First Existent or First Cause, (2) the second intellects, (3) the active intellect, (4) the soul, (5) form, and (6) matter. His theory of human nature is dualistic. Al-Farabi stated that body and soul have no essential connections with each other. Al-Farabi affirms that each faculty has a ruling organ and others that are auxiliaries and subordinates. The scholar maintains that the ruling organ in the human body is the heart, whilst the brain is a secondary ruling organ subordinated to the heart; however, all the other organs and limbs are subordinated to the brain. He suggests that the heart rules sensation, and its subordinates are the five senses. The imaginative faculty is located in the heart and has no auxiliaries distributed in other organs, but it controls what is provided by the five

---

[141] Baker D., The Oxford Handbook of the History of Psychology: Global Perspectives, Oxford University Press, 2012, p.445.

[142] Alwishah A., Aristotle and the Arabic Tradition, Cambridge University Press, 2015, p.216.

[143] *Ibid*

[144] http://plato.stanford.edu/entries/al-farabi-psych/, consulted on 01.07.2016

senses.[145] Al-Farabi claimed, "The sensations we have once experienced are not utterly dead. They can reappear in the form of images. The power by which we revive a past sensible experience without the aid of any physical stimulus is called imagination (el-motakhayilah)." Therefore, in his view, the imaginative function is to retain the memory of impressions and reproduces them. Reproductive imitation (muhakat) implies the capacity of the imaginative faculty to imitate a series of stored elements in it. This is why the imagination has the capacity to stimulate particular emotions, humors, desires, and temperaments that move the body and put it into action.[146] When a person enjoys powerful imaginative capacities, then the experience of extreme beauty by means of imitation becomes possible. Its highest rank is the awareness of present and future events, which Al-Farabi calls the most perfect attainment of vision. In his treatise "On the Cause of Dreams", which appeared as chapter 24 of his "Principles of the Opinions of the Citizens of the Ideal City", he distinguished between dream interpretation and the nature and causes of dreams.[147] The appetitive faculty activates the will (irada) as soon as the sensitive, the imaginative, or the rational faculties have detected something. In terms of the reproductive system, he believed that the female prepares the matter while the male prepares the form.

Ibn Sina (980-1037)

Ibn Sina, known in the West as Avicenna, was born in the village of Afshana, which today is located on the territory of Russia. His major works The Cure (al-Shifa) and The Canon (al-Qanun fil-Tibb) have had a decisive impact on the European academia. Since his childhood, he already mastered the recitation of Quran, Arabic literature, Islamic jurisprudence, psychology, philosophy, natural science and other subjects. Ibn Sina was the first one to attribute definition to numerous neuropsychiatric terms, such as dementia, epilepsy, hallucination, insomnia, mania, nightmare, melancholia, paralysis, stroke, vertigo, and tremor. On the basis of his researches, the modern psychosomatic medicine was born. He created a system for associating changes in the pulse rate with inner feelings, which

---

[145]   http://plato.stanford.edu/entries/al-farabi-psych/, consulted on 01.07.2016

[146]   Al-Farabi, Mabadi ara ahl al-madinah al-fadilah (al-Farabi on the Perfect State), Oxford: Clarendon Press, 1985, p. 216-219.

[147]   Amber Haque, Psychology from Islamic Perspective: Contributions of Early Muslim Scholars and Challenges to Contemporary Muslim Psychologists, Journal of Religion and Health, 2004, 43 (4), pp. 357-377.

---

can be considered as a preconception of an association test by Carl Jung. Ibn Sina is said to have tested a patient by "feeling the patient's pulse and reciting aloud to him the names of provinces, districts, towns, streets, and people."[148] His attention was drawn by the fact that the patient's pulse was increasing each time the certain names were mentioned. One story related that a Prince in Jurjan was laying sick for a long time and whose malady local doctors did not know to define. So, with the above-mentioned technique, Avicenna deduced that the patient was in love with a girl who, Ibn Sina advised the patient to marry her. Not surprisingly, that after the marriage the patient soon recovered. So, love sickness counts among those psychological diseases, to which Ibn Sina gave a name. Avicenna's ideas on the reasons for mental illnesses widely opposed the widely accepted beliefs of jinn's and demon's possessions. He aimed at constructing a comprehensive system, which would explain the contingency of one's self-existence in relation to the universe and accord with the religiosity of the Muslim culture. Avicenna gives a proof for the substantiality of the soul that renders it capable of existing by itself apart from the body.[149] Being essentially immaterial, the soul does not perish with the body, and even retains its individuality, i.e. the images and intelligible ideas it amassed during its sojourn on earth.[150] The assertion of self-consciousness, which exists apart from the body, is the basis to claim that the soul is a purely spiritual substance, and this revokes his famous "proof of the suspended man." This argument was later refined and simplified by Rene Descartes in epistemic terms when he stated: "I can abstract from the supposition of all external things, but not from the supposition of my own consciousness."[151] In metaphysics, Avicenna (Ibn Sina) defined truth as: "What corresponds in the mind to what is outside it."[152] Avicenna elaborated on his definition of truth in his Metaphysics: "The truth of a thing is the property of the being of each thing which has been established in it."[153]

---

[148] Baker D., The Oxford Handbook of the History of Psychology: Global Perspectives, Oxford University Press, 2012, p.445.

[149] http://www.iranicaonline.org/articles/avicenna-vi, consulted on 01.07.2016

[150] http://plato.stanford.edu/entries/arabic-islamic-mind/#Avi, consulted on 01.07.2016

[151] Nasr S., Leaman O., History of Islamic Philosophy, Routledge, 1996, p. 315.

[152] Osman A., Influence of Muslim Philosophy on the West, Monthly Renaissance, 2007

[153] Aertsen J., Nature and Creature: Thomas Aquinas's Way of Thought, BRILL, 1988, p. 152.

Avicenna claims that knowledge comes about by abstraction.[154] Just as there are five external senses (vision, audition, touch, taste, and smell), the scholar believed that there also exist internal senses. So, he elaborated a system of five internal senses, which are: (1) common sense (al-hiss al-mushtarak), (2) imagination (al-khayal), (3) the imaginative faculty (at-takhayul) which is capable of producing new images, (4) estimation (wahm) that gives meaning to the perceived image, (5) a sense, which does not store the images themselves, but their meanings. The common sense and (one aspect of) the imaginative faculty comprise the first pair, located in the front ventricle of the brain[155]. The middle ventricle is the location of "estimation". Avicenna stated that there were three cognitive types of causes for death anxiety. This included the following types of disordered thinking: (a) ignorance as to what death is, (b) uncertainty of what is to follow after death and (c) supposing that after death, the soul may cease to exist. He stated that the degree of anxiety one experiences is directly related to the level of knowledge one has about the idea of death.[156] His idea of free will epitomize the strong capacity of the thought to influence the physical state, which, in the end, influenced the views of the modern psychologists. Also, Ibn Sina was favouring the music therapy, as a treatment for the spirit.

Avicenna was a pioneer of psychophysiology and psychosomatic medicine. He was studying human consciousness, in particular, thoughts, feelings, sensations, perception and memory. He recognized "physiological psychology" in the treatment of emotional troubles and developed a system for associating changes in the pulse rate with inner feelings. In his legendary work, the Canon of Medicine (Al-Qanun-fi-il-Tabb), he provided symptomatic definitions and treatments for such conditions as insomnia, mania, vertigo, paralysis, epilepsy, depression, as well as male sexual dysfunction. Avicenna was also a pioneer of neuropsychiatry. His works in this field were dedicated to degenerative diseases, mood disorders, neurotic disorders, sleep disorders and many others. Avicenna was often referring to deductive reasoning, that is to say, going from general to specific in philosophy, as well as medicine. Ibn Sina was extensively using inductive logic when working with a syndrome. In his medical writings, Avicenna was the first to describe the methods of agreement, difference

---

[154] Rahman, Fazlur, Avicenna's Psychology, Oxford: Hyperion Pr, 1952, p.38

[155] http://plato.stanford.edu/entries/arabic-islamic-mind/#Avi, consulted on 01.07.2016

[156] Avicenna, Metaphysics of The Healing Provo,UT: Brigham, 2005, p.118

and concomitant variation which are critical to inductive logic and the scientific method.[157]

Avicenna's works on metaphysics, who was himself influenced by Al-Farabi, make distinction between essence and existence. Whereas existence is the domain of the contingent and the accidental, essence endures within a being beyond the accidental.[158] Some scholars believe that Avicenna was the first to view existence (wujud) as an accident that happens to the essence (mahiyya). Avicenna posited the concept of essentialism per se, given that existence (al-wujud) when thought of in terms of necessity would ontologically translate into a notion of the Necessary-Existent-due-to-Itself (wajib al-wujud bi-dhatihi), which is without description or definition, and particularly without quiddity or essence (la mahiyya lahu).[159] Consequently, Avicenna's ontology is "existentialist" when accounting for being qua existence in terms of necessity (wujub), while it is "essentialist" in terms of thinking about being qua existence (wujud) in terms of contingency qua possibility (imkan; or mumkin al-wujud: contingent being).[160] Some argue that Avicenna anticipated Frege and Bertrand Russell in "holding that existence is an accident of accidents" and also anticipated Alexius Meinong's view about nonexistent objects.[161] He also provided early arguments for "a necessary being" as cause of all other existents.[162] The idea of "essence precedes existence" is a concept which dates back to Avicenna[163] and his school of Avicennism as well as Shahab al-Din Suhrawardi and his Illuminationist philosophy. The opposite idea of

---

[157] Goodman L., Islamic Humanism, Oxford University Press, 2003, p. 155.

[158] Kennard F., Thought Experiments: Popular Thought Experiments in Philosophy, Physics, Ethics, Computer Science & Mathematics, Lulu, 2015, p.105.

[159] A one-day colloquium on Heidegger's legacy to religious thought in a global perspective "Heidegger and the Contemporary Religious Situation", Oxford University Faculty of Theology: Centre for Theology and Modern European Thought

[160] El-Bizri N., Avicenna and Essentialism, The Review of Metaphysics, Vol. 54, June 2001, pp. 753-778.

[161] Alejandro H., La distinción entre esencia y existencia en Avicena, Revista Latinoamericana de Filosofía 16, 1990, pp. 183–195.

[162] Fadlo H.,Ibn Sina on necessary and possible existence, Philosophical Forum 4, 1972, pp. 74–86.

[163] Irwin J., Averroes' Reason: A Medieval Tale of Christianity and Islam, The Philosopher, LXXXX (2), 2002

"existence precedes essence" was thus developed in the works of Averroes[164] and Mulla Sadra's transcendent theosophy. Also Avicenna and Ibn Al-Nafis had their own theories on the soul. They both considered the soul and the spirit as two separate entities. Avicenna contributed immortality to the soul as a consequence of its nature, and did not consider it as a final goal. In his theory of The Ten Intellects, he viewed the human soul as the tenth and final intellect.[165] Also, he placed anger as a factor in the progression of melancholia to mania. He hypothesized that happiness increases the breath, leading to the uncontrolled increase in brain moisture and resulting in mental disorders. Avicenna also discovered a condition resembling schizophrenia and described it as Junun Mufrit (severe madness) with characteristic symptoms such as agitation, behavioral and sleep disturbance, giving inappropriate answers to questions and occasional inability to speak.

Al-Ghazali (1058-1111)

Imam Al-Ghazali, also known as Algazelus, was a Muslim theologian, jurist, philosopher, and a mystic. Al-Ghazali was working on an all-in definition for the concept "self" and the causes of its misery and happiness. He viewed the self existing in four terms: qalb (heart), ruh (spirit), nafs (soul) and aql (intellect). He stated that "the self has an inherent yearning for an ideal, which it strives to realize and it is endowed with qualities to help realize it."[166] He claimed that the self has propensities and impulses to satisfy its needs. Among the propensities, there are two types: appetite and anger. He supposed that impulse resides in the muscles, nerves, and tissues, and moves the organs to "fulfill the propensities". Al-Ghazali identified five external senses (hearing, sight, smell, taste and touch) and five internal senses: common sense (hiss mushtarik); imagination (takhayyul); reflection (tafakkur); recollection (tadhakkur); and the memory (hafiza). Al-Ghazali attributed to the internal senses different locations inside the brain. He also maintained that the memory is located in the hinder lobe, imagination - in the frontal lobe, and reflection -in the middle folds of the brain. He assumed

---

[164] *Ibid*

[165] Nahyan A., Pulmonary Transit and Bodily Resurrection: The Interaction of Medicine, Philosophy and Religion in the Works of Ibn al-Nafïs (d. 1288), Electronic Theses and Dissertations, University of Notre Dame, 2006, pp. 209-210.

[166] Baker D., The Oxford Handbook of the History of Psychology: Global Perspectives, Oxford University Press, 2012, p.448.

that "the self carries two additional qualities, which distinguishes man from animals enabling man to attain spiritual perfection[167]", which are aql (intellect) and irada (will). Al-Ghazali affirmed that knowledge can either be innate or acquired. He drew a line between phenomenal (material world) knowledge and spiritual (related to God and soul), and, therefore, divided acquired knowledge into imitation, logical reasoning, contemplation and intuition. He believed human nature consists simultaneously of spirits of four creatures: the sage (intellect and reason), the pig (lust and gluttony), the dog (anger), and the devil (brutality).

Based on the Quranic verses, Al-Ghazali gave the following conceptions of nafs:

- nafs ammarah (sura 12, ayat 53) which "exhorts one to freely indulge in gratifying passions and instigates to do evil."[168] It is a primitive self that pushes a person up to commit evil acts. It also manifests itself when a person expresses dissatisfaction. In this regard, the sura Yusuf narrates: "I do not exculpate myself. Lo! the (human) soul enjoineth unto evil, save that whereon my Lord hath mercy. Lo! my Lord is Forgiving, Merciful";
- nafs lawammah (sura 75, ayat 2) which is "the conscience that directs man towards right or wrong";
- nafs mutmainnah (sura 89, ayat 27) which is "a self that reaches the ultimate peace". It is a positive and wise self. Its example can be found in sura "Al-fajr": "He will say: Ah, would that I had sent before me (some provision) for my life! None punisheth as He will punish on that day! None bindeth as He then will bind. But ah! thou soul at peace! Return unto thy Lord, content in His good pleasure! Enter thou among My bondmen! Enter thou My Garden!".

He ascribed the cause of spiritual diseases to the deviation from the God's path. Al-Ghazali suggested to apply the following methods in psychotherapy, such as mahasaba for improving the children's memory, while mujhahida and muraaqba implement as therapeutic interventions.

---

[167] http://www.academia.edu/19298899/Psychology_from_islamic_perspective, consulted on 31.04.2016

[168] Haque A., Psychology from Islamic Perspective: Contributions of Early Muslim Scholars and Challenges to Contemporary Muslim Psychologists, Vol. 43, No. 4 (Winter, 2004), p. 363.

Ashraf Al Thanvi (1873-1943)

Ashraf Al Thanvi, an eminent Islamic physician and sufi, who was considered as "Physician of the Muslims" (Hakim al-ummat) and "Reformer of the Nation" (Mujaddid al-Millat).

Among his most famous books there are Behishti Zaiver and Tarbiyyat-ul-Shalik. His other psychological works are entitled as follows:

1. Personality Theory. According to Thanvi, a child's life starts from a clean sheet. He appropriates good and bad things from the surrounding people. On these grounds, he may develop one of three types of "nafs", which are: (a) Nafs ammara (manifestation of evil), (b) Nafs lavvama (cursing after sin) and (c) Nafs mutmainna (following divines).

2. Causes and Classification of Disease. Ashraf Ali Thanvi described the causes of mental diseases as follows: When a person goes astray from God he becomes worthless, which, consequently leads to the mental sufferings. The scholar stated that a human being possesses two types of forces: constructive force and destructive force. He believed that correct education has the biggest impact on a person's future life.

Ali Thanvi differentiated between organic and functional diseases. The organic diseases may be cured by medical drugs, while psychological diseases are to be cured by individual and group therapies. In the individual therapy, a patient should achieve full self-expression and self-realization through insight. Whilst the group therapies were organized by Maulana Thanvi at his "Khanqah", where he would read a sermon on a relevant topic, and each member of the group would make sure to do as advised under close supervision of the spiritual leader. The group was living together during a certain period of time.

3. Treatment or Therapies. Ali Thanvi considered it essential that the patient expresses his own will and effort in the cure of disease. So, before starting treatment, he made sure that the patient was well aware that his therapeutic techniques would not lead to the following:
   • Miracle and "Kashf"
   • Guarantee for forgiveness on the day of judgment
   • Promise of material gain or better prospects in life
   • Automatic cure through counselor's attention

- Possibility of action without will
- Promise or surely for inner experiences

As for another type of remedial treatment, he was using reading therapy, which initiated from the exchange of letters between a doctor and a patient, in which a patient was talking about his problem. This technique helped to establish an essential link between them, after which the main treatment started. All treatment of Ali Thanvi was fully based on Quranic tradition.

Ibn Rushd (1126 –1198)

Ibn Rushd, also known as Averroes. He wrote on logic, philosophy, theology, Islamic jurisprudence, psychology, political and Andalusian classical music theory, geography, mathematics, mediæval sciences of medicine, astronomy, physics, and celestial mechanics. Ibn Rushd viewed the studying of the mind as a part of physics science. In his own words, "[metaphysics] surpasses all other sciences, except for divine science [...] and so we must hold that the science of the soul comes before the other sciences; and for this reason, we placed it in a position of priority among all subjects of inquiry." His Short Commentary on De anima exemplifies a summary of Aristotle's work. Ibn Rushd also made some studies regarding Active intellect and Passive intellect, both of the following were formerly regarded subjects of Psychology.[169] Ibn Rushd's views on psychology are amply expressed in his Talkbis Kitab al-Nafs (Aristotle on the Soul). Here Ibn Rushd, as M. Fakhry comments, divided the soul into five faculties: the nutritive, the sensitive, the imaginative, the appetitive and the rational.[170] The primary psychological faculty of all plants and animals is the nutritive or vegetative faculty, passed on through sexual generation, as noted above. The remaining four higher faculties are dependent on the nutritive faculty and are really perfections of this faculty, the product of a nature urging to move higher and higher.[171] Ibn Rushd approved of Themistius' position that "material intellect is a single incorporeal eternal substance that becomes

---

[169] Jayyusi S., The Legacy of Muslim Spain, Brill, 1992, p. 330.

[170] http://plato.stanford.edu/entries/arabic-islamic-mind, consulted on 31.04.2016

[171] http://www.iep.utm.edu/ibnrushd/#H7, consulted on 01.07.2016

attached to the imaginative faculties of individual humans."[172] He believed that the human soul is a separate substance alike the active intellect; and when this active intellect is embodied in an individual human it becomes the material intellect. Therefore, the human mind consists of the material intellect and the passive intellect, which makes up the third element of the intellect. The passive intellect is incarnated with imagination. When the material intellect is actualized by incoming information, it is described as the speculative (habitual) intellect. In one of his minor essays on the topic, Averroes portrays the fully realized acquired intellect of a person as losing its identity upon attaining conjunction with the Agent Intellect being totally absorbed in it.[173] He concluded that knowledge could, therefore, be gained by looking at causes of objects and events. Ibn Rushd thought of recollection (tadhakkur) as of a process of joining new images with already existent images in the mind. Averroes thus understands recollection as a three-fold operation: the cogitative faculty employs the intentions of an imagined form retained in memory, and combines them with the original sensory image to collect a full recollection of the thought image. The scholar believed that good memory mainly relies on dryness in the front and back of the brain.

Muḥammad ibn Aḥmad Al-Biruni (973 -1048)

Muhammad ibn Aḥmad Al-Biruni, born in Kath (Uzbekistan) is a Muslim scholar and polymath. He contributed with his researches to the field of physics, mathematics, astronomy, natural sciences, history, astrology, chemistry, comparative sociology, geology, medicine, philosophy, pharmacology, physics, psychology, geodesy and indology. He is a Founding Father of anthropology and experimental psychology. Al-Biruni pioneered experiments that helped him identify the concept of reaction time,[174] which he described as follows: "Not only is every sensation attended by a corresponding change localized in the sense-organ, which demands a certain time, but also, between the stimulation of the organ and consciousness of the perception an interval of time must elapse,

---

[172] Davidson H.,Alfarabi, Avicenna, and Averroes, on Intellect: Their Cosmologies, Theories of the Active Intellect, Theories of Human Intellect, Oxford University Press, 1992, p.295.

[173] http://plato.stanford.edu/entries/arabic-islamic-mind, consulted on 31.04.2016

[174] Baker D., The Oxford Handbook of the History of Psychology: Global Perspectives, Oxford University Press, 2012, p.445.

corresponding to the transmission of stimulus for some distance along the nerves."[175] It was clear to Al-Biruni that the measuring equipment, as well as the human observers, tend to errors and bias conclusions, therefore, he started conducting the same experiment many times until a "common average" was reached. Thus with Al-Biruni the history of experiment as a scientific method started. He later entered upon written communication with ibn Sina regarding Aristotelian natural philosophy and Peripatetic school of thought. His book dedicated to psychology is called Translation of the Yoga`s Sutra`s".

Muhyid-Din Ibn Ali (1164–1240)

Muhyid-Din Ibn Ali (Ibn Arabi), born in Murcia (Spain). Ibn Ali influenced the field of psychology with his writings on the soul, perception, imagination, dreams and the nature of desire. He believed that the human heart is an independent acting machine of esoteric nature, which interacts closely with mind and soul. He thought of the heart as a rational part of the body.He was influenced by Aristotelian ideas and believed the human soul has three aspects—rational soul, animal soul and vegetative soul. Souad Hakim once said about Ibn Arabi:"...it is the heart which is the place and instrument of knowledge...[yet Ibn Arabi] makes no separation between the heart and the intellect... [For] if the Sufi does not state his knowledge in intelligible form then the intellect will not accept it, and no-one will pay any attention to what he says... He will be unable to state his knowledge in intelligible form insofar as he has not brought his knowledge across from the heart to the intellect, or else receives an understanding developed in the image of reasoned theory, as did Ibn Arabi... The heart is drunkenness (sukr), the intellect is lucidity (sahw) [and]... the "knowing" Sufi, although he has tasted all states of knowledge, does not omit to return to the sensory in order to give a line of conduct to disciples."

Ibn Arabi provided an extensive description of human faculties- dhawq, imagination, reason and sensory perception - operate and interrelate. Ibn Arabi debated about the meaning of human perfection, and he concluded that a man can perfect only if he is in unity with God. Since God is One, the Reality is also One Reality. And nothing else exists beyond God. The whole world is the continuation of Divine Revelation. The beginning of Fusus al-Hikam exemplifies the main idea as follows: "God (al-haqq) wanted to see the essences of His most perfect Names whose number

---

[175] Iqbal M., The Reconstruction of Religious Thought in Islam, Stanford University Press, 2013, p.187.

is infinite - and if you like, you can equally well say, God wanted to see His own Essence in one global object which having been blessed with existence, summarised the Divine order so that there he could manifest His mystery to Himself. For the vision that a being has of himself and in himself is not the same as another reality procures for him, and which he uses for himself as a mirror; (in this, he manifests himself to his self in the form which results from the 'place' of the vision...) So the Divine order required the clarification of the mirror of the world, and Adam became the light itself of this mirror and the spirit of this form."

For Ibn Arabi, the final goal of a man is not to reunite with God; but to become the place of God's self-revelation to Himself. Ibn Arabi says in the Futahat:"...the Prophet reported that God created Adam in His form, and the human being is the place where the whole cosmos is brought together. God's knowledge of the cosmos is none other than the knowledge of Himself, since there is nothing in existence but Him. So inevitably, the cosmos is in His Form.Thus, for Ibn Arabi the important thing about our knowledge of the external world - the only important thing - is that it is an indicator of something in ourselves."[176] He added, "He made you a sign (or a demonstration) (dalil) [of your Lord]. That is, he made your knowledge of yourself a "sign" (dalîl) to your knowledge of Him. This is either by way of the fact that He describes you with the same essence and attributes with which he describes Himself, and He made you His vice-regent and deputy upon the earth. Or it is that you have poverty and need for Him in your existence, or it is the two affairs together...

...He mentioned the horizons... lest you imagine that something remains in the horizons giving a knowledge of God that is not given by yourself. Hence he turned you over to the horizons...[Then he] turned you over to yourself alone, because he knew that the Real would be your faculties and that you would know Him through Him, not through other than Him... When you know Him and you attain to Him no-one will have known and attained to Him save Himself... for the door to knowledge of Him is shut, unless it comes from Him. Ibn Arabi reflected upon the names of God, which indicated to His true nature, which he called as manifestations (mazahir) of the Divine attributes or actions by which the Divine is known. In this regard Ibn Arabi narrated:

"'Allah" is the name of the divine Essence as it is in Itself absolutely. "Al-Rahman" is He Who causes existence and perfection to flow upon all things in accordance with the dictates of [divine] wisdom and according

---

[176] Chittick W., Self-Disclosure of God, The: Principles of Ibn al-'Arabi's Cosmology, State University of New York Press, 1998, p.28.

to the capacities of the receivers to bear it in their primary stages.[177] Al-Rahim is He Who causes ideal perfection [in the Platonic sense] to flow upon the human species, which is proper to it in its final stages. For this reason, it is said [in invoking God], "O Rahman of this world and the next and Rahim of the hereafter!" This means, in the perfect human all-encompassing form, general and specific mercy, which is the manifestation of the divine Essence as well as of the Truth of supreme exaltation with all His attributes. It [the name of Allah] is the greatest name of God; it is to this name that the Prophet referred when he said, "I have been given comprehensive speech [jawami al-kalim – The Quran, which is of a finite number of words but infinite number of meanings}, and I was sent to complete the excellences of morals". That is why Jesus was called "a Word from God". The excellence of morals are the states of existents and the special properties which are the sources of their actions and which are all contained in the comprehensive human microcosm. Prophets placed words side by side with the ranks of existence. I found things at the time of Jesus and that of the Prince of the Faithful ['Ali] and some of the Companions which point to this truth."

According to Ibn Arabi`s doctrine of "Tajdid alkhalaq Filanat" (the renewal of creation at each instant), everything in the universe is the manifestation of Divine Creation[178]. In his famous Meccan Revelations, Ibn Arabi proposed his science of imagination, which had a profound impact on the theory of imagination in Sufism with important implications for Analytical Psychology[179]. In his voluminous treatise, Ibn Arabi gave a detailed analysis of his experiences in active imagination including a profound dialogue that he had with an anima figure, who was the earthly manifestation of Sophia Aeterna, during active imagination circumambulating the Kaaba in Mecca[180].

---

[177] Ayoub M., The Qur'an and Its Interpreters, State University of New York Press, Vol. 1, 1984, p.50.

[178] Kiehl E., Copenhagen 2013 - 100 Years On: Origins, Innovations and Controversies: Proceedings of the 19th Congress of the International Association for Analytical Psychology, 2015, speech by Steven Nouriani

[179] *Ibid*

[180] Kiehl E., Copenhagen 2013 - 100 Years On: Origins, Innovations and Controversies: Proceedings of the 19th Congress of the International Association for Analytical Psychology, 2015, speech by Steven Nouriani

The notion of Mundus Imaginalis, coined by Ibn Arabi, is different from the concept of imagination in western psychology.[181] Mundus Imaginalis [...] is thought to go beyond the unconscious and the psychoid to include levels of the spirit world and imagination, which are independent of the psyche and include the superconscious.[182] Imagination at the level of Mundus Imaginalis has a noetic function and is capable of the creative act of producing images that have mental and subtle bodies in which the thoughts and the will of the soul are carried.[183] At its lower levels, Mundus Imaginalis is similar to the psychoid level of the imaginal world as an in-between realm which emerges out of an area of the soul called "Nakoja Abad" (Nowhere Place), and is described as an intermediary level between spirit and body, which is neither dark, nor light neither matter nor spirit[184]. In Ibn Arabi`s system, the organ for the perception of Mundus Imaginalis is the symbolic heart which provides the function of active imagination through which mental and sense perceptions as well as theophanies are transformed into symbolic forms and various levels of soul and spirit can be perceived to bring healing and harmony with the Anima Mundi.[185] The first stage of Creation is described of as the One (Ahadiyyah) or Absolute, which is inconceivable and beyond all attributes, moving towards Oneness (Wahidiyyah) or Absolute possessing characteristics (equivalent perhaps to the Vedantic distinction between nirguna (qualityless) and saguna (possessing qualities) Brahman). For Ibn Arabi, the characteristics of the Absolute are the Divine Names.

The ayan thabita are the "fixed prototypes" or "latent realities of things". Before a thing materializes in the real world it exists as a potential in the divine Essence of God; as ideas of His future becoming, the content of His eternal knowledge, which is His knowledge of Himself. As summarized by A. Affifi: "God revealed Himself to Himself" in His "First Epiphany or Particularisation (al tayyun al awwal) in which He saw in Himself and for Himself an infinity of a`yan as determinate "forms" of His own Essence, which reflected and in every detail corresponded to His own eternal ideas of them."[186]

---

181 *Ibid*

182 *Ibid*

183 *Ibid*

184 *Ibid*

185 *Ibid*

186 Afifi A.,The Mystical Philosophy of Ibnul Arabi, Cambridge University Press, 1939, p.47.

Ahadiyya
> One or Essence or Absolute
>> |
>> \|/
>> Wahadiyya
>> Multiplicity in One;

the Divine Names
>> |
>> \|/

ayan thabita
> "fixed archetypes"
>> |
>> \|/
>> Khalq
>> "appearance"

The Divine Names are active in relation to the ayan al thabita (the archetypes of the phenomenal world), and these in turn are active in relation to the external world. In each case the higher is active in relation to the lower and passive in relation to the higher.[187]

Above all, Ibn Arabi insists on the central role and privileged status of the Human Self, or at least each individual`s potential status as a possible exemplar of the archetypal human, known as insanu-al-kamil, the complete or perfect human being.[188]

All knowledge for Ibn Arabi is necessarily a form of self-knowledge.[189] To put the matter in contemporary existentialist terms Ibn Arabi`s is a participatory view of knowledge which recognizes that in every act of knowing stands the knower.[190] All knowledge for Ibn Arabi necessarily a form of self-knowledge.[191]

---

[187] Affifi A., The Mystical Philosophy of Ibnul Arabi, Cambridge University Press,1939, p.46.

[188] Coates P., Ibn Arabi and Modern Thought: The History of Taking Metaphysics Seriously, Anqa Publishing, 2002, p.3.

[189] *Ibid, p.4.*

[190] *Ibid*

[191] *Ibid*

Abu Bakr Mohammad ibn Zakariya Al-Razi (865 – 925)

Abu Bakr Mohammad ibn Zakariya Al-Razi, known as Razi by the Arabs, and Rhazes in the West, was an influential scholar and psychologist, who among the first in the world wrote on mental health and psychotherapy. He occupied a post of chief physician at Baghdad hospital, and a director of one of the first psychiatric wards in the world. This type of clinics did not exist in Europe at that time. But for his two works Al-Mansuri and Al-Hawi, which are dedicated to the treatment of mental illnesses, Razi authored more than two hundred books. His analytic work Al-Hawi, typifies a detailed medical encyclopedia in twenty-five volumes with the full definition of symptoms and methods of treatment. This book has been widely consulted by doctors and students all around the globe since the 15th century. He was an active advocate of psychotherapeutic treatment. The discussion on mental health was published in his book entitled Al Mansuri in Al Tibb al-Ruhani. Such psychiatric clinics did not exist in Europe during that time for fear of demonic possessions.

Razi was considered the first person to apply psychological methods alongside with medical treatment. Oftentimes Razi was curing the caliphs and ministers, e.g. once he was asked to treat a famous caliph who was suffering from severe arthritis. Razi prescribed a hot bath and, while the caliph was bathing, Razi approached him and threatened to kill him. The shock, which a caliph lived through, increased the blood pressure, and, therefore, created proper conditions for dissolution of the softened humours. The caliph got up from the bath, raised on his knees and ran after Razi.

A special feature of his medical approach was the correct usage of food, which he applied to healing even mentally ill people. Besides alcoholism, he attributed to the excessive consumption of wine such illnesses as epilepsy, paralysis, visionary distortions, debility, impotence, as well as mental disorders. He believed that wisdom arises not from the thought of death, but from overcoming that thought. He affirmed that a thought of death undermines the state of happiness. Al-Razi explained it: "As long as the fear of death persists, one will incline away from reason and toward passion (hawa)." The scholar claimed that the sexual drive is provoked as much by the fear of death as by natural appetite. The fear of death may never be vanished from a human soul unless a person is certain that after the death follows a better state. And this leads to conclusion that it "would require very lengthy argumentation if one sought proof rather than just allegations (khabar)." All in all, he maintains that there is no need to fear death if the soul is immortal. Al-Razi also believed that ordinary men are fully capable of independent thinking and do not need guidance from another, which is a critical point in understanding the place of a human in between the prescribed destiny and a free will. Also, the religious rituals he viewed as the obsession, through which a human tries to cleanse oneself from impurity. He also supports the idea that in this world the pain and suffering prevail over peace and well-being. He affirmed that life as a whole and bodily existence, in general, represent a fall for the life-giving principle, the Soul. But the fall is broken by the gift of intelligence.

Abu Zayd Ahmed ibn Sahl Al-Balkhi (850-934)

Abu Zayd Ahmed ibn Sahl Al-Balkhi, a Muslim polymath: a geographer, mathematician, physician, cognitive psychologist, and scientist. He developed the basic concepts of mental health, as well as was among the first to raise awareness on necessity of "mental hygiene". In his Sustenance for Body and Soul (Masalih al-Abdan wa al-anfus), he demonstrated the existent deep influence between the state of body and soul. He alleged that "if the nafs [psyche] gets sick, the body may also find no joy in life and may eventually develop a physical illness."[192] Al-Balkhi left his impact on the development of psychotherapy, psychophysiology, and psychosomatic medicine. He acknowledged that both a body and a soul can suffer, or be "balanced or imbalanced". By his practice he demonstrated that mental illness can have both psychological and physiological causes. As an example of imbalance in body he referred to a headache, while imbalance of a soul brings on anxiety, sadness, and other mental symptoms. Al-Balkhi advanced an idea of treatment of the body with respect to the imbalance. Later Joseph Wolpe introduced this idea as "reciprocal inhibition". He distinguished between two types of depression: the causes of the first are known (such as nervous breakdown), which responds to psychological treatment, while the factors of the other are unknown, probably, those of physiological nature, and, therefore, can be treated with drugs and physiotherapy. Further Al-Balkhi categorized depression into sadness— normal depression—reactive depression and endogenous depression[193]. What makes Al-Balkhi`s categorization of types of depression outstanding is the differentiation between the second and the third type: the endogenous and reactive depression. His reflections on depression follow: "Huzn,

---

[192] Baker D., The Oxford Handbook of the History of Psychology: Global Perspectives, Oxford University Press, 2012, p.449.

[193] Haddad Y., The Muslims of America, New York: Oxford University Press, 1991, p.78.

---

sadness or depression is of two kinds. The (environmental) causes, for one of them is clearly known, such as the loss of a loved relative, bankruptcy or loss of something the depressed person values greatly. The other type has no known reasons. It is a sudden affliction of sorrow and distress ghummah, which persists all the time to prevent the afflicted person from physical activity or from showing any happiness or enjoying any clear reasons for his lack of activity and distress. This type of huzn or depression with no known reasons is caused by bodily symptoms such as impurity of the blood and other changes in it."[194] Also, Al-Balkhi believed that through therapy the patient must realize the physical psychosomatic harm which the depressive mood is causing to his health, and since his own self should be the thing the dearest to him, it will indeed be greatly irrational to harm the most the most beloved for losing things that can be substituted.[195] Al-Balkhi suggests that a depressed person should ask himself which of the two groups he would want to identify with and belong to, "the failed" or "the successful?"[196] According to Al-Balkhi, losing one`s perseverance is a greater catastrophe than losing what one is depressed about.[197] Al-Balkhi also states that "One can heal oneself [...] when feeling peaceful and when the faculties of the soul are in a tranquil state, one should convince the heart (mind) that this world dunya has not been created to give people whatever they wish or desire without their being subjected to anxieties and worries or harmful unwelcome symptoms [...] A person should train himself not to overreact to the minor incidents or things that he hears or sees. In doing so he will be analogous to one who (gradually) trains himself to tolerate the painful effects of a slight increase in temperature, heat or cold, as well as other minor bodily pains without showing impatience or tension until this becomes part of his usual habits. This will then help him to endure the test of greater pain if he were to encounter it."[198] Al Balkhi was the first to differentiate between neuroses and psychoses. The scholar categorized neuroses into four emotional disorders: anxiety, fear, aggression and anger,

---

[194]   Badri Malik, Abu Zayd al-Balkhi's Sustenance of the Soul: The Cognitive Behavior Therapy of a Ninth Century Physician, 2013, Herndon: International Institute of Islamic Thought, p.21.

[195]   Badri Malik, Abu Zayd al-Balkhi's Sustenance of the Soul: The Cognitive Behavior Therapy of a Ninth Century Physician, 2013, Herndon: International Institute of Islamic Thought, p. 22.

[196]   *Ibid*

[197]   *Ibid*

[198]   *Ibid, p.31.*

depression and sadness, and obsessions.[199] Al-Balkhi strongly believed that the best way to achieve good health is to maintain the balance between the mind and body. He was very critical of the medicine of his time, which placed too much of importance on the physical illness, and not the mental. He claimed, "since man's construction is from both his soul and his body, therefore, human existence cannot be healthy without the ishtibak [interweaving or entangling] of soul and body." Al-Balkhi`s approach to the mental health stems from the Quran, which says in particular: "In their hearts is a disease." (sura 2, ayat 10). Abu Zaid al-Balkhi is most likely to be considered as the first cognitive psychologist. In his book, Al-Balkhi claims that "man`s stamina is a combination of both his body and soul and one cannot imagine that he can exist without this dual combination which causes him to act as a human being. Their combination gives to man his ability to respond to threatening issues and painful symptoms." Moreover, he considered a mental disorder as a learned habit, which could not divide people into healthy and ill.

Najab Uddin Muhammad (10th century)

Najab Uddin Muhammad precised detailedly a definition of a number of mental diseases. He was observing mentally ill patients, in particular, those suffering from agitated depression, neurosis, periapism and sexual impotence, and arranged his notes in a book that "made up the most complete classification of mental diseases theretofore known."[200]

Ibn Al-Haitham (965-1040)

Ibn Al-Haitham is considered to be the founder psychophysics, for his pioneering work on the psychology of visual perception, which is called The Book of Optics. Ibn al-Haitham argued that vision occurs in the brain, and not in the eyes, as it was widely believed at the epoch. He pointed out that numerous subjective factors, such as personal experience etc., influence the way people see and perceive the things. He writes, "The act of vision is not accomplished by means of rays emitted from the visual organ"; rather, "vision is accomplished by rays coming from external objects

---

[199] Haque A., Psychology and Religion: Their Relationship and Integration from Islamic Perspective, The American Journal of Islamic Social Sciences, 15, 1998, pp. 97–116.

[200] Baker D., The Oxford Handbook of the History of Psychology: Global Perspectives, Oxford University Press, 2012, p.446.

and entering the visual organ"[201]He asserts that "Truth is sought for itself" but "the truths," he warns, "are immersed in uncertainties"[202] and adds, "Therefore, the seeker after the truth is not one who studies the writings of the ancients and, following his natural disposition, puts his trust in them, but rather the one who suspects his faith in them and questions what he gathers from them, the one who submits to argument and demonstration, and not to the sayings of a human being whose nature is fraught with all kinds of imperfection and deficiency. Thus the duty of the man who investigates the writings of scientists, if learning the truth is his goal, is to make himself an enemy of all that he reads, and, applying his mind to the core and margins of its content, attack it from every side. He should also suspect himself as he performs his critical examination of it so that he may avoid falling into either prejudice or leniency."[203]

Ishaq bin Ali Rahawi (9th century)

The standards and ethics that Muslim doctors should follow in their work were first laid down in the 9th century by Ishaq bin Ali Rahawi in his book The Conduct of a Physician (Adab al-Tabib). He regarded physicians as "guardians of souls and bodies", and wrote twenty chapters on various topics related to medical ethics, including:[204]

- What the physician must avoid and beware of
- The manners of visitors
- The care of remedies by the physician
- The dignity of the medical profession
- The examination of physicians
- The removal of corruption among physicians

In Adab al-Tabib, Al-Ruhawi also suggests the possible penalties for incompetent treatment. Al Rahawi was the first to raise the topic of the ethics of a Muslim doctor.

---

[201] Alhazen, Opticae Thesaurus: Alhazeni Arabis Libri Septem Nunc Primum Editi, Eiusdem Liber De CrepusculisEtNubiumAsensionibus, New York: Johnson Reprint Corp, 1972, p.17.

[202] http://harvardmagazine.com/2003/09/ibn-al-haytham-html, consulted on 01.07.2016

[203] *Ibid*

[204] http://www.muslimheritage.com/article/islamic-science-scholar-and-ethics, consulted on 01.07.2016

Ibn Al-Wardi (1290-1349)

Ibn Al-Wardi in his Al-Lubab fi Ilm al-Irab studied and analysed the manifestations of psyche, associated with emotional shocks, which were forgotten and deeply suppressed to unconscious. The therapies, which they applied, aimed at letting a patient recall without censorship the emotional experience, thus enabling, the patient's liberation. They stated that the dreams, in fact, were elements of the functioning of unconscious processes.

Abu Bakr ibn Bajjah (1095–1138)

Abu Bakr ibn Bajjah, known in the West as Avempace, was a physician, philosopher, and scientist. His psychological theories were based on physics.[205] Ibn Bajjah, like Aristotle, bases his psychology on physics. Ibn Bajjah's writings focused on active intelligence and believed it was the most important ability humans possessed.[206] He was also interested in sensations and imaginations and believed that knowledge cannot be obtained by both senses and active intelligence, which is the governing intelligence of nature.[207] He believed that matter, form and intelligence are key components of the "soul". The appetitive soul consists of three faculties: (1) The imaginative appetite through which progeny are reared, individuals are moved to their dwellings, and have affection, love, and the like.[208] (2) The intermediate appetite through which there is a desire for food, housing, arts, and crafts. (3) The appetite that makes the speech and, through that, teaching possible and, unlike the other two, is peculiar to man. The appetitive soul desires a perpetual object or an object in so far as it is perpetual.[209] He believed sound knowledge could only be acquired through intelligence, which permits humans to acquire success

[205] Haque A.,Psychology and Religion: Their Relationship and Integration from Islamic Perspective, The American Journal of Islamic Social Sciences, 15, 1998, pp. 97–116.

[206] Hamarneh K.,In M.A. Anees (ed.), Health Sciences in Early Islam: collected Papers, Vol. 2, Blanco, TX: Zahra Publications, 1984, p.353.

[207] Haque A., Psychology and Religion: Their Relationship and Integration from Islamic Perspective, The American Journal of Islamic Social Sciences, 15, 1998, pp. 97–116.

[208] https://www.al-islam.org/history-muslim-philosophy-volume-1-book-3/chapter-26-ibn-bajjah, consulted on 01.07.2016

[209] *Ibid*

and construct characters.[210] He explained the knowledge as a two-step process. First, (i) the human intellect analyses concrete substances and separates forms from matter.[211] Second, (ii) it analyses forms themselves in their constituents.[212] In fact, Ibn Bajah speaks not so much of "forms" as of "intentions" (maana), which are, in turn, rendered as quiddities (quidditas) in the Latin translation of Averroes`s Long Comentary on the De Anima.[213] His writings also emphasized on the connection of the rational soul and the individuals identity with the virtue of its contact with the active intelligence become one of those lights that gives glory to God.[214] Moreover, Ibn Bajjah believed that with spiritual knowledge, Active intelligence and Divine intervention humans could acquire freedom.[215] "Agent Intellect" designates the active power involved in the conceptualization, which resides in a self-subsistent form separate from matter.[216] "Potential Intellect" is the potentiality to receive intelligible notions, and it is located in man`s soul or, more precisely, in his imagination.[217] Intelligible notions are like forms that have as their matter the forms of imagination.[218] When all intelligible are acquired, the potential intellect turns into an "acquired intellect" (al aql al mustafad).[219] The sensibles or the natural accidents are of two kinds: either they are particular to the natural bodies or common to the natural and the artificial bodies; and they are, again, either mover or moved.[220] They are always moved towards the species since a mover causes motion in them only in so far as they are particular species, and not because they

---

[210] Badri M.,The Dilemma of Muslim Psychologists, MWH Publishers, 1979

[211] Marenbon, John, The Oxford Handbook of Medieval Philosophy, Oxford: OUP USA, 2012, p.110.

[212] *Ibid*

[213] *Ibid*

[214] Haque A., Psychology and Religion: Their Relationship and Integration from Islamic Perspective, The American Journal of Islamic Social Sciences, 15, 1998, pp. 97–116.

[215] Badri M., The Dilemma of Muslim Psychologists, MWH Publishers, 1979

[216] Marenbon, John, The Oxford Handbook of Medieval Philosophy, Oxford: OUP USA, 2012, p.110.

[217] *Ibid*

[218] *Ibid*

[219] *Ibid*

[220] https://www.al-islam.org/history-muslim-philosophy-volume-1-book-3/chapter-26-ibn-bajjah, consulted on 01.07.2016

possess matter. The five senses -- sight, hearing, smell, taste, and touch are five faculties of a single sense- the common sense[221]. His original treatises include Tadbir al-Mutawahid (Rule of the Solitary), Risala al-Wada" (Letter of Farewell) and Risala al-Itisal al-Aql bi Insan (Epistle on the Conjunction of the Intellect with a Man).

Abu Bakar ibn Tufail (1110-1185)

Abu Bakar ibn Tufail, well-known in the West under the name of Abubacer, was a Spanish physician and scholar whose work emphasized the concept of human's spiritual and philosophical abilities and treatment of the soul.[222] Ibn Tufail's discoveries influenced many Western philosophers and writers, in particular, Daniel Defoe, who later wrote Robinson Crusoe. Ibn Tufail believed that Active intellect is guided by divine intervention. He suggested that culture; language and religion are unnecessary and could hinder the development of the mind.[223] According to Ibn Tufail, the First Cause is incorporeal and can be known, accordingly, through annihilation of the body, and, ultimately, of the self.[224] Ibn Tufail's work is remarkable for the peculiar way in which the indigenous tradition is reinterpreted in at least three respects:[225] (i) the naturalistic conception of the relationship between reason and revelation; (ii) the reflection on the social role of the philosopher; (iii) the interpretation and appreciation of mysticism. If revelation agrees with reason, it is because (i) revelation adds nothing to the results of rational investigation and the positive contents of the science.[226] A key element of Ibn Tufail's views on human essence played fitra (inborn nature). Ibn Tufail insists that the content of this

---

[221] https://www.al-islam.org/history-muslim-philosophy-volume-1-book-3/chapter-26-ibn-bajjah, consulted on 01.07.2016

[222] Haque A., Psychology and Religion: Their Relationship and Integration from Islamic Perspective, The American Journal of Islamic Social Sciences, 15, 1998, pp. 97–116.

[223] *Ibid*

[224] Marenbon, John, The Oxford Handbook of Medieval Philosophy, Oxford: OUP USA, 2012, p.113.

[225] *Ibid*

[226] *Ibid*

ecstatic experience transcends the ordinary language or logic, also it can be alluded to by symbols (mithal) hints (ishara).[227]

Ali ibn Sahl At-Tabari (838-870)

Ali ibn Sahl At-Tabari, a Persian physician, who converted to Islam in his youth, was mostly working in the field of child development. His most influential book called Firdaus al Kikmah on medical writings discussed psychotherapy that were ideas derived from ancient Indian writings on medicine.[228] At-Tabari insisted on a strong correlation between usage of psychotherapy and efficiency of general medical treatment. He believed the importance of psychotherapy to cure illness, especially the illness due to delusive imagination.[229] He believed that with through counseling and appropriate treatment options patients can be cured. At-Tabari was the first to demonstrate the importance of medicine and psychology.[230] He was writing that oftentimes the patients suffer not so much of the physical symptom itself, as of an imaginative one, which is due to delusions and illusions. He believed that wise counseling can cure such patients. According to Michael Dols, "At-Tabari used the tripartite division of the brain to locate psychic disorders". His book Firdous al-Hikma is one of the first medical Islamic encyclopedias. It consists of 7 sections and 30 parts, which are:

Part I. Introduction to the main philosophical concepts, the categories, natures, elements, genesis. It is subdivided into 12 chapters, in particular:

- On the Name of the Book and its Composition.
- On Matter Shape, Quantity, and Quality.
- On Simple and Compound Temperaments.
- On the Antagonism of these Temperaments and the Refutation of the Opinion of those who allege that the Air is cold (of Temper).
- On the Genesis of Temperaments One from Another.

227 Marenbon, John, The Oxford Handbook of Medieval Philosophy, Oxford: OUP USA, 2012, p.114.

228 Hamarneh K.,In M.A. Anees (ed.), Health Sciences in Early Islam: collected Papers, Vol. 2, Blanco, TX: Zahra Publications, 1984, p.353.

229 Haque A., Psychology and Religion: Their Relationship and Integration from Islamic Perspective, The American Journal of Islamic Social Sciences, 15, 1998, pp. 97–116.

230 Hamarneh K.,In M.A. Anees (ed.), Health Sciences in Early Islam: collected Papers, Vol. 2, Blanco, TX: Zahra Publications, 1984, p.353.

- On Metamorphosis.
- On Genesis and Decay.
- On Activity and Passivity.
- On the Genesis of Things from the Elements, the Action of the Celestial Sphere and the Luminous Bodies therein.
- On the Effects of the Action of the Elements on the Air and Subterranean Conditions.
- On Shooting Stars and the Colors which are Generated in the Air. (Rainbows).

Part II. Embryology, pregnancy, the functions and morphology of different organs, ages and seasons, psychology, the external and internal senses, the temperaments and emotions, personal idiosyncrasies, nervous affections, tetanus, torpor, palpitation, nightmare, the evil eye, hygiene and dietetics (in total 5 books).

Part III. Treats of nutrition and dietetics.

Part IV is the longest one, even though each chapter is no longer than one page.

Book 1 (9 chapters) describes general pathology, the signs and symptoms of internal disorders, and the therapeutic principles.

Book 2 (14 chapters) is dedicated to the diseases and injuries of the head; and diseases of the brain, including epilepsy.

Book 3 (12 chapters) is focused on the diseases of the eyes, ears, nose, face, mouth and teeth.

Book 4 (7 chapters) is about nervous diseases, including spasm, paralysis etc.

Book 5 (7 chapters) narrates about the diseases of the throat, chest, including asthma.

Book 6 (6 chapters) is concentrated on the diseases of the stomach.

Book 7 (5 chapters) encompasses the diseases of the liver.

Book 8 (14 chapters) relates to the diseases of the heart, lungs, gall-bladder and spleen.

Book (19 chapters) concerns the diseases of the intestines, the urinary, and genital organs.

Book 10 (26 chapters) recounts the symptoms of fevers, pleurisy, erysipelas, smallpox etc.

Book 11(13 chapters) pays attention to rheumatism, leprosy, elephantiasis, scrofula, lupus, cancer, tumours, gangrene, wounds and bruises, shock, and plague. The last four chapters deal with anatomical matters, including the numbers of the muscles, nerves, and blood vessels.

Book 12 (20 chapters) describes phlebotomy, cupping, baths and the indications of the pulse and urine.

Part V explores the senses, tastes, scents and colors.

Part VI includes medical and toxicological material.

Part VII gives an account of specificities of climate and geographical conditions and their influence on health.

His other books comprise: Tuhfat al-Muluk (The King's Present describes the proper use of food, drink, and medicines); Hafzh al-Sihhah (The Proper Care of Health compares Greek and Asian health-care traditions; Kitab al-Ruqa (Book of Magic or Amulets investigates the influence of magic on the human behaviour); Kitab fi Tartib al-Ardhiyah (Treatise on the Preparation of Food provides healthy recipes and recommendations on healthy eating, etc.

Ali ibn Abbas Al-Majusi (982)

Ali ibn Abbas Al-Majusi discussed how the psychosocial state of a person can have direct impacts on the immune system and vice versa in his celebrated book Complete Book of the Medical Art. He found a correlation between patients who were physically and mentally healthy and those who were physically and mentally unhealthy, and concluded that "joy and contentment can bring a better living status to many who would otherwise be sick and miserable due to unnecessary sadness, fear, worry and anxiety."[231] He is also the first person to discuss in detail such mental disorders as sleeping sickness, memory loss, coma, meningitis, vertigo, epilepsy, and hemiplegia. Moreover, he emphasized the preservation of health through diet and natural healing as much as on medication or drugs[232]. He also emphasized the importance of doctor-patient relation and its impact on the patient's healing. He was also raising the topic of moral conduct of a doctor.

Yakub Ibn Miskawayh (941-1030)

Miskawayh was an Islamic thinker. Even though the scholar was vividly passionate about psychology, he is more remembered as an ethics

---

[231] Deuraseh N., Abu Talib M. Mental health in Islamic medical tradition. The International Medical Journal. 2005, 4, pp.76-79.

[232] Haque A., Psychology and Religion: Their Relationship and Integration from Islamic Perspective, The American Journal of Islamic Social Sciences, 15, 1998, pp. 97–116.

writer. His book Taharat al-Araq (Purity of Dispositions) also known as Tahdhib al-Akhlaq (Cultivation of Morals) became a comprehensive sourcebook on ethical conduct. He suggested a human being needs to control oneself and learn the resistance of thinking and behaviour. He is the first known Muslim scholar, who introduced the concept of "self-reinforcement" and response cost. Ibn Miskawayh narrated that a Muslim, who feels guilty about doing something pleasurable to his al-nafs al-ammarah, should learn to punish himself by psychological, physical or spiritual ways such as paying money to the poor, fasting, etc.

Al-Jahiz (766–868)

The earliest works on social psychology and animal psychology were written by Al-Jahiz, an Afro-Arab scholar who studied the social organization of ants and animal communication and psychology[233].

We can conclude that during the golden era of Islamic civilization, the Muslim scholars were profoundly discussing the concept of psychology, psychiatry, psychotherapy, and their relationship to mental health. The greatest Arab physicians were treating both a body and soul, and not just one disease. They were already aware of somatization disorder, in which a patient had a preoccupation with physical state, and, in fact, its cause is psychological. Already at the epoch, a notion of psychoanalysis termed ilaj-il-nafsani, or psychotherapeusis, was no stranger to the Arab doctors. Razi was among the first, who introduced the method of bringing a patient back to an incident of his/her past life, which was now forgotten, hidden from consciousness, however, was the cause of physical and psychological sufferings. Islamic scholars also elaborated ethical responsibilities pertaining to a medical professional based on Greek, Indian and Persian teachings as well as the pillars of Islam. Among early books on the subject was Literature of Medicine (Adab al-Tibb) by Ishaq ibn Ali al-Ruhawi. He stressed on the significance of good doctor-patient communications and proper conduct of physicians, which would correspond to high ethical standards. To ensure compliance with the rules, an office was created in early 9th century to deal with overcharging, profiteering, extortion and fraud in medical practice, as well as to control medical staff and administer a special oath to doctors.

---

[233]   Haque A., Psychology and Religion: Their Relationship and Integration from Islamic Perspective, The American Journal of Islamic Social Sciences, 15, 1998, pp. 97–116.

In essence, even 1,000 years ago Islamic medicine was the most advanced in the world with a wide range of diagnostic and therapeutic methods in numerous specialities. Ten centuries after, the achievements of Islamic medicine still remain relevant.

Development of Psychology Science during the Ottoman Empire

By the end of the 15th century, the Arabo–Islamic Empire was divided into three distinct parts: the Safavid Empire in Persia (modern Iran), the Mughal Empire in India, and the Ottoman Empire. At various periods the Ottoman Empire comprised Arabic lands such as, Egypt, Tunisia, Syria and many others. The study, research and practice of modern psychiatry in the Empire were institutionalized by Dr. Rasit Tahsin at the end of 19th century. Tahsin offered practical psychiatry education, which was diverse from various points of view, by establishing the Neurology and Psychiatry Service (Asabiye ve Akliye Servisi) in the military medical school (Askeri Tıbbiye) in Gulhane, Istanbul in 1896.[234] However, the "treatment" of the mentally ill dated back to centuries ago, all the way back to the Seljuk Period*. The historic archives certify an emerging human attitude toward the insane (mecnun) in the Seljuk and earlier Ottoman periods. Traditionally, during the Ottoman era "mad" people, who could not be kept at home, were admitted to small asylums (bimarhane) adjacent to religious complexes (külliye). These interconnected buildings consisted of a mosque, public kitchen, medreses, caravansary, mausoleums, and were funded by foundations (vakıf). In Istanbul, Fatih, Haseki Sultan, Sultanahmed and Suleymaniye Darussif as started admitting the insanes in the 15th century.

While the mental patients were subjected to intense physical and mental tortures and inhuman treatment, since they were considered as possessed by the Western medicians during the Middle Age, mentally ill were receiving psychotherapy and musicotherapy at the Darüşşifa (mental hospital) section of the institution in Edirne. For example, Toptasi Asylum became the major public mental institution in the whole Ottoman capital after the mental patients were moved from Suleymaniye Asylum on the

---

[234] * The Seljuk Empire controlled the territories stretching from the Hindu Kush to eastern Anatolia and from Central Asia to the Persian Gulf.
**At the 15th century the Ottoman Empire, but for other territories, comprised Baghdad, Mesopotamia and attained a naval access to the Persian Gulf.
http://www.turkishculture.org/architecture/hospitals-964.htm, consulted on 31.04.2016

8th of November 1873. At the time Dr. Louis Mongeri was the senior responsible of the asylum. Dr. Mongeri improved the conditions, in which a patient was receiving treatment in the asylum and began the timeline of the modern development of psychiatry in the Empire. He also initiated the first ethical regulations of the asylums in 1876.

Toptasi Asylum in Üsküdar, also known as Valide-i Atik Bimarhanesi or Toptaşı Nurbanu Valide Sultan Darüşşifası was part of the Nurbanu Valide Sultan Külliyesi. This religious complex includes mosque, medrese, tekke, sıbyan mektebi (primary school), darülhadis, darülkurra, imaret (public kitchen and caravansary), hospital and a public bath (hamam). Toptasi Asylum was administered by Dr. Mongeri (1873-1882, until his death), Kastro (1882-1909), Dr. Avni Bey, and Mazhar Osman.[235]

The first hospital wards for the treatment of the mentally ill in Turkey were established in the 15th century**, and care was based on the precepts of the Islamic medicine; mentally ill people were usually treated kindly and with respect, and psychotic individuals were considered to have a particular closeness to God.[236]

Role of Sharia Law in the Management of Psychological Disorders

The literal meaning of sharia is "to introduce" or "prescribe." Shariah is more than just rules about religious rituals, and civil and criminal matters—it also includes ethical and moral principles[237]. In Islam Sharia signifies "the path" and it refers to the life path that Muslims should follow. It lays basis for requirements in relations between (a) people and Allah (worship); (b) person to person(social transactions). Much of the sharia was revealed in Medina, and Muhamed elaborated on the Islamic rituals. The main sources of sharia comprise the Quran and suna. Reliance on Allah leads to better psychological functioning. The citation of the following suras confirms this common belief of Muslims:

"… And whosoever puts his trust in Allah, then He will suffice him…"
(sura 65, ayat 3)

---

[235] http://www.turkishculture.org/architecture/hospitals-964.htm, consulted on 01.07.2016

[236] Scull A., Cultural Sociology of mental illness, an A-to-Z Guide, University California Press, vol.1, 2014, p. 904.

[237] Ahmed S., Counseling Muslims: Handbook of Mental Health Issues and Interventions, Routledge, 2012, p.6.

"So, verily, with every difficulty, there is a relief: Verily, with every difficulty, there is relief." (sura 94, ayat 5-6)
"And for those who fear Allah, He always prepares a way out, and He provides for him from sources he never could imagine. And if anyone puts his trust in Allah, sufficient is Allah for him. For Allah will surely accomplish His purpose: verily, for all things has Allah appointed a due proportion." (sura 65, ayats 2-3)

One of the hadiths in this regard narrates: "One day I was behind the prophet and he said to me: "Young man, I shall teach you some words (of advice): Be mindful of Allah, and Allah will protect you. Be mindful of Allah, and you will find Him in front of you. If you ask, ask of Allah; if you seek help, seek the help of Allah. Know that if the Nation were to gather together to benefit you with anything, it would benefit you only with something that Allah had already prescribed for you, and that if they gather together to harm you with anything, they would harm you only with something Allah had already prescribed for you. The pens have been lifted and the pages have dried.""[238]

Islam established sharia as a law for all, including medical personnel, who comply with it on personal and professional levels. As such, sharia requires them to be sincere, humble, and constantly strive to seek the pleasure of Allah.

Meaning of Psychological Health in Sharia

On the basis of Quran and suna, Muslim scholars made the following conclusions about the meaning of mental health for a Muslim. In particular, sharia describes mental health in the following terms:

1. Strong faith in Allah, and ability to perform one's ibaada (worshipping) to Allah.
2. The absence of any negative states, such as, anxiety, envy, jealousy, aggressiveness, hatred etc; avoidance of any evil that degrades one's own ability to carry on with the challenges of life in high spirits, for example, laziness, arrogance, pessimism, vanity, extravagance, etc.
3. Capacity to control one's own emotions, words, actions.

---

[238] Jamaal al-Din, Zarabozo M., Hadith, Al-Basheer Publication & Translation, pp. 729-730.

4. From the social side: love to one`s parents, sociability, love to one`s children, help to those in need, faith, avoidance of those, who disrespect the others through the lie, fraud, adultery, theft, murder; friendship with those, who love truth, work, responsibility.

5. From the biological side: sustaining body in a healthy state, care for one`s own health.

6. From the psychological side: maintain one`s thoughts clear and heart clean, maintenance of morality, sincerity, achieving skillfulness in a certain profession.

Definition of Insanity on Sharia

Insanity in Islamic law it is not considered as a separate or distinct category in legal textbooks.[239] It is discussed as a cause of legal disability or interdiction (bajr) and as a particular disability within such broad areas as taxation, marriage, divorce, inheritance, contracts, and religious obligations[240]. The most profitable manner of gaining an understanding on insanity in Islamic law is to look closely at bajr, or legal interdiction, which designates both the imposition of restriction and the status of restricted individual.[241]

The Approach to Mental Health in Sharia

There exist three approaches as such:

1. Strengthening of one`s own spirit through worshipping Allah.
2. Piety, which is manifested in reliance on Allah, truthfulness, faith, proper behavior, and constant attempts to moral improvement.
3. Devotion to Allah, which includes regular prayers, remembrance of Allah (zikr), teaching the other about Allah, seeking for knowledge about Allah, gaining virtues in front of Allah and avoiding sins, helping the other to reinforce his/her faith in Allah.

---

[239] Dols M., Historical Perspective. Insanity in Islamic Law, Journal of Muslim Mental Health, 2, 2007, pp. 81-99.

[240] *Ibid*

[241] Dols M., Historical Perspective. Insanity in Islamic Law, Journal of Muslim Mental Health, 2, 2007, pp. 81-99.

Recognizing and establishing control over one's own impulses constitute an integral part of one's own mental health, in accordance with sharia, which helps a Muslim to grow. Seeking refuge from one's own internal impulses a Muslim can through Quran and Prophet's suna, the reading of which brings relief. Belief in qadr and (destiny) and maktoub (fate), and also sabr (patience) to overcome the obstacles and follow what is prescribed by Allah.

Various Islamic scholars have expressed their views on one or more of the following issues: management of family conflicts, divorce, parenting, and the roles and responsibilities of spouses. Sometimes during a counseling session, family members can present conflicting views, which may be confusing for a psychologist without solid knowledge of legal code. That is why understanding sharia is an essential requirement for a psychotherapist practicing in the Islamic milieu. The clinician allows the patients to share their perspectives in a comfortable and nurturing environment and assists in enhancing the understanding of each other.

For the matters, which are not explicitly treated by the Quran or the Prophet's sayings, Islamic scholars apply juristic consensus (ijma) or analogy (qiyas). Ijma is achieved by consensus on a certain issue by Muslim scholars. Qiyas implies editing laws by analogy to the laws, which already existed during the Prophet's times. For example, wine is forbidden in Islam due to its intoxicating effects, so by analogy other intoxicating drugs are also forbidden by Islamic law. When other jurists do not admit qiyas, they can use juristic preference (istihsan) between two analogies, which might also lead to different scholarly interpretations. Islamic law also does not prohibit the inclusion of local social norms and customs into consideration, as long as the local norms and customs do not contradict the Quran and suna. Islamic jurisprudence started covering mental health issues in the beginning of the 7th century. Islamic laws addressed patient's confidentiality, insanity defense, involuntary hospitalization and treatment, mental competencies, family laws related to the mentally handicapped, child custody issues, child abuse, child as a witness, etc.

Given these points, the Islamic law is, probably, one of the oldest of its kind in the world. Sharia as a main legal source gives direct instructions on dealing with a mentally ill person. Specifically, Quran mentions the category of the mentally disabled as those, who stay closer to God, and prescribes caring attitude towards them.

Roots of Psychoanalysis in Islam

Psychoanalysis had been known in the Islamic world even earlier before it was discovered by Freud, even though it was not called as such then. Meddeb explains that the symbolic power of Islam lays in the "incarnation" of the voice of God in the text.[242] Echoing Lacan's teachings in his The Instance of the Letter in the Unconscious, he goes on to explain that when the letter then migrates out of the page (when it is read and as such interpreted), the letter is "celebrated" as a pure signifier, cut off from its supposed signified.[243] While Meddeb does not throw into question the authenticity of the letter and its meaning, he rejects, with Lacan, the concept of literal, solitary meanings and as such favors interpretation of the letter and sees in Islam the capacity to change as a religion through interpretation and the movement of the letter from the text into life. This explanation resonates with one earlier in the text in which, like Lacan explains about the unconscious, religion is structured like a language.[244] Like a language, religion can be employed for violence, for tolerance, for love. Meddeb's use of Lacan's instance of the letter means that Islam, like language, like the unconscious, shifts through time, and it is through the instance of the letter, or interpretation of the word, that this shift occurs, that systematic change hauls its way into being.

There are three stages of revelation in the Islamic tradition: veiling; unveiling; reveiling. These stages echo the creation of the cosmos: the blinding light; the darkness that allows one to see; and the screen that blinds the seen object.[245] This chapter will review dream interpretations and Sufism, as two primary sources of modern psychoanalytic practice, which are accepted by Islamic tradition.

Once Ibn Arabi said, "The only reason God placed sleep in the animated world was so that everyone might...know that there is another

---

[242] Meddeb A., Face à l'islam,Textuel, 2004, p.142.

[243] Lacan J., The Instance of the Letter in the Unconscious, or Reason Since Freud, in Écrits: A Selection, trans. B. Fink, W. W. Norton, 2002, pp.142-143.

[244] Lacan, Jacques. The Instance of the Letter in the Unconscious. Ecrits. Trans. Bruce Fink. New York: W. W. Norton & Company, 2006, c. 1970, pp. 412-441.

[245] Tutt D., Psychoanalysis and the Veil in Islam: Rethinking Truth and Liberation, Berfrois, 2013, p.1-8.

world similar to the sensory world."[246] He also stated that "Dreams have a place, a locus, and a state. Their state is sleep, which is an absence from manifest sensory things that produce ease because of weariness which overcomes the soul in this plane in this state of wakefulness."[247] Also Ibn Arabi was often evoking the Prophet`s saying: "People are asleep, and when they die they awake."

Premodern Muslims viewed dreams as the only way to get to know the world, which cannot be known otherwise than in dreams. Quran accorded particular significance to true dreams of prophets. For example, the figure of Abraham with the symbolic sacrifice of his sons (Ishmael for Muslims and Isaac for Jews and Christians) is made possible through the manifest content to discover or highlight his latent content, which represents the realization of desire or aspiration, or, on the contrary, angst, neurotic trouble linked to the repression.

Interpretation of dreams in Islam is one of the 46 parts of prophecy.[248] The truthfulness of the dream is related to the sincerity of the dreamer. Those who have the most truthful dreams are those who are the most truthful in speech.[249] Once Imaam al-Baghawi said, "Know that the interpretation of dreams falls into various categories. In accordance to Sharh al-Sunnah, dreams may be interpreted in the light of the Quran or in the light of suna, or by means of the proverbs that are current among people, or by names and metaphors, or in terms of opposites. On many occasions, Prophet Muhammad after finishing the morning prayer in the mosque, would face the companions and ask, "Who amongst you had a dream last night?" So if anyone had seen a dream he /she would narrate it. The Prophet would say, "Mashaallah" (God has willed it) and he would start interpreting the dream. Thus dream interpretation had a special place in the Prophetic wisdom. And this tradition is preserved in Islamic society, as well as practiced in many sufi orders. Sahih Al-Bukhari reported that Prophet Muhamed had said, "Nothing is left of Prophethood except glad tidings." Those with him asked, "What are glad tidings?" He replied, "True dreams." The Prophet Muhamed warned that after he was gone prophecy would come only through true dreams. Based on this and other

---

[246] Chittick W., The Sufi Path of Knowledge: Ibn Al Arabi`s Metaphysics of Imagination, SUNY Press, 1989, p.119.

[247] *Ibid, p.120.*

[248] http://hadithcollection.com/sahihbukhari.html, consulted on 01.07.2016

[249] Muslim S., Being Traditions of the Sayings and Doings of the Prophet Muḥammad as Narrated by His Companions and Compiled Under the Title Al-Jamil al sahih, Volume 4, Kitab Bhavan, 2000, hadith 4200

statements, early Muslims developed an Islamic approach to oneirology, the study of dreams. There existed a belief that Allah speaks to a person in a dream, which became a commonly accepted especially after the death of Prophet. Abu Hurayrah narrated that Messenger of God, Muhamed said, "There are three types of dreams: a righteous dream which is glad tidings from Allah, the dream which causes sadness is from Shaitan, and a dream from the ramblings of the mind." Thus based on suna, dreams can be of three types: 1. ruyaa - good dreams; 2 hulum - bad dreams; 3. dreams from one's own psyche. Abu Bakr, one of the closest companions of Prophet Muhamed, was also considered as the most accurate dream interpreter after the Prophet. As an Islamic tradition narrates, the Holy Prophet said that he God told him to relate his dreams to Abu Bakr. Whenever the Prophet Muhamad had a dream, he would recount it to Abu Bakr. The Prophet said, "Never was anything revealed to me that I did not pour into the heart of Abu Bakr." Whenever Abu Bakr had a dream, he would share it with the Prophet. They would then come to a common conclusion on a final interpretation about the dream. In early Islam, the practice of dream analysis was viewed as a spiritual exercise. It was believed that only those who were in a pure state could go to the heart of the deep meaning of a dream and start interpreting it.

Till nowadays the Islamic tradition has preserved the dreams of the Prophet and those of his people, which were sent to predict the major events in the whole Islamic umma. They can be narrated as follows:

Black and white sheep. Once, the Holy Prophet saw in a dream that he was driving a herd of black sheep. Then he found himself driving a herd of white sheep. After some time the two herds were inextricably intermingled and all attempts to separate them were of no avail. Interpreting the dream, Abu Bakr said that the black sheep signified the Arabs while the white sheep signified the people of other regions. The dream indicated that Islam would spread to other regions beyond considerations of color and creed[250].

Christ and Anti-Christ. Messenger of God said, "I saw myself (in a dream) near the Kaaba last night, and I saw a man with whitish red complexion, the best you may see amongst men of that complexion having long hair reaching his earlobes which was the best hair of its sort, and he had combed his hair and water was dropping from it, and he was performing the Tawaf (circumambulation) around the Kaaba while he was leaning on two men or on the shoulders of two men. I asked, "Who is this man?". Somebody replied, "(He is) Messiah (Christ), son of Mary." Then

---

[250] http://dreams-interpretation-in-islam-1728.hargaponsel.info, consulted on 31.04.2016

I saw another man with very curly hair, blind in the right eye which looked like a protruding out grape. I asked, "Who is this?" Somebody replied, "(He is) Messiah, Ad-Dajjal (Anti Christ)."[251]

Battle of Uhud. On the eve of the Battle of Uhud, the Holy Prophet saw in a dream, that he was driving some cows, and some cows out of these were slaughtered. He also saw a dent on his sword.[252] Abu Bakr interpreted that the dent on the sword signified that one of the relatives of the Prophet would be martyred.

Siege of Taif. When after the fall of Mecca, Taif was besieged, the Prophet saw in a dream that he had with him a bowl of butter. A cock pecked at it and spilt it. Abu Bakr interpreted the dream to mean that the siege of Taif would have to be raised without actual conquest.[253]

Expedition against Banu Jadhima. When Khalid was sent on an expedition against Banu Jadhima of Kinana, the Prophet saw in a dream that he swallowed a morsel of dates mixed with butter and enjoyed their taste. Some of them, however, stuck in his gullet when he tried to swallow them. Then Ali thrust in his hand and pulled them out. Abu Bakr interpreted the dream to mean that something would happen in the campaign against Banu Jadhima at which the Prophet would be happy as well as unhappy, and that he would send Ali to put matters right. In the campaign against Banu Jadhima, the tribe was overpowered, and at this, the Prophet felt happy. Muhamed, however, felt unhappy when he learnt that Khalid had killed some Muslims as well. The Prophet said, "O God I am innocent before Thee of what Khalid has done." Ali was then sent to the tribe to pay blood money.[254]

Drawing water from a well. On another occasion, the Prophet saw in a dream that he was drawing water from a well. Then he stepped aside and asked Abu Bakr to draw water. Abu Bakr was able to draw water for two to three rounds only, and then he showed signs of exhaustion. Umar then took up the job, and he was able to complete ten rounds. Abu Bakr interpreted the dream to signify that after the passing away of the Prophet; the caliphate would vest in Abu Bakr whose period of office would be two

---

[251] http://www.myislamicdream.com/dying_kaaba_tawaf.html, consulted on 31.04.2016

[252] http://theislamicjournal.com/battle-of-uhud/, consulted on 31.04.2016

[253] http://www.alim.org/library/biography/khalifa/content/KAB/17/pdf/4, consulted on 31.04.2016

[254] *Ibid*

to three years only. He will be succeeded by Umar whose period of office will be ten years.[255]

Wading through night soil. Once Abu Bakr saw in a dream that he was wading through the night soil of the people. He related the dream to the Holy Prophet who interpreted it to mean that after the death of the Holy Prophet, Abu Bakr would be called upon to undertake apostasy campaigns.[256]

Three moons. Once, Ayesha saw in a dream three moons descend on her house. She related the dream to Abu Bakr, and he interpreted it that her house would be the burial place of three luminaries of the world. Subsequently, the Holy Prophet, Abu Bakr, and Umar were buried in her house.[257]

Urinating blood. Once a person waited on Abu Bakr and asked for the interpretation of his dream. In the dream, he had seen himself urinating blood. Abu Bakr addressing him said, "God curse you. It appears that you go to your wife even when she is with the monthly course. Desist from that".[258]

Opening of the sky. Mahrz b Nuzlah, a companion saw in a dream that the sky had opened for him and that he had reached the seventh heaven. Abu Bakr interpreted the dream to signify that he would meet the death of a martyr and that his abode would be in paradise.[259]

As mentioned earlier, Islam distinguishes between the true and false dreams. Muslims are warned against the false dreams, which can be manifested in seven different forms, among which there are:

1. Confused dreams, which are usually caused by distress, exaggerated hopes, and personal thoughts.
2. Sexual dreams that require one to take a ritual ablution (ghusul) if they end in the ejection of semen and they have no interpretation.
3. Warnings from shaitan or nightmares.
4. Dreams evoked by jinn spirits, thus, they are judged as senseless.

---

[255] http://sunnah.com/search/Search-%E2%80%A6I-was-offering-my-prayer-in-the-mosque-and-Abdullah-b, consulted on 01.07.2016

[256] http://www.alim.org/library/biography/khalifa/content/KAB/17/pdf/4, consulted on 31.04.2016

[257] Al-Bukhari S., Volume 9, Book 87, Interpretation of Dreams

[258] http://www.alim.org/library/biography/khalifa/content/KAB/17/pdf/4, consulted on 31.04.2016

[259] *Ibid*

---

5. Dreams, where devil appears, and this type is not considered to be a dream.

6. Dreams, which derive from one's own desires, confusion or stress situation.

7. Dreams, which are caused by physical suffering.

Among the true dreams Islam distinguishes:

1. A clear vision by a faithful person, which is considered to represent one of forty-six branches of a prophecy, including the dream of God's Prophet entering Mecca or the dream of God's prophet Abraham sacrificing his son, etc. A dream interpreter once said: "Blessed is he who sees a true dream, for they come directly from God Almighty and without an intermediary."

2. Direct warning from Allah. God's Prophet once said, "The best of dreams are the ones where you see your Lord, or your prophet, or your Muslim parents." Someone asked, "O, Messenger of God, can one see his Lord?" He replied, "The king represents God, and God is the king in one's dream."[260]

3. A dream from the angel of dreams, whose name is Siddiqun. This blessed angel may come into one's dream and, by God's leave, reveal some of what Allah made known to him from what is already written. Such dreams usually come in enciphered symbols, however, decodable for a dreamer.

4. Dreams of allegories, apotheosis, or symbols one can decipher. This type comes through good spirits, blessed souls, angels.

5. True dreams that include a true witness. In it, such a witness will manifest one's own prevailing presence in the dream.

So, the main particularity of dream interpretation in Islam is that it shall be made based on Quranic tradition and Muslim wisdom, since dreams shape, and are decisively shaped by personal and collective notions of self and society.[261] Here are just a few examples of dream meaning in islam[262]:

Athaan (call to prayer): Seeing oneself giving the call to prayer may indicate one's plans for Hajj will succeed.

---

[260] http://www.myislamicdream.com/hugging_god.html, consulted on 31.04.2016

[261] Zeevi D., Producing Desire, University of California Press, 2006,p.106.

[262] http://www.naseeb.com/journals/dream-interpretation-through-islam-191228, consulted on 01.07.2016

Bathing: Dreaming of oneself bathing in cool water may refer to Allah`s forgiveness, and soon recovery for a sick person.

Dates: If one sees fresh Ibn Taab dates in a dream, it indicates that one`s practice of the religion will become better. Based on: Anas ibn Malik quoted Prophet Muhamed saying, "Last night I dreamt that we were in the house of Uqbah ibn Raafi and were brought some Ibn Taab fresh dates. I interpreted it as meaning that eminence in this world will be granted to us, a blessed hereafter and that our religion has become good."

Garden: Seeing a garden in a dream indicates the abundance of Islam. Based on: Abdullah ibn Salaam said, "(In a dream) I saw myself in a garden, and there was a pillar in the middle of the garden, and there was a handhold at the top of the pillar. I was asked to climb it. I said, I cannot. Then a servant came and lifted up my clothes and I climbed (the pillar), and then got hold of the handhold, and I woke up while still holding it. I narrated that to the Prophet who said, "The garden symbolizes the garden of Islam, and the handhold is the firm Islamic handhold which indicates that you will be adhering firmly to Islam until you die."

Laughing: is a positive sign of receiving good news.

Mecca: Seeing oneself in Mecca in a dream may indicate entering into a state of security and peace. Based on: Whoever enters Mecca will be secure.

Marriage: Dreaming of oneself getting married may indicate an approaching marriage. If there are no marriage plans, one may soon get married with the person seen in the dream. Based on: Aisha said: Allah`s Apostle said to me, "You were shown to me twice (in my dream) before I married you. I saw an angel carrying you in a silken piece of cloth, and I said to him: Uncover (her), and behold, it was you. I said (to myself), "If this is from Allah, then it must happen. Later I dreamt of the angel carrying someone in a silken piece of cloth, and I said (to him), Uncover (her), and behold, it was you. I said (to myself), If this is from Allah, then it must happen."

Milk: Receiving milk in a dream means religious knowledge. Based on: Abdullah ibn Umar said, "Allah`s Apostle said, "While I was sleeping, I was given a bowl full of milk (in the dream) and I drank from it (to my fill) till I noticed its wetness coming out of my limbs. Then I gave the rest of it to Umar bin Al-Khattab. The persons sitting around him, asked, "What have you interpreted (about the dream) O Allah`s, Apostle. He said, "It is (religious) knowledge."

Sufis explore dreams even more seriously, since, for them, it is not only a proxy for spiritual symptoms but a particular way of receiving mystical knowledge. The interpretation of dreams, including dreams that comprise dialogues with one's spiritual teachers, have played a significant role in some Sufi orders since the earliest days. The Sufi Najm ad-din Kubra (1145-1220) was discovering the dreams` symbols, citing the "constant direction of a shaykh who explains the meanings of one's dreams and visions." And Baha ad-din Naqshband of Bukhara (died in1389), after who Naqshbandi Order of Sufism was named, became a celebrated dreams interpreter. It is even said that he would accept a dervish only after he had had a dream indicating that the person was an appropriate disciple[263]. In this regard, Sufi teacher Vaughan Lee says, "If you have a really important dream, you will remember it. The Higher Self within you will make you remember it."[264] He also claims that "much of the work on Sufi path is psychological"[265] and that "sometimes many people will have ancient Sufi symbols in their dreams without consciously realizing from where they`ve come."[266] For this reason, exploration of Islamic mysticism is one of the priority steps towards the deeper comprehension of Muslim unconsciousness.

Etymologically, the word "sufism" is derived from a word "sufi", which is translated from Arabic as as "wool". The first generation Muslim ascetics used to wear woolen garments and as these Dervishes traveled around they gradually became known as Sufis.[267]

Islamic mysticism, as a road (tariqa) has endured three phases:

- the moral phase in the first three centuries (asceticism of the 1st century, Rabia al-Adawiya and Al-Hasan Al-Basri in the 2nd and Thu Al-Nun and Al-Junaid in the 3rd);
- the ethico-psychological phase in the 4th and 5th centuries (Al Hallaj in the 4th century, and Al Gazali in the 5th);
- the metaphysical phase in the 6th and 7th centuries (Al Suhrawadi, Ibn Al-Farid and Ibn Arabi and Ibn Sabin in the seventh).[268]

Mystics used to establish their own closed societies (sufi order) with their own practices and rituals, withdrawn from society. The old mystical

---

[263] Yoga Journal, jan.-feb. 1997, p.65.

[264] *Ibid*

[265] *Ibid*

[266] *Ibid*

[267] Nurbakhsh J., The Crucible of Light, Khaniqahi-Niamtullahi Publications, 2009, p.35.

[268] Hanafi H.,Islam in the modern world. Religion, Ideology and Develoment, Dar Kebaa Bookshop, Heliopolis, vol. I, p.33.

solution was the spiritualization of rituals, the interiorization of movements, the transformation of the acts of the organs to the acts of the heart[269]. In development, what is needed is social action, the transformation of rituals to social contents as they were originally conceived in the law: unity of utterance as political opposition by the double act of negation (la ilaha), and of affirmation (ilya Allah), included in the witness (shahada); prayers as the sense of time; alms as social action and symbolic redistribution of wealth; fasting as social cohesion; pilgrimage as mutual community, and the unity of umma. The organization of mystic orders in the contemporary Muslim world is even stronger than that of political parties. Moreover, sufis are respected greatly by common people.

Mysticism does not deal anymore with the external dimension of human's acts, but with the internal essence. What matters is not the body, but the purity of the heart. Quran states that one hour of reflection about oneself and the universe equals seventy years of prayers. Therefore, Islamic mysticism is rather a way of communication with the heart. It is also a science, which includes two aspects: morality (muqawamat) and psychology (ahwal).

Poverty (faqr) in classical mysticism was not considered as something negative. On the contrary, it was viewed as a manifest spirit of strong opposition to the desires of the materialistic world. The sufi was not looking for avaricious consummation. He was on the side of the spiritual enrichment, and, thus approaching Allah even closer.

Asceticism (zuhd) in old mysticism is an extreme poverty, poverty of the soul. In an affluent society, everybody takes and desires. Asceticism is believed to purify a soul from desire.

Reliance (tawakul) in Islamic esoterism also signifies strong faith in Allah to the point that a man entrusts one's fate completely in Allah's hands.

Resignation (taslim) means complete acceptance of whatever comes from Allah. It follows reliance and expands to the final acceptance, without questioning or contesting anything. Taslim in the Quran means complete and free acceptance of revelation by the believers or complete surrender of the unbelievers, the general consensus of the believing community.

Eros (mahabba) and Agape (shawq). Given the significance of these one or two steps, mystical love became a synonym to mysticism itself. Given its abundance, it is everywhere at the beginning of the mystical road, the moral phase in the middle (ethical-psychological phase) and at the end (metaphysical phase). Al shawq is an outmost degree of love (mahaba) and its dynamic power. If love is only a state of affection between one another,

---

[269] *Ibid, p.30.*

al-shawq is the sense of direction from the one to another. The shawq is born from a lack. It is an everlasting attempt to reach an unattainable goal, which induces a constant request. The shawq corresponds to a desire: it demands unceasingly to renew the desire, and this is the most essential point to address something, which is absent in sufism, likewise in psychoanalysis. The Quranic term refers to love and hate in the same register, as two opposing sides of one. God loves pious and does not love the impious.

Taweel is a meditative process that involves the transformation of visions and mental images into from Active Imagination into symbols and their reproduction in a different dimension of reality. In other words, the function of taweel is to make evident the hidden essence.

However, some mystical steps need transformation from the individual level to the social level, such as good intention (al-niyya), sincerity (al-ikhlas), trustfulness (al-sidq), self-surveillance (al-muraqaba), and self-discipline (al-muhasaba).

Strangeness (hayba) denotes a state of anxiety and uneasiness regarding the hidden sides of the spirit. It is a sense of smallness in the world of greatness, a sense of loss in the world of fullness. When the mystic gets used to this new world of strange happenings, he becomes familiar with them and he moves from the state of strangeness to the state of familiarity (uns). While the term Hayba is not Quranic, the term Uns is.

Contraction (qabd) and relaxation (bast) refer to the double pump function of the heart. Contraction follows an insight. When a mystic is accustomed to it his heart begins to expand. Then another impulse arrives, and like this the cycle recommences.

Separation (farq) is a psychological state in which the mystic experiences the far distance between his goal and him. However, unexpectedly, the far becomes near (qurb) and the separation between the subject and the object ends by the unification (jam) between the mystic and his goal. Farness is a motivating factor on the mystic's way, which makes him more active and resolute in achieving one's own goal.

Annihilation (faqd) is a very powerful state of complete self-absorption in the other. Mystic existence is reduced to nothingness in order to gain another mode of everlasting life. The new state of existencialization emerges from nothingness at the image of creation ex nihilo. In the Quran the term Faqd means only to loose something or not to find a bird, but never that kind of self-destruction. On the contrary, the term Wajd exists as verb which means simply to find a thing, a person, but never in the sense of self-creation, that is making oneself or somebody else exist since existence is the self-evident experience.

Self-absorption or disappearance (fana) is the highest level of self-metamorphosis. Once the mystic's essence is completely transformed, the positive state appears, self-sustenance or eternal existence (baqa). And this is an end of a sufi's way, since mysticism oriented itself to the other world as a final refuge.[270]

The main difference between Christian and Muslim mystics is that the former is most frequently practiced by unmarried, withdrawn from the outside world, people, whereas the latter is chosen by men and women al-Hallaj, death by crucifixion.[271]

We have observed that Sufism is a precursor of psychoanalysis in the Islamic world. Sufism represents a symbolic castration. In other words, the necessary destruction so that to continue living. Like in psychoanalysis, one needs to let go of everything that is too heavy for ego to carry as a threat to superego so that a real ego resurrects. Like at the psychoanalytic session, where sudden acquaintance appears from the unconscious through the liaisons, which we can make in the chain of signifiers, Sufism believes that the heart is given to love and language to dialogue between the divine subject and the sufi. The divine silence, which does not equate with nothingness, like in psychoanalysis: the silence of a psychoanalyst, which encourages more free associations, does not mean his absence. Regarding the sufi's relation to the image of Allah, it is shaped by one's own relation to Him; in psychoanalysis, this dimension is called projection.

All things considered, the elements of psychoanalysis were well known in the premodern Islamic world, e.g. dream interpretations; muhasiba (self-analysis); zuhd (asceticism), as a form of symbologenic castration. However, the period between the 7th and 13th centuries has been commonly neglected, despite the remarkable developments of the biomedical science of the Arabic-Islamic world with the resultant flowering of knowledge that influenced medical practice throughout Europe[272]. While the Muslim scholars were among the first to explore the domain of mental health, the European Renaissance took up the responsibility of the flame of medical development.[273]

---

[270] Hanafi H., Islam in the modern world. Religion, Ideology and Develoment, Dar Kebaa Bookshop, Heliopolis, vol. I, p.54-56.

[271] http://www.cairn.info/revue-topique-2010-1-page-117.htm, consulted on 01.07.2016

[272] Falagas M., Zarkadoulia E., Samonis G., Arab science in the golden age (750-1258 C.E.) and today. FASEB J, 2006, pp. 1581-1586.

[273] http://ibro.info/wp-content/uploads/2012/12/Arab-and-Muslim-Contributions-to-Modern-Neuroscience.pdf, consulted on 01.07.2016

CHAPTER 6

COLONIAL PERIOD

Colonial period ranges between the 18th and 20th centuries when the Islamic region fell under the rule of European imperial powers. Following World War I, the former territories of the Ottoman Empire were divided between Britain, Germany, France, Italy, Portugal, Spain, Belgium, Russia, Austria-Hungary and the Netherlands in the capacities of European protectorates. There has been no major widely accepted claim to the caliphate since this time (which had been last claimed by the Ottomans). Despite this political partition and the great progression of modern medicine, Greco-Arab medicine was still very popular in Europe and beyond.

Geographically the Arab world is divided into two parts: Maghreb, the North Africa and Mashriq, the Arab East. Historically both parts have developed differently owing to the colonial division. The Mashreq region remained under the British control (e.g. Egypt, Iraq, etc.) whereas the Maghreb region (e.g. Algeria, Morocco, Tunisia) was administered by French metropolia.

In the Western scientific world, psychotherapy was introduced in the 18th century by Pinel – in a form of human assistance (in contrast to drugs and medications), and later by Leuret and psychiatrists of the 19th century, in a form of advice accorded to the patient, later by Dubois, who brought in a notion of "moral psychotherapy". Care for mental patients deteriorated after the decline of the Ottoman Empire, and modern methods of treatment were only consistently established after the founding of the republic in 1923.[274]*

The colonial period put "on pause" the development of psychology for less than one hundred years on the lands, where the science of human mind was previously flourishing. During the times of protectorate, no researches in psychology domain were conducted. If psychotherapy existed, it was practiced in rural areas in a form of magical-religious rituals by brotherhoods or marabouts. Oftentimes traditional therapy was the only available source of remedy and hope for curing the diseases, like infertility, diabetes,epilepsy, psychosomatic disorders, etc. The previously glorious mental hospitals, maristans, became no more than half-destructed buildings with unsupportable and inhuman living conditions. Therefore, at the beginning of the XXth century, in the Arab world, there was no modern establishment for mental health care.

In the beginning of the 19th century during the French occupation of Egypt, the director of medical services in the Egyptian Armed Forces, a French physician named Claude, approached the Egyptian ruler regarding the appalling state of mental patients in Cairo.[275] At that time, all medical hospitals were controlled by the military, so mental patients in Cairo were transferred to a military hospital in the middle of the City (Al Azbakia). A few years later a separate hospital was constructed not far from Bolaque. In 1880, a great fire demolished one of the palaces of the prince except for a two-story building. This was painted yellow and became the first mental hospital in Cairo in 1883. It was called the Yellow Palace (El Saray El Safra) located in Abbassia, which is the Cairo`s suburbs. Now it is located in the middle of a cosmopolitan city. In 1912 another state mental hospital was built in Khanka, in the north of Cairo, with more than 300 acres of total space. In 1967 a third mental hospital was established in Alexandria (Al Mamoura) and in 1979 another was founded in Helwan, a suburb south of Cairo.[276]

In what it concerns the Maghreb countries, from time to time they were visited by French psychiatrists and psychoanalysts, such as Gaetan de

---

[274] *Here it refers to Egypt, when the UK unilaterally declared Egyptian independence on 28 February 1922

Scull A., Cultural Sociology of mental illness, an A-to-Z Guide, University California Press, vol.1, 2014, p. 904.

[275] http://scholarworks.wmich.edu/cgi/viewcontent.cgi?article=1980&context=jssw, consulted on 01.07.2016

[276] http://scholarworks.wmich.edu/cgi/viewcontent.cgi?article=1980&context=jssw, consulted on 01.07.2016

Clarambault in 1915, in their capacity of private mental health practitioners. That is when psychoanalysis started penetrating into Morocco. Also, the unique Spanish psychiatrist, Alfonso Turegano, opened a private practice in Morocco. The mental health care system was split into two services: the fist line service, which was located at the public hospitals and was dealing mainly with emergency cases; and the second line service, based at the psychiatric hospitals, which was predesignated for the chronic patients.

Colonialism left deep traces in the mind of the Islamic world with its ideological division into "race" and "culture". The colonial discourse was treating the question of the human capacity, pathology, and identity from the standpoint of the above-mentioned factors. Colonialism is a specific form of oppression. Colonial regimes are exclusively maintained within two signifiers: the colonizer's "superior" way of life and the colonized people's "inferior" way. The psychiatrist and an extraordinary thinker Franz Fanon highlighted the brutal influence of inhuman conditions of colonial exploitation on the psyche of native people. Michel Foucault was also analyzing the colonial power through the very emergence of particular kinds of "modern" selves. Originating from the Foucault's conception of the nexus of power and knowledge, Said's Orientalism became a cornerstone research on postcolonial studies. In Orientalism, Said detailed the various ways European colonial powers created the image of the Arabic Orient as primitive, uncivilized and in need of Western intervention. All in all, the colonial past is not only a historical attribute but a fresh and alive memory in the minds of many contemporary Muslim people.

In studying the matter of the restoration of a traumatized soul, Jung described the normative psyche as a hierarchically organized psyche, dominated by a one-sided ego and collectively identified persona. Such a hierarchy sweeps to the margins everything that is inferiorized by the culture (the shadow) and preserves a sense of power via identification with the collective norms. Dissociation, denial, repression, projection were the most common defenses that maintained the psychological balance during the colonial epoch. History was viewed by the autochthones, as a prescribed by God natural evolvement, a "destiny". In this fantasm, much was silenced, which has just begun to manifest today.

CHAPTER 7

POST-COLONIAL PERIOD

When we talk about the evolution of psychoanalysis and clinical psychology in Arab countries we talk about similar and at the same time totally different historical contexts. From one hand, they are alike, as all Arab countries have a common colonial past, whilst certain of them, have also inherited the culture of psychotherapeutic practice. From the other hand, different, because each country has undergone its unique way in the formation of psychoanalysis, as well as psychological services.

In the Arab and Islamic world, "three countries constitute, by their history, the pioneers, if not to say, the pillars, of psychoanalysis in this part of the world: Egypt, Lebanon, and Morocco.[277] Certainly, there exists a psychoanalytic movement in other countries, such as Tunisia, and to a lesser extent, in Algeria and Syria.[278] However, in the first three cited countries the psychoanalytic activity was the most important, and, particularly, they have known the foundation of psychoanalytic societies", in accordance to Jalil Bennani.[279] One should also note that colonization-decolonization of the Arab countries is one of the key points to be taken in consideration in the history of psychoanalysis. True, that the psychoanalysis appeared late in these countries, however, that is not a

---

[277] http://lavieeco.com/news/societe/psychanalyste-le-therapeute-qui-ne-fait-que-vous-ecouter-21495.html#pL4gKmejL1qC35Ds.99, consulted on 01.07.2016

[278] *Ibid*

[279] *Ibid*

---

case for Egypt, which became a sovereign state in 1936. Certainly, other factors matter for the institutionalization of psychoanalysis, notably, the modernist thinking, democracy, and a free political life. However, even one hundred years after the foundation of psychoanalysis, fifty years after the Freud`s death, the entire Arabo-Islamic world remains resistant at the same to the psychoanalytic thought, as well as to the therapies of psychoanalytic inspiration, and this, despite an attempt undertaken by certain intellectuals, who received their education in the West, to introduce a little bit, through the intervention of university education, the Freudian system.[280] The socio-cultural facts speak for themselves: in the immense Arabo-Islamic context of about two hundred millions of citizens, there are only six psychoanalysts. Some renowned psychoanalysts, of Arabic and Muslim origin, are based in Europe or in both Americas.[281]

Ultimately, even after gaining independence, the Muslim countries were maintaining a tight connection with the metropolias, which had a substantial impact on the development of scientific psychology, and a psychoanalytic movement in this region. Therefore, psychoanalysis was made possible only within the frame of the Western thought. And the newly appeared psychoanalytical societies were more of a replica of the Western school, rather than an independently functioning organism.

EGYPT

Egypt got to know the psychoanalytic experience very early, to be precise, in the years 1930, or, before the World War Two, which means, earlier than Italy, Spain and Belgium. The first lectures on psychology for women started in 1911. And Freud himself was particularly passionate about Egypt. He considered that Akhenaton was the first Ruler who worshiped the One God. However, with the death of Akhenaton, Amon came back to power and the adepts of monotheism were obliged to practice their religion in secret, or to flee the kingdom.

In the history of psychoanalytic movement, the case of Egypt is exceptionally particular. From one side, this is the first Arab country, where psychoanalysis has been practiced by local people, since the beginning of 1930, and taught at the University since 1950, the date of foundation

---

[280] https://www.monde-diplomatique.fr/1989/10/CHAMOUN/42092, consulted on 01.07.2016

[281] *Ibid*

by Mustapha Ziwer (1907–1990).[282] This means that psychoanalysis was finally available in Arabic language, and analytic concepts, relating to the Muslim unconsciousness, were coined in Egypt, without the Western intermediate. In 1929 Ziwer graduated from the department of psychology at the University Ain-Shams. In 1959 the military campaign unleashed a wave of repression against the intellectuals from the left, accusing them of supporting the pan-Arab regime of Jamel Abdennasser. Two disciples of Ziwer were striken by this authoritarianism, in particular: Kadari Hifni, who was sentenced from 59 to 64; and Ahmed Faik. He was one of the first psychologists and was sentenced from 69 to 69.[283] The years 1936 and 1943 were known as dark year of Egyptian psychoanalysis, since the first local psychoanalyst, Shoukri Efendi Guirguiss (died in 1945) was charged with the criminal accusation of illegal practice of medicine. He left numerous thematical publications. Also, Guirguis was accused by public opinion for his link with the British Psychoanalytic Association, that is to say, an institution of a colonizing country. In 1939 the publication Moses and Monotheism blew up another scandal. Fethi Ben Slama narrates it as follows: "When in May 1939 in the famous daily Egyptian Al-Ahram information appeared from its London correspondent about the Freud's book The Man Moses and Monotheism there were many protests and responses coming from academia contesting the Freud`s conception about the Egyptian origin of Moses. One of these Egyptian scholars wrote: "The professor Freud is the one, who stands out among the scientists by this strange and marginalized thesis. The books of history and revealed books maintain the belief among the scholars since thousand of years, according to which Moses was Jewish by his father and ancestors, even though he was brought up at the palace of Egypt. He revolted with his brother Aron to defend his Jewish brothers against the Pharaoh, then decided to help them escape from Egypt". Following these debates Sabri Guirguiss, a psychiatrist, published a book called The Jewish-Zionist Heritage and Freudian Thought in 1970, where he pointed to the Zionist origins of the Freud`s thought. Kadari Hifni, published articles such as Freud between Science and Sionism or Israeli Personality. On the 8th of September 1968 Mustapha Ziwer edited his studies named The Clarifications about the Israeli Society: a Psychoanalytic Study at Al-Ahram newspaper.

Moustapha Safwan was born in Alexandria on the 17th of May 1921. Having accomplished his studies he moved to Paris, where he became

---

[282] http://www.cairn.info/revue-topique-2010-1-page-83.htm, consulted on 31.04.2016

[283] *Ibid*

a strong adherent of Jacques Lacan. In 1949 Safouan met Lacan as his control analyst. He published an analytical essay Why the Arab World is Not Free, first in Arabic language, in Egypt, in total discretion from mass media. Later it was edited in English and French languages.

Notions of the unconscious had seeped into Arabic writings in Egypt since at least as far back as the 1920s and through a myriad of sources, including Pierre Janet, Sigmund Freud, Carl Jung, and Alfred Adler.[284] The imprint of Freudian psychology, in particular, was becoming increasingly visible in the 1930s and 1940s in the focus on unconscious sexual impulses as translations of Freud began to appear.[285] For example, a 1938 article in Al-Hilal noted that a generational shift had taken place and that Egyptian youth were avidly reading Freud and were familiar with his ideas on the unconscious, the interpretation of dreams, psychoanalysis, and the sexual instincts.[286] As the exemplar of modern science, Freud, it was argued, could help the East move forward.[287] By the mid-1940s a burgeoning popular literature on psychology was so well developed that scholarly journals felt compelled to critique the unscientific literature "drowning the marketplace"—a testament to the increased salience of psychology to popular public discourse.[288] Psychology, as an academic discipline, was initially taught at the Egyptian University in the philosophy department as soon as the University was founded in 1908. By mid-century the academic psychologists were teaching in the major universities in Cairo and Alexandria, among them there were the Higher Institutes of Education and Ibrahim University. When Yusuf Murad and Mustafa Ziywar returned to Cairo in 1940s after their studies and work in France, the discipline received a new life. They founded the Jamaat Ilm al-Nafs al-Takamuli (Society for Integrative Psychology) and the Egyptian Majallat Ilm al-Nafs (Journal of Psychology) in 1945. Another Arabic edition Sikulujiyyat al-Jins combined in itself both psychology and sexology. Murad was applying an integrative approach to psychology, and in 1948 he edited a popular handbook of psychology, which endured at least seven editions. The journal comprised Freudian and anti-Freudian concepts

---

[284] Musa S., Al-Aql al-Batin, aw Maknunat al-Nafs, Al-Hilal, 1928

[285] Tafsir al-Ahlam, trans. Mustafa Safwan, Dar al-Maarif, 2004

[286] NajiI., "Al-Shabab al-Misri wa-l-Mushkila al-Jinsiyya," al-Hilal 47, 1 November, 1938, pp. 57–60.

[287] *Ibid*

[288] Mustafa Ziywar's book review of Ilm al-Nafs al-Amali, Majallat Ilm al-Nafs 1, 1945, pp. 75–78.

alike, which ascertained its openness to a psychoanalytic thought in Egypt in the 1940s. The journal was explaining the meaning of psychology to an educated audience, and in particular the need to create its applicability to Egyptian and Arab contexts. In 1945, the inaugural year of Majallat Ilm al-Nafs Yusuf Murad proposed a research agenda for the study of adolescent psychology in Egypt and the Arab world. Murad was an active advocate for creation of an Arabic-speaking space for the development of psychology, which would consider the Arab cultural factors. He was regularly contributing with the publication of new psychological terms to the dictionary in Majallat Ilm al-Nafs. He was also a member of the Academy of Language for the committee on psychological terms and thus was the main figure in the standardization of an Arabic psychological vocabulary. He claimed that psychology was a special science, because each single clinical case creates its own laws, and, therefore, is not subjected to general laws. Yusuf believed that the particularity of culture can be fully explored only while studying the adolescents. In particular, European and Egyptian youths were brought up in different contexts, and this has a deep impact on their psyche. To cover the wide area of researches focused on youth, the Egyptian psychoanalyst was applying the Freud's stages of sexuality, even though they were culturally more relevant to the European young people. In his researches Yusuf specifically insisted on the role of cultural exposure in shaping the contours of psyche. The analyst expressed in Majallat Ilm al-Nafs his conceptualization about adolescence, as of period of knowledge seeking about oneself, high vulnerability, sharp rise of awareness and manifestation of sexual impulses, which were previously lodged in unconscious.[289] The interest in the psychology of adolescents was not typical for Egypt only. It was also arising in parallel with the researches of the European psychoanalyst Maurice Debesse, a student of Henri Wallon. The writings of Wallon, from whom Lacan borrowed the concept of the mirror stage,was in high demand in postwar Egypt. By the late 1930s, the topic of juvenile delinquency became so pertinent that the major lectures at the Cairo School of Social Work (CSSW) during the 1937–38 years were mainly dedicated to it. In addition to that, the school's parent organization, the Egyptian Association of Social Studies, dedicated its most fundamental researches to the same topic in 1940. The authors of Majallat Ilm al-Nafs were among the first in Egypt to underline not only the social component of the juvenile delinquency but also its aberrant psychosexual origins. Al-Miliji's discussion focused more on understanding the juvenile delinquency as a symptom of maladjustment, and not just

---

[289] AlAlawnaA.,Zeelalialyam, IslamKotob, DarAlmanaralinashrwtawzi, p.210.

ethical regression. On Friday mornings in Cairo in the mid-to-late 1940s and the 1950s, scholars and students of all disciplines would assemble at the house of psychology professor Yusuf Murad.[290] Having presented the Freud's theory of the unconscious to the Egyptian audience, Murad was, undoubtedly, the pioneer in his homeland. Murad also introduced the Arabic term for the "unconscious", which is la-shour, a term previously used by Sufi philosopher Ibn Arabi. In 1943 Murad edited a book Shifaal-Nafs (Healing the Self), which familiarized the Egyptian audience with the principal theories and basic knowledge about psychology. During his analytical practice Murad was devotionally concentrated on finding resolutions to the existing psychosexual problems in the Egyptian society. In keeping with his theoretical emphasis on integrative psychology, he focused on conflicts that emerged between different parts of the self, or between conscious and unconscious impulses. The revolution, which Murad incited in the realm of Egyptian and Arabic psychoanalysis influenced not only the review of the patient's treatment, but the theorization of a unique Islamic approach to unconscious. Notions of the unconscious had seeped into Arabic writings, albeit in an imprecise and lay fashion, since at least as far back as the late 1920s through a myriad of sources, including Sigmund Freud, Alfred Adler, and Carl Jung.[291]

In what it concerns, the evolution of the state mental health system in post-war Egypt, the last piece of relating legislation was enacted in 1944, which focused on: (a) access to mental health care including access to the least restrictive care; (b) competency, capacity and guardianship issues for people with mental illnesses; (c) voluntary and involuntary treatment; (d) law enforcement and other judicial system issues for people with mental illnesses; (e) mechanisms to oversee involuntary admission and treatment practices; and f) mechanisms to implement the provisions of mental health legislation.[292]

Starting from 1949, outpatient facilities have been extended by central hospitals in almost all governorates of Egypt.[293] Thirteen medical schools have been functioning in Egypt and each has a psychiatric unit

[290] Al Shakry O., The Arabic Freud: the Unconscious and the modern subject", Modern Intellectual History, Volume 11, Issue 01, April 2014, p.90.

[291] Al Shakry O., The Arabic Freud: the Unconscious and the modern subject", Modern Intellectual History,Volume 11 Issue 01, April 2014, p.91.

[292] http://arabpsynet.com/Archives/OP/TopicJ20NumanGharaibeh2.pdf, consulted on 01.07.2016

[293] http://scholarworks.wmich.edu/cgi/viewcontent.cgi?article=1980&context=jssw, consulted on 01.07.2016

with inpatient and outpatient psychiatric services. The largest mental hospital, Abbassia, is more than 100 years old and Khanka is about 80 years old. They experience serious challenges regarding care, finances, treatment, and rehabilitation while accommodating about 5,000 patients, which might lead to accumulating difficulties in future. The new policy of deinstitutionalization and provision of community care may reduce the number of hospitalized psychiatric patients but will not solve the problem.[294]

A national mental health programme was formulated in 1986.[295]

The Supreme Council for the Control of Drug Addiction and Abuse, chaired by the Prime Minister, is a leader in this direction.[296] Legislation for drug control has been promulgated, such as the law on drugs passed by the People`s Assembly (1989), the President`s Decree establishing the National Fund for the Control of Drug Addiction and Abuse, the joint decisions of the ministers of justice, social affairs and health establishing sanitaria and departments for the treatment of drug abuse and addiction.[297]

Oedipus and the Sphynx

The story of Oedipus and the sphynx strengthens the link between the Ancient Egypt and psychoanalysis. It says that the sphynx was sent by Hera in Beotie following the death of the king Thebes: Laios. She starts devastating the fields and terrorize the populations. Having heard from the muses one enigma, she declares that she would not leave the province unless somebody resolves it, adding that she would kill anybody who failed. The regent Creon promises a hand of a widowed Queen Jocaste and the crown of Thebes to whoever helps Beotie to get rid of this flaw.Many candidates have been trying, however, all have died by the arrival of Oedipus. The sphynx asks him, "Which creature has one single voice, at first four legs, then two legs, and three legs afterwards ? It relates to a man. In fact, when he is a child, he has four legs, since he moves on four legs; when he is old, he has three legs, since he leans on his stick…" Furious at seeing oneself being drilled through, the sphynx throws himself from the top of his mountain (or the walls of Thebes, according to the authors) and dies every day. So, Creon kept his promise, and Oedipus contracted with his mother Jocasta

---

[294] *Ibid*

[295] Mental Health Atlas, WHO, 2005

[296] http://arabpsynet.com/Archives/OP/TopicJ20NumanGharaibeh2.pdf, consulted on 01.07.2016

[297] *Ibid*

an incestuous union. This confrontation between Oedipus and the sphynx is fundamentally different from most of other mythological myths. In fact, if Hercules, Perseus and Theseus beat their opponents by force, Oedipus, like Ulysses, triumph above all owing to his cunningness and sagacity. Oedipus was able to resolve the Sphynx's enigma, however, did he really save his skin in view of the end of his own life story? The legend tells us that he blinded himself; regarding his mother-wife Jocasta, and their daughter Antigone, they hanged themselves. Certainly, Oedipus missed his initiation, his rite of passage with the sphynx. Oedipus did not kill the monster, that is the sphynx who killed oneself. Which is rare in mythology.

Altogether, the Egyptian sphynx has rather a funeral vocation, while the Greek sphynx represents intellectual confrontation. In fact, the sphynx's question concerns the existence of the subject: where do we come from, and where are we going? However, surprisingly, the Oedipus complex is such does not appear in Arabic folklore. Moreover, even published collections of psychiatric case descriptions from private practices[298] do not include the Oedipal situation.

Egypt was the gateway of modern psychology to other Arab countries, owing to the inquiry spirit inherited from the great Pharaonic era, which settled an example for the development of psychoanalysis in the whole Islamic world.

MAGHREB COUNTRIES

In the Islamic world, after Egypt, there follows the Maghreb region, in particular, Morocco and Tunisia, where the psychoanalytic practice was actively introduced after gaining independence. However, it was possible only in Morocco to establish the first analytic institution. In Algeria, the psychoanalytic practice was suspended, whereas in other countries (Libya) it has never existed.

ALGERIA

The period of French rule in Algeria expanded from 1830 until 1962. The whole way to the independence was permeated with sufferings and blood. For every Algerian, this had a crucial impact on the perception of oneself, collective consciousness and ethnical identity.

---

[298]   El-Rakhawi, Yehia. 1972 When Man is Denuded: Cases From A Psychiatric Clinic. Cairo: Dar Al-Ghad, p. 83.

In the absence of democracy, the rule of law is an essential mininum for the introduction of psychoanalysis in this country, like in any other country.[299] The rule of law was previously absent in Algeria, during and after the decolonization, which took a form of extremely violent conquest starting from 1830 so that to terminate around 1871, the date of the first great, so to speak "tribal", revolt.[300] It took many years for psychoanalysis to stand in the row with other reputable disciplines in Algeria. And there existed numerous reasons for that. First of all, in the 1970s the population was mostly concerned with issues of rebuilding the country, strengthening one's own infrastructure after the colonial rule, and other practical tasks. Secondly, the philosophical debates centered mostly around the questions of "origin" and "identity", which severely weakened during colonization time. Thirdly, psychoanalysis, as anything coming from the West, was avoided, or handled with suspicion, since it could have been another maneuver to return to neo-colonialism. However, France was not preparing its return. Moreover, the Psychoanalytic Association of Paris, which hosted the second French university in Alger, did not even have a fixed policy for psychoanalysis promotion in Algeria. Frantz Fanon, a psychiatrist from the Carribean, played a crucial role at the Blida hospital from 1953 to 1956, where he introduced the institutional psychiatry, alternatively, psychoanalysis, which gained certain sensibility of the local audience owing to the clinical work and introduction of groups for studying Freudian texts.On a more general level, the psychoanalytic studies were becoming gradually popular. And in the 80s Professor Boucebci, a psychiatrist trained in France, and others attempted to introduce both in their teaching and care institutions, references to psychoanalysis. The mental health law was included in the Law on Health Protection and Promotion of 1985. In 1987 SARP was created (Société Algérienne de Recherche en Psychologie) by teachers from the Alger's university, who organized studying and research groups. Its work had a great interest for psychosomatic medicine. Every year the psychoanalysts from S.P.P such as R. Perron, P. Marty and others were invited to the conferences, organized in Algeria. The study of Freudian metapsychology was made necessary for the specialists of psychosomatic medicine, which enabled a larger outlook for psychoanalysis in Algeria. In 1989, following the uprising of October 1988, the Association of Continuing Education in Mental Health was created. It organized work groups, seminars of psychoanalytical training,

---

[299] http://www.cairn.info/revue-topique-2010-1-page-23.htm, consulted on 01.07.2016

[300] *Ibid*

to which French colleagues (mostly Lacanian) were invited and this until 1994, the date when violence installed for long in the Algerian society. Among other initiatives, it shall be noted the creation of the Center for Autistic Children in Alger at the district Bab-El-Oued; the introduction of the child and adolescent psychiatry in Blida; and a practice inspired by a team of Basaglia (Italy).

For the most part, the minimum conditions for the establishment of psychoanalysis did not exist in Algeria. The hard time when the country was rigorously fighting for its independence, could not have been dedicated to nothing else, but to gaining and maintaining one`s own liberty. Only with individual efforts, psychoanalysis could have been included as a part of psychiatry course or mental health program.

MOROCCO

There has been a psychiatric tradition in Morocco since the Middle Ages – "The Moristans" (health care places for the mentally ill) were psychiatric hospital precursors of the public sector.[301] Psychiatry was founded during the Protectorate era at the beginning of 1920. Starting from 1956 it became widely expanded at the hospitals. The first psychiatric institution in Morocco was built in 1920.[302] Berrechid Hospital was the first functioning, asylum-like, the clinic with 2,000-bed capacity (near Casablanca). Later Til Mellil Psychiatric Hospital (in the Casablanca region) was constructed. Then regional psychiatric hospitals, with capacity varying from 80 to 100 beds, were opened in Casablanca (Tit Mellil Hospital, 1924 and le Pavillon 36), Meknes (Moulay Ismail Hospital, 1923), Marrakech (1935), Fes (1947), Tetouan, Tangiers, and Oujda. In Rabat, the temporary psychiatric service was established at the military hospital Marie-Feuillet, which in 1963 moved to Arrazi Hospital in Salé. The main feature of the development of psychoanalysis in Morocco was its diverse nature, which comprised organic, pharmacological and psychological elements. Such openness was particularly beneficial for the further progress of psychoanalysis in this country. Also, the absence of a well-organized psychiatric school may have prompted a group of French psychoanalysts to settle in Morocco in 1948 and to introduce psychoanalysis. Later, two Psychiatric University Centres were established

---

[301] http://psychologyinafrica.com/profiles/2013/6/23/morocco-mental-health-profile, consulted on 01.07.2016

[302] http://www.who.int/mental_health/evidence/morocco_who_aims_report.pdf, consulted on 31.04.2016

in Salé in the 1960s and in Casablanca in the 1970s. According to mental health policy of the Ministry of Health, several mental health services are being created each year in the general hospitals. The goal is to have sectorized coverage of mental needs of the population in the entire country.

The Central Mental Health office was created in 1959. It became fully "operational" in 1988. Currently, this office is named Mental Health and Degenerative Diseases Service and has the following responsibilities:[303]

- Developing plans and programmes for the prevention and treatment of mental illnesses as well as the protection of the mentally ill;
- Supervising medical care institutions (public and private), health centres and psychiatric institutions;
- Coordinating different sectors involved in mental health care and with national and international nongovernmental organizations;
- Overseeing continuing education of health professionals;
- Furthering the goal of mental health;
- Participating in the fight against drug addiction in coordination with other sectors.

The development of psychiatric field would not have been possible without the crucial contribution of the Moroccan practitioners, trained in the West, who returned home in the 70s. And the formation of psychiatrists and psychologists in Morocco followed soon after.

A mental health policy was initially formulated in 1972. The components of the policy are promotion, prevention, treatment and rehabilitation. Decentralization is also a component of the policy. Since 1972, the mental health policy has been reviewed several times with the help of the Moroccan Society of Psychiatry. The legislation on mental health, which was formulated in 1959 by Dahir, is the highest legislation form in the country. There is also present a substance abuse policy, which was initially formulated in 1972.[304] Likewise, a national mental health programme is available. The programme was formulated in 1973. The mental health programme was revised several times, in 1992 and 1995. The programme was composed according to the Dahir. The programme has also been reviewed numerous times. There exists a national therapeutic drug police, which was formulated in 1972. The list of new and old drugs

---

[303]   *Ibid*

[304]   http://psychologyinafrica.com/profiles/2013/6/23/morocco-mental-health-profile, consulted on 01.07.2016

(e.g. neuroleptics, antidepressants, mood-regulators) is re-examined every year.

In 1974 the Circulaire (Ministerial recommendations document) launched a process of regionalization and "deinstitutionalization". This was the start of a strategic policy to reduce the number of beds in psychiatric hospitals, to create smaller units with fewer beds (20-40 beds) and to integrate mental health into general hospitals.[305] In the 1960s, a demand for psychiatry kept growing, and not only at hospitals but also in ambulatory practice, consultations and psychotherapies. Besides chemotherapy, the consultations without prescriptions started appearing: they proved the growing influence of psychotherapies and later psychoanalysis. Gradually, the other answer was given to suffering: that of listening to the symptoms for a resolution of psychic conflicts, by other than chemical means. The answer commenced from simple support, and specialized techniques, such as analytical, psychotherapy of analytical inspiration, family therapy, behavioral therapy. The Moroccan practitioners knew well that it was not enough for the therapist to listen and sympathize with the patient so that the treatment was theoretically and ethically satisfactory. The Moroccan psychoanalysts were aware that they were ought to position themselves differently from the healers, magicians or marabouts. The psychoanalytic practice itself became possible only owing to the psychiatric and psychological funds. The requests, addressed to a psychoanalyst, concerned a big variety of symptoms. During these years the psychiatric practice was flourishing.

In fact, in Morocco, there exist, from one side, psychiatrists, psychologists, psychotherapists and psychoanalysts, and from another, the fusion of traditional therapies. The magical-religious therapies remain very present in Morocco and no practitioner can escape from a risk of being reminded about this reality by his/her patients, many of who have been going back and forth between the traditional practices and those related to modernity. Traditional therapies constitute a memory of cultural heritage. Sometimes condemned, sometimes valued, their role was the subject of numerous debates, various interpretations, and rarely that of rigorous theories.

Practitioners, psychiatrists, and psychologists, who practice psychotherapy, that is to say, treatment operating by an impact of patient-therapist relationship, and whose common denominator is the absence of any physicochemical process, has reduced, both in medical and psychiatric

---

[305] http://arabpsynet.com/Archives/OP/TopicJ20NumanGharaibeh2.pdf, consulted on 01.07.2016

institutions. By developping their practice, popularizing it for the users and the population, the psychotherapists have operated true sensibilization to their discipline, to the extent of popularizing it among all those who had an access to the information, and making it indispensable in certain milieux. Therefore, there happened inevitable drifting towards psychologism, which outpasses the ethical limits of the profession. Morocco was the only country who knew the psychoanalytical influence during the colonial period. It was René Laforgue who introduced psychoanalysis in the 48s. He exiled with a group of sympathizers, friends, and analysants, who joined in the practitioners already working in Morocco (J. Bergeret, M. Igert, M. Foissin, L. Clément). Laforgue postulated a radical and structural difference between peoples, ethnic groups, religions, and races. These theories, segregating and remote from the Maghreb concerns, were rejected by the North African practitioners. Some of his students had hospital responsibilities (Igert Clement, Rolland) and contributed to introduce Moroccan psychopathology. As the first movements for independence of Morocco started, René Laforgue preferred to return in France. Some members of a group left progressively, and some remained, which is the case of L. Clément et de M. Legrand. During the 1970s, the psychoanalytic practice was proceeding very quietly in rare private practice. The biggest part of French psychoanalysts left Morocco and Moroccan psychiatrists-psychoanalysts continued their formation in France.

The Moroccan psychoanalyst Leila Sherkaoui, who was practicing at the Medicopsychological Centre before settling down at the other office of another psychoanalyst Smiljka Sif after the 1970s. Starting from 1980 new practitioners, graduated from France, have reintroduced psychoanalysis in the private and public sectors, these were, in particular, M. Kasbaoui, G. El Khayat and M. Benchekroun.

The evolution and development of demand, on one hand, the presence of Moroccan psychiatrists and psychoanalysts favoring the listening in Arabic on the other hand, allow psychiatry and psychoanalysis in Morocco to leaf a new page. The Moroccan doctors-psychoanalysts and non-doctors, reintroduce psychoanalysis in their private and public practice. The psychoanalytic discourse took its place, amidst certain psychiatric institutions in Rabat and Casablanca, in particular. In other non-medical institutions, the psychoanalysts were asked to participate in the meetings or works. During the two following decades, working groups and individuals working in private or public sector reintroduced psychoanalysis and contributed to its development in private practice, and to a much lesser extent, in institutions. Practitioners belonged to different psychoanalytic currents, however, were not affiliated with any international organization.

The Freudian Text

The Association The Freudian Text (Le Texte Freudien) was created in 1985, and it gathered together all the practitioners, who were interested in the Freudian texts. Even though there were too little of practitioners, the enlarged format of these meetings allowed to focus on theory and to launch a series of psychoanalytic debates. In the framework of this association, there were organized numerous seminars, conferences and a colloquium called Freudian Circle (Le Cercle Freudien). Four years later this association was dissolved by a joint decision, since its objectives were achieved.

As has been noted, psychoanalysis was brought in Morocco by French psychoanalysts, who settled in its sea-coast cities and started gradually introducing their practice on the Arab land. Morocco has always been open to diversity, so the conditions for developing a new practice were more than favourable. After a while, they were replaced by the native Moroccan analysts, who were returning home after graduation in the West. With time Morocco unfolded a solid base for an operational analytic field.

TUNISIA

A mental health policy is present. The policy was initially formulated in 1986.[306] The policy includes advocacy, promotion, prevention, treatment, and rehabilitation. There are specialized committees and subcommittees for the training of personnel, preparation of manuals for physicians, visits of specialists to outpatient departments, review of drug list, radio and television programmes and research. The top priorities of the policy are the integration of mental health into primary care, training of non-psychiatric medical professionals in psychiatric care, the creation of psychiatric services in general hospitals and separation of the services. Tunisia promulgated a law regulating mental health care in 1992.[307] Involuntary admission and treatment of persons of in mental health facilities are to take place if the following conditions are fulfilled: a) the person suffers from mental disorders necessitating immediate care, b) the person is unable to give informed consent, and c) the person poses a risk to his or her own safety

---

[306] http://psychologyinafrica.com/profiles/2013/4/5/tunisia-mental-health-profile, consulted on 01.07.2016

[307] http://arabpsynet.com/Archives/OP/TopicJ20NumanGharaibeh2.pdf, consulted on 01.07.2016

or that of other people[308]. Decisions are made and reviewed by a judicial authority and are based on the recommendations of two doctors, at least one of whom is a psychiatrist. Involuntary admission is limited to three months only[309]. This Law guarantees a right to exercise all civil, economic and cultural rights to people with mental disorders unless they are placed in the care of a guardian.

Law 92-83 of 3rd of August 1992, relative to mental health and to the conditions of hospitalization for mental disorders requires that the hospitalization is done with the respect for individual liberties and human dignity.[310] A person affected by mental disorders cannot be hospitalized without his (or her) consent except where it is impossible to obtain an informed consent or if the state of mental health of the person concerned requires urgent care or threatens his (or her) security or the security of others.[311]

According to Pr. Sleim Ammar, in Tunisia, the scarcity of data written in the field of psychoanalysis, without any allusion to psychoanalysis in publications or history of Arab, Muslim and, specifically, Tunisian medicine and psychiatry pretends as if, until then "officially" there was no trace, or passage, or introduction of foreign or Tunisian psychoanalysis on Tunisian soil.[312] The social schema of the Arabic society favoured the preoccupations much more over the interests of nations, groups, tribes, clans rather the personal ones. That is why there could not be any particular demand to this way of seeing.[313] Cultural resistance of Tunisian society to psychoanalysis was caused by the perception of the Freudian theories as pan-sexualist, immoral, individualistic and marked by Freud`s Jewishness. Starting from the years 1960 the movement of antipsychiatry and humanization of treatment at the mental hospitals (Lacanian psychoanalysis, in particular, and anti-psychiatry) marked the Tunisian experience. The first contact of Tunisia with psychoanalysis seems to have been realized by Hesnard. After his studies at l'École de Santé navale de Bordeaux, from 1905 to 1910 or

---

[308] *Ibid*

[309] http://arabpsynet.com/Archives/OP/TopicJ20NumanGharaibeh2.pdf, consulted on 01.07.2016

[310] *Ibid*

[311] *Ibid*

[312] Journal 3-4that reproduces "Rencontres Franco-Maghrébines de Psychiatrie" organized in Alger on 22- 24 April1983

[313] https://www.cairn.info/revue-topique-2010-1-page-41.htm, consulted on 01.07.2016

1912, Angelo Hesnard (1886-1969) was assigned on naval vessels and was named in Bizerte in 1917 (he was 31 years old) and he remained there 2 or 3 years. According to Guy Darcourt, he had already become interested in psychoanalysis. When he discovered the writings of Freud in 1913 (in German) he published with Régis three articles in L'Encéphale about The Doctrine of Freud and His School. Then in 1914 he published, again with Regis, a book Psychoanalysis of Neuroses and Psychoses.[314] Hesnard was also a founding member of the Paris Psychoanalytic Society (PPS) since 1926, which was the first psychoanalytic society in France. He remained there until the first split that would hit the association in 1953 in order to give birth to the French Psychoanalytic Society (FPS), of which he was the President from 1959 to 1960. In 1963, during the second split, he happened to be in the ranks of l'École freudienne de Paris side by side with Jacques Lacan. He also has the merit of having written the first book on psychoanalysis, which appeared in France in 1914. He published many other books soon after. Despite the fact that Hesnard was challenged for his distances regarding Freud's theories and his refusal of a didactic analysis, he enjoyed great fame for the mere fact that he was a pioneer. According to Guy Darcourt, he was a clinician open to all forms of psychotherapies and who tried to confront the research of eventual synthesis. This allowed him to train several psychoanalysts throughout France, especially in the South, where he was for a while, only to practice psychoanalysis. In accordance to Jalil Bennani, at the end of his military career, he had to stay in Morocco, make the clinic and introduce psychoanalysis in 1943-1945. We must admit that we can not, a priori, build the foundations of psychoanalysis in Tunisia from this contact.[315] The second meeting of psychoanalysis with Tunisia seems to have been that of Carl Gustav Jung (1875-1961). According to Hachim Dauoi, between 1920 and 1925, this psychoanalyst of the first generation performed a series of research trips and explorations in North Africa and passed through Tunisia. Reading of Jung's testimony reflects the state of someone who was exploring himself much more than that of others. His observations and reflections were marked by ethnocentrism and hasty judgments, as Najib Djaziri stated. It is, therefore, understandable that Jung could not offer psychoanalytic services to Tunisians.[316]

Frantz Fanon (1925-1961), later known as Ibrahim Omar Fanon, is a psychiatrist, who practiced at first in Algeria in 1953, then in Tunisia in

[314] https://www.cairn.info/revue-topique-2010-1-page-41.htm, consulted on 01.07.2016

[315] *Ibid*

[316] *Ibid*

April 1957 at the hospital Manouba (current Razi) and then at Charles Nicolle Hospital. During his Tunisian period, Fanon was also teaching at the Faculty of Medicine of Tunis. Rejecting Freudian psychoanalysis, however, he introduced the "psychoanalytic psychotherapy of support" and "psychodrama". He borrowed the theory of "mirror stage" from Lacan and introduced the current "institutional psychotherapy". He contributed in his way by helping to prepare the grounds for psychoanalysis, which was in critical anticolonial position. The first psychoanalytic text published by a Tunisian in Tunisia is that of a university sociologist and associate philosopher, Abdelwahab Bouhdiba The Notebooks of Tunisia. The official journal of the University of Tunis refused to publish Hammam. Contribution to a psychoanalysis of Islam. Then this text appeared in the first issue of the Tunisian Social Science Journal (TSSJ), publication of the Center of Studies and Economic and Social Research of Tunis affiliated to the University of Tunis.

However, the introduction of psychoanalysis Tunisia owes to Lydia Torasi. The whole process was occurring in an irregular manner starting from 1975, and then steadily from 1980. However, in October 1984 Lydia Torasi decided to leave Tunisia. And after years of hesitation, in 1989, Torasi eventually published her book Matrix, Psychoanalytic Modeling of Regulating Laws of Cellular Genetics. Nejia Zemni was also engaged in psychoanalysis with Dr. Torasi while at the same period (1975-1980), going regularly to attend the seminars of Lacan in Paris.

Mohamed Ghorbal (1940-2005), trained at Razi hospital during 1970-1971 and analyzed by Salomon Resnik, has the merit to have introduced in 1980 the course of "child psychopathology" and "psychoanalysis" in the curriculum of graduate students of psychology faculty. At that time, for students and teachers of the Faculty of Humanities and Human Sciences it was the first academic encounter with psychoanalysis. Moreover, Ghorbal was launching a seminar "Al Kindi" every Wednesday night at the Razi hospital with a single purpose to introduce the "psychoanalytic approach of neuroses in Tunisia". This seminar was conducted together with Saida Douki, and gathered psychiatrists and psychologists. In addition, Ghorbal made the effort to theorize about "The North African personality" in his numerous publications and psychoanalytic interventions[317]. He personified the "beautiful years of psychoanalysis" in Tunisia.

Mohamed Halayem, having graduated from Paris started his practice as child psychiatrist and psychoanalyst in 1982 at the Hospital of Tunisian

---

[317]   https://www.cairn.info/revue-topique-2010-1-page-41.htm, consulted on 01.07.2016

Chidren (l'Hôpital d'Enfants de Tunis). He introduced a psychoanalytic reading through various publications on the relevant topics, such as masked depression, psychoses of children, stuttering, abandoned children etc. He was leading on his own two seminars every week on child psychopathology and psychoanalysis. Several young psychologists and psychiatrists were assiduously following these seminars. Among them there were: Salem Hamza Raja Labbane, Hajer Karray, Houda Hamza, Feika Bagbag, Boutheima Bellamine and many others. The same year Halayem founded a Society of Studies and Research in Psychoanalysis (Société d'Études et de Recherches en Psychanalyse, SERP), the first psychoanalytic society in Tunisia.

It becomes evident that after the departure of Lydia Torasi, only Mohamed Ghorbal and Mohamed Halayem occupied the field of psychoanalytical theorization and practice in Tunisia. The latter one belonged to the orthodox psychoanalysis, while the former pertained to the Lacanian currents. The debates between the representatives of both movements were actively ongoing. While other psychiatrists, of analytical education, were not participating in these dual discussions. It concerns Slaheddine Gallali, Professor of Medicine and Doctor-Colonel, who has introduced psychoanalysis into the psychiatric military milieu. This also concerns Jouda Ben Abid, Professor of Psychiatry, Head of Centre's services, who was mostly working in the area of addiction.Some disciples of Halayem opted for independent work. Thus, Hamza Salem decided to leave Tunisia to settle in France while Fadhel Mrad was continuing to introduce psychoanalytic practice in the psychiatric hospital Razi.[318] During the years 1995, the Tunisian Association of Psychiatry (la Société Tunisienne de Psychiatrie) was tightly collaborating with Psychoanalytic Association of Paris (la Société Psychanalytique de Paris) in order to assure the training seminars and seminars of initiation into psychoanalysis in Tunis. During this short experience, such psychoanalysts as Paulette Letarte, Paul Denis, Paul Israel, and others were coming in Tunisia to give conferences and lead control groups. However, this practice was not meant to last long.

In 1979 Lilia Labidi, a psychologist and psychoanalyst, trained at the school of Bonneuil, created by Maud Mannoni, introduced the psychoanalytical listening at the Children's Hospital in Tunis. For her part, Khedija Besbes introduced a psychoanalytic listening within the carcinology Institute of Tunis in 1981. The Social and Pediatric preventive unit invited F.Dolto in March 1984 to deliver her speech on Irreplaceable

---

[318] *Ibid*

Role of Communication, Serge Leclaire in March 1985 to talk about The Teenager: Figure, Myth and Reality, Michel Polo and Chaudra Kovindassamy.

To sum up, the development of psychoanalysis in Tunisia is linked with certain names, such as Hesnard, Fanon, Bouhdiba, Torasi, Ghorbal and others. Those people were the active promoters of a psychoanalytic approach, whose enthusiasm and non-stop work made possible the introduction of psychoanalytic thought in the medical domain of Tunisia.

MASHRIQ COUNTRIES

At the epoch, the Mashriq region was not as much favoured by the attention of foreign analysts as the Maghreb region due to numerous reasons, among which there are: the distance, the absence of democracy, the political conditions and others. Despite this, Lebanon was the only country, which succeeded in providing the necessary basis for the expansion of psychoanalysis, and, furthermore, in inspiring the neighbor countries.

IRAQ

As mentioned earlier, in Iraq, the first mental hospital in the world was established (705 AD). It is one among few countries, which has inherited rich traditions in the field of mental health. In 1927-the Baghdad Medical School was established, which was modelled in accordance to the UK system. In 1950s mental health services were offered in Iraq at two psychiatric hospitals in Baghdad, in particular, Al-Rashad Hospital, a 1200 bed chronic care facility and Al-Rashid Hospital (now Ibn-Rushid Hospital), and a 74-bed facility for acute psychiatric care. During the period of 1960s-1970s-the mental health centres and mental health units were extensively introduced in hospitals, school mental health programmes and mental health promotion efforts.

The mental health legislation was achieved with the collaboration of Ministry of Justice and was reviewed by most psychiatrists in the country.[319]

Chapter 4. Section 1 of Iraq`s 1969 penal Code entitled "Criminal liability and exemptions from it" reads "Loss of reason and volition: Paragraph 60 – Any person who, at the time of the commission of the offence, is suffering from a *loss of reason* or *volition due to insanity* or infirmity of mind or because he (or she) is in a state of intoxication or under

---

[319] http://arabpsynet.com/Archives/OP/TopicJ20NumanGharaibeh2.pdf, consulted on 01.07.2016

the influence of drugs resulting from the consumption or intoxicating or narcotic substances given to him against his (or her) will or without his (or her) knowledge or due to any other reason which leads one to believe that he has lost his (or her) reason or volition is not criminally liable. However, if he (or she) is not suffering from any *infirmity of mind* nor is under the influence of intoxicating, narcotic or other substances but only from a defect of reason or volition at the time of the commission of the offence, then it is considered a mitigating circumstance."[320]

In the 1960s and 1970s, Iraq's health care system introduced a significant variety of services and was considered as an example for the entire region. The hospitals had a well-established infrastructure with proper sanitary conditions, water-supply, logistics, communication system and a road network. As the WHO`s statistics states, prior to 1991 the health care system served 97% of the urban and 79% of the rural population. Health care, including mental health services, was mainly reliant on oil revenues and to a lesser extent taxation. Usually, its services were free of charge to the public. During the 1960s, and 1970s mental health services were established in general hospitals, and school mental health programmes and public awareness campaigns were developed.[321] However, Iran-Iraq war (1980-88), Iraq's invasion of Kuwait (1990) and the subsequent UN imposed sanctions negatively affected the health care system in Iraq, which led to the reduction in public spending on the health care. Based on statistics of Iraqi MOH, health expenditure fell from 3.72% of GDP in 1990 to 0.81% in 1997 and health infrastructure also deteriorated. The mortality rate for infants and children more than doubled between 1984-9 and 1994-9[322].

Generally speaking, prior to the war, the Iraqi mental health services were set as an example to the whole region, which, what is more, were free of charge. Conversely, as a result of aggressive foreign politics, the Iraqi health system became its primary victim, which suffered from the reduction of costs, and, thereupon, the quality of offered services diminished sharply.

---

[320] *Ibid*

[321] Sharma S., et al., Mental Health Policy in Iraq since 2003, a Post-Invasion Analysis, p. 5.

[322] Ali M., Shah I., Sanctions and childhood mortality in Iraq. Lancet, 2000, p. 355.

LEBANON

The Lebanon Hospital for the Insane, Asfuriyeh, was founded in 1898 by Dr Theophilus Waldmeir (1832-1915), a Swiss Quaker, to provide care for the mentally afflicted of the Lebanon, Syria and the Middle East.[323] On 17th of April 1896 Dr Henry Jessupmade public his intentions to found "the first Home for the insane in Bible Lands". For these means, Waldmeier travelled to Europe and the USA to collect funds, and the Beirut Executive Committee was founded. On 11th of March 1897 London General Committee (LGC) was inaugurated at the Bethlem Royal Asylum and its Medical Superintendent, Dr Percy Smith, was elected as Chairman. The Asfuriyeh opened its doors on the 6th of August 1900, and the first 10 patients were admitted. The Hospital's Constitution and Rules were formally drawn up in 1907. Under the Constitution, the Beirut Committee officially became the local executive committee in Beirut of the London General Committee, which retained overall authority over the Hospital. On the basis of Law of Lebanon in 1912 the building became a religious foundation on a condition that the Hospital should be made international.The Lebanon Hospital for the Insane was presumably capable of accommodating over 150 people by 1924; 350 by 1935; and 410 by 1936. By 1949, 14,000 patients had been treated since the opening of the Hospital. In 1938 the Hospital was renamed the Lebanon Hospital for Mental and Nervous Disorders. In addition to clinical work, the Hospital organized training in the field of psychiatry. In 1922 it was affiliated with the American University of Beirut and became the Psychiatric Division of the University Hospital. In 1939 it was recognized by the Royal Medical/Psychological Association as a Training Centre for the Mental Nursing Certificate. In 1948 it opened a School of Psychiatric Nursing, the first one in the Middle East, where the World Health Organisation used to organize its training of specialized personnel. Treatment at the Hospital followed worldwide medical advances, and included insulin coma therapy, cardiazol convulsion therapy, occupational therapy and electric convulsion therapy. Chemotherapy was used for the first time in 1952. In the period between 1941 and 1946, a substantial part of the Hospital passed under the control of the British Military Authorities. It was reported that by 1972 the Hospital was experiencing financial hardship. It was decided to sell the existing building and to re-build the Hospital in a more modern style. A new site was chosen at Aramoun, near Beirut Airport. Asfuriyeh was sold in April 1973. The construction did not commence until summer 1977. Despite

---

[323] http://www.mundus.ac.uk/cats/4/1065.htm, consulted on 01.07.2016

appeals for funds, by early 1981 negotiations had commenced between the London General Committee and the Beirut Executive Committee to close the Hospital and to dispose of the property in accordance with the legal terms of the "Wakf". The Hospital at Asfuriyeh was officially closed on the 10th of April 1982. Aramoun did not cease functioning, although some its parts were largely destructed. The LGC eventually resigned control of the Hospital itself to the Beirut Committee. The Hospital's founder, Theophilus Waldmeier, published The Autobiography of Theophilus Waldmeier, Missionary, being an account of ten years life in Abyssinia and sixteen years in Syria (1886).[324]

In brief, the history of a psychology field in Lebanon is rigidly connected with the Hospital Asfuriyeh, which, besides, being the first mental hospital in the region, in years to come turned into a sanctuary for practitioners, medicians, professors and international guests, who were contributing to the institutionalization of scientific psychology.

SYRIA

The rules governing mental health and psychiatric treatment in the Syrian Arab Republic are derived from the health legislation issued in 1981 by the Ministry of Health.[325] Until today, in public and private psychiatric hospitals in Syria there only exist drug treatments and electric shock therapy, without any psychological approach. The arrival of a young doctor with an open mind allows to introduce the psychological approach but avoiding carefully the psychoanalysis and, instead, relying on mixed methods marked by behaviorism.[326]

Lebanon played a significant role in the introduction of Syrian psychoanalysis when Adnan Houbballah and his wife Mouzayan Osseiran and others were invited to organize the training seminars. Also, Dr. Nashed has worked as a psychoanalyst in Syria since 1984. She completed her degree in clinical psychology at the University of Paris-Diderot in France. In 2000, she founded the Damascus School of Psychoanalysis. She is married to Dr. Faisal Mohammed Abdullah, a professor of ancient history at Damascus University, who is a specialist in Sumerian writing.

---

[324] http://www.mundus.ac.uk/cats/4/1065.htm, consulted on 31.04.2016

[325] http://arabpsynet.com/Archives/OP/TopicJ20NumanGharaibeh2.pdf, consulted on 01.07.2016

[326] Nached R., "Histoire de la psychanalyse en Syrie.", Topique 1/2010, issue 110, pp. 117-127.

In the final analysis, we can speak of some episodes of psychoanalytic appearance in Syria, which were fugitive, irregular, and, deriving, chiefly, from the mere enthusiasm of single analysts.

GULF COOPERATION COUNTRIES

When former Egyptian president Hosni Mubarak was on a visit to the United States, renowned American host Charlie Rose asked him, "Why is there no democracy in Egypt?", "Simply because the people are not ready yet," Mubarak answered. The same can be stated about GCC region in terms of psychoanalysis. The whole region, like no other part of the modern Muslim world, is dependent on father`s figure, a strong political leader. If psychoanalysis enters as a usual remedy of Gulf nationals, it risks destroy the statal foundations. The tribe`s society will risk dissolution, and new order might come to this part of the world.

SAUDI ARABIA

In KSA the start of modern psychiatry is associated with the building of Shahr Hospital in Taif in 1962. On the whole, no other psychological event is known to have taken place at this period in KSA.

In conclusion, psychoanalysis could have only developed in Muslim countries such as Morocco, Lebanon, Egypt and Syria. Psychoanalysis was not able to take the roots in the whole Islamic world, because of the absence of the rule of law, as well as the context of intense destructiveness and slaughter during the conquest and decolonization times, or simply because the local society was not yet ready for it. Until now it remains largely unknown for a Muslim patient in the countries like Algeria, Djibouti, Lybia, Somalia, etc. Disregarded and oftentimes mistaken for psychiatry. Unknown and, therefore, tabooed.

CHAPTER 8

MODERN PERIOD (1990-)

This chapter summarizes the current situation of mental health services in the Arab world. The Arab world includes 22 countries, with total population 385.3 million.[327] The region has the largest proportion of young people in the world: 38% of Arabs are under 14.[328] Life expectancy has increased by 15 years over the past three decades,[329] and infant mortality has dropped by two-thirds. Around 12 million people, or 15% of the labor force, are unemployed.[330] The quality of education has recently deteriorated, and there is a severe mismatch between the labor market and the education system. Adult illiteracy rates have declined, but are still very high: 65 million adults are illiterate,[331] almost two-thirds of them women. Some 10 million children still have no schooling at all. Out of 20 countries for which information is available, six do not have a mental health legislation and two do not have a mental health policy (see Table 8.1.) The first Arab

---

[327] http://data.worldbank.org/region/ARB, consulted on 01.07.2016

[328] Zdanowski J., Middle Eastern Societies in the 20thCentury, Cambridge Scholars Publishing, 2014, p.26.

[329] *Ibid*

[330] Rosenberg J., Aftermath of the Arab Uprisings: The Rebirth of the Middle East, Hamilton Books, 2012, p.16.

[331] Selvik K., Stenslie S., Stability and Change in the Modern Middle East, I.B.Tauris, p.14.

country to have a mental health act in 1944 was Egypt which was updated in 2009 by a new mental health Act "The care of psychiatric patients."

There are no projections on the burden of mental disorders specific to the Arab world. Only two countries (Lebanon and Iraq) so far conducted national studies using the comparable methodology, based on the World Health Organization (WHO) World Mental Health Surveys. Two other studies were conducted in Morocco and Egypt using different methodologies. The lifetime prevalence of any anxiety disorder among adults was 16.7%[332] in the Lebanese study and 13.8%[333] in the Iraqi survey; that of any mood disorder was, respectively, 12.6%[334] and 7.5%.[335] The study carried out in Morocco reported a point prevalence of 9.3% for generalized anxiety disorder and 26.5% for major depressive disorder,[336] while the Egyptian study reported a point prevalence of 4.8% for anxiety disorders and 6.4% for mood disorders.[337]

Three countries (Lebanon, Kuwait, and Bahrain) had in 2007 more than 30 psychiatric beds per 100,000 population, while two (Sudan and Somalia) had less than 5 per 100,000.[338] Total hospitals beds were highest in Libya 370/100.000, then Lebanon 345/100.000, Saudi Arabia 217/100.000, Algeria 210/100.000 then Tunisia 209/100.000, and Emirates 193/100.000.[339]

---

[332] Jabbour S.,Public Health in the Arab World, Cambridge University Press, 2012, p.179.

[333] http://www.cdc.gov/immigrantrefugeehealth/profiles/iraqi/health-information/mental-health.html, consulted on 01.07.2016

[334] Jabbour S.,Public Health in the Arab World, Cambridge University Press, 2012, p.179.

[335] http://www.cdc.gov/immigrantrefugeehealth/profiles/iraqi/health-information/mental-health.html, consulted on 01.07.2016

[336] http://www.ncbi.nlm.nih.gov/pmc/articles/PMC3266748, consulted on 01.07.2016

[337] Jabbour S.,Public Health in the Arab World, Cambridge University Press, 2012, p.179.

[338] http://css.escwa.org.lb/SDPD/3572/4-Social.pdf, consulted on 01.07.2016

[339] http://www.who.int/whosis/whostat/EN_WHS2011_Full.pdf, consulted on 01.07.2016

Table 8.1 Mental Health Policies in the Arab Countries[340]

Country	Mental health policy (year)	Substance abuse policy (year)	National mental health programme (year)	Mental health legislation (year)
Algeria	Yes (?)	Yes 1990	Yes 2001	Yes 1998
Bahrain	Yes 1993	Yes 1983	Yes 1989	Yes 1975
Djibouti	No	No	No	An old French legislation
Egypt	Yes 1978	Yes 1986	Yes 1986	Yes 2009
Emirates (UAE)	Yes (?)	Yes (?)	Yes 1991	Yes 1981
Iraq	Yes 1981	Yes 1965	Yes 1987	Yes 1981
Jordan	Yes 1986	Yes 2000	Yes 1994	Yes 2003
Kuwait	Yes 1957	Yes 1983	Yes 1997	No
Lebanon	No	No	Yes 1987	No
Libya	Yes (?)	No	Yes 1988	Yes 1975
Morocco	Yes 1972	Yes 1972	Yes 1973	Yes 1998
Oman	Yes 1992	Yes 1999	Yes 1990	Yes 1999
Palestine	Yes 2004	Yes 2004	Yes 2004	Yes 2004
Qatar	Yes 1980	Yes 1986	Yes 1990	No
Saudi Arabia	Yes 1989	Yes 2000	Yes 1989	No
Somalia	Yes (?)	Yes (?)	Yes (?)	No
Sudan	Yes 1998	Yes 1995	Yes 1998	Yes 1998
Syria	Yes 2001	Yes 1993	Yes 2001	Yes 1965
Tunisia	Yes 1986	Yes 1969	Yes 1990	Yes 2003
Yemen	Yes 1986	No	Yes 1983	No

There are 2,387 psychologists working in the Middle East. The highest number of psychiatrists is found in Qatar, Bahrain, and Kuwait, while seven countries (Iraq, Libya, Morocco, Somalia, Sudan, Syria and Yemen) have less than 0.5 psychiatrists per 100,000 population (see Table 8.2.) Although there is a mental hospital in Djibouti, yet there are no psychiatrists, and general practitioners with special interest in mental health look after those patients. The number of psychiatrists decreased

---

[340] http://www.ncbi.nlm.nih.gov/pmc/articles/PMC3266748, consulted on 01.07.2016

with respect to the 1998 survey in Libya, Saudi Arabia, and Sudan, while there was a substantial increase in several other countries.Psychiatric nurses per 100,000 population range from 23 in Bahrain and 22.5 in Emirates to 0.09 in Yemen and 0.03 in Somalia.[341] The number of nurses increased in almost all countries compared to the 1998 survey. The same applies to psychologists and social workers, with the most substantial increase observed in Bahrain, Emirates, Jordan, Egypt, Kuwait, Libya, Saudi Arabia and Yemen.

Table 8.2 Mental Health Resources in the Arab Countries[342]

Country	Psychiatric beds per 100,000	Psychiatrists per 100,000	Psychiatric nurses per 100,000	Psychologists per 100,000	Social workers per 100,000
	1998	2007	1998	2007	1998
Algeria	14	25	1.1	2.2	1.1
Bahrain	33.8	33	3.7	5	13.3
Djibouti	N.A.	7	0	0	0
Egypt	12.5	13	0.9	0.9	2
Emirates (UAE)	N.A.	14	0.9	2	N.A.
Iraq	7	6.3	0.1	0.7	0.1
Jordan	20	15.7	1.1	1	0
Kuwait	47	34	2.6	3.1	16.2
Lebanon	47	75	1.2	2	0.9
Libya	56	10	0.3	0.2	N.A.
Morocco	7.6	7.8	N.A.	0.4	N.A.
Oman	5.5	4.9	0.2	1.4	0.2
Palestine	14.2	8.8	0.8	0.9	3.2
Qatar	37.9	9.7	0.8	3.4	7.4
Saudi Arabia	6.5	11.8	2.4	1.1	6.3

---

[341] https://www.researchgate.net/publication/221796187_Mental_health_services_in_the_Arab_world, consulted on 01.07.2016

[342] http://www.ncbi.nlm.nih.gov/pmc/articles/PMC3266748/table/T2, consulted on 01.07.2016

Somalia	N.A.	4	0.5	0.06	0.03
Sudan	0.1	2	0.2	0.09	N.A.
Syria	7.8	8	N.A.	0.5	N.A.
Tunisia	9.6	11.3	0.8	1.6	3.3
Yemen	N.A.	18.5	0.1	0.5	N.A.

In the majority of Arab countries, there is no interaction between the medical profession and the traditional healers. In Jordan, there is some kind of a relationship, which remains informal and unorganized. In Saudi Arabia, however, they constitute part of the staff, using religious text and recitation in management.[343]

Although a majority of the countries of the region have agreed in principle to integrate mental health into the primary health care delivery system, implementation so far has been limited. Globally, the mental health infrastructure and services in most countries is grossly insufficient for the large and growing needs. Recent years have seen significant changes in the field of mental health in the countries of the Arab region. Psychiatric services, which were earlier totally confined to a few large mental hospitals, are now gradually being replaced by psychiatric units with both inpatient and outpatient facilities in general hospitals. In some countries, the process of decentralization has been taken still further, and psychiatric services are being provided at district hospitals and smaller peripheral units, along with other general health services. Training programmes in mental health for general practitioners, non-physicians and health personnel working at primary health care level have started in a large number of countries as a part of in-service skills enhancement programmes.

The budget allowed for mental health as a percentage from the total health budget, in the few countries where information is available, is far below the range to promote mental health services. According to the WHO World Health Report (2010) the health expenditure estimated as percentage of gross domestic product is the highest in Lebanon (11.3%) followed by Jordan (8.8%), Tunisia (5.3%) and Bahrain (5%).[344] Health services in all Arab countries are provided by public (government) and private sector facilities and out of pocket (this last category representing

---

[343] http://www.ncbi.nlm.nih.gov/pmc/articles/PMC3266748/, consulted on 01.07.2016

[344] https://www.aub.edu.lb/fm/shbpp/ethics/Documents/Brigitte-Khoury-mental-health-research-arab-region.pdf, consulted on 31.04.2016

58.7% in Egypt, 58% in Yemen, 56.1% in Morocco and 54.9% in Syria).[345] In some countries insurance systems contribute to the provision of the service. Non-governmental organizations (NGOs) have come to be recognized as active partner in the provision of health services, especially in countries with internal instability (in particular, Lebanon in late 1980s and Palestine now). None of the remaining Arab countries fulfilled the WHO recommendation of a minimum expenditure of 5% of GDP on health.[346]

Arab Regional Center for Research and Training in Mental Health joined WHO advisory group for revision of ICD-10 in 2009. The topics of the published papers related to mental health research in the Arab world from 1996 until July 2007[347] are given in the Table 8.3.

Table 8.3 Publications Related to Mental Health in the Arab Region

Topic	Number
Child	698
Depression	529
Anxiety	432
Addiction	208
Suicide	106
Affective	89
Classification	55
Psychosis	52
Organic	41
Somatoform	22
Psychopharmacology	20

Accordingly, this chapter covers the national mental health field in the following order:

- Historical timeline and chronology of mental health sector;
- National legislation on mental health;

---

[345] http://www.ncbi.nlm.nih.gov/pmc/articles/PMC3266748, consulted on 01.07.2016

[346] https://www.aub.edu.lb/fm/shbpp/ethics/Documents/Brigitte-Khoury-mental-health-research-arab-region.pdf, consulted on 31.04.2016

[347] https://www.aub.edu.lb/fm/shbpp/ethics/Documents/Brigitte-Khoury-mental-health-research-arab-region.pdf, consulted on 31.04.2016

- Common mental disorders;
- Mental health hospitals;
- Education and trainings for psychologists;
- National budget for mental health expenditure;
- Researches on mental health (if available);
- Strengths and weaknesses.

In summary, in the last ten years there has been an increase in all aspects of mental health services in the Arab region. The total number of psychologists and social workers have increased in all Arab countries (in particular, in Bahrain, Emirates, Jordan, Egypt, Kuwait, Libya, Saudi Arabia and Yemen).

EGYPT

In 1993 the first Encyclopedia of Psychology and Psychoanalysis was published. In 2004 Egyptian Psychoanalytic Association was finally created, however, this association, through its objectives and activities, did not identify psychoanalysis as a specific discipline. The first objective assigned by this association is organization of training sessions for psychological testing (projective tests, personality tests, intelligence test, etc.) Following a situation appraisal in 2001, a six-year mental health reform programme (Egymen) 2002-7 was initiated by an Egyptian-Finnish bilateral aid project at the request of a former Egyptian minister of health and the work was incorporated directly into the Ministry of Health and Population from 2007 onwards. The Egymen project also recruited expert assistance to capacity build specialist expertise and develop services for forensic psychiatry, rehabilitation, and child psychiatry, and continued support was given by the Finnish government, 2000-9, WHO Collaborating centre, Institute of Psychiatry, London 2000-9 and the RCPsych 2006-9.[348] This comprised visits to Egypt of the Finnish and UK experts, Egyptian study tours to Finland, England and other European countries, and specifically tailored placements in the UK. Funding for service developments from the Finnish government, and the MOHP has continued to access expert assistance from the UK for forensic psychiatry and legislation.

Dedicated mental health legislation exists and was initiated, or most recently revised, in 2009. Mental health is also specifically mentioned in

[348] http://www.who.int/mental_health/evidence/atlas/profiles/egy_mh_profile.pdf, consulted on 01.07.2016

the general health policy.[349] A mental health plan exists and was approved or, most recently revised, in 2008. The mental health plan components include:

- Timelines for the implementation of the mental health plan;
- Shift of services and resources from mental hospitals to community mental health facilities;
- Integration of mental health services into primary care;

Legal provisions concerning mental health are also covered in other laws (e.g. welfare, disability, general health legislation, etc.). The new mental health law includes the following provisions:

- Strict legal criteria specifying the circumstances in which a person can be detained in mental health institutions;
- The right of a detained patient to have the lawfulness of detention reviewed by a local court;
- The establishment of both national and regional mental health commissions;
- A requirement that doctors document and periodically review treatment plans;
- A more restrictive definition of circumstances in which solitary confinement and physical restraints can be used;
- A bill of rights for patients inside mental health facilities and the obligation of mental health facilities to inform patients of their rights;
- The creation of a patients' rights committee in every mental health facility in order to monitor the human rights of people receiving treatment in those institutions;
- A range of sanctions for service providers who violate patients' rights;
- Monitoring bodies providing an independent review of involuntary admissions.

On the 18th of May 2009, the Egyptian Parliament adopted a new law entitled the "Law for the Care of Mental Patients."[350] Mental health law reform is particularly timely in Egypt given the country's ratification in April

---

[349] *Ibid*

[350] http://www.mdac.info/en/news/new-mental-health-law-egypt, consulted on 01.07.2016

2008 of the UN Convention on the Rights of Persons with Disabilities, which includes rights provisions for persons with mental health disabilities. The civil society organization, the Egyptian Initiative for Personal Rights (EIPR) led a vigorous advocacy campaign to ensure that the new law protects the rights of people with mental health disabilities. The new law includes the following new provisions, specifying the circumstances in which a person can be detained in mental health institutions:

- The right of a detained patient to have the lawfulness of detention reviewed by a local court;
- An obligation upon mental health institutions to notify the public prosecutor within 24 hours of involuntarily admitting a patient;
- A right to consent to treatment for "voluntary" patients;
- A requirement that doctors document and periodically review treatment plans;
- A more restrictive definition of circumstances in which solitary confinement and physical restraints can be used;
- A bill of rights for patients inside mental health facilities;
- An obligation on mental health facilities to inform patients of their rights;
- The creation of a patients' rights committee in every mental health facility to monitor the human rights of people receiving treatment in those institutions;
- An explicit stipulation of the participation of civil society organizations in these patients' rights committees;
- A range of sanctions for service providers who violate patients' rights;
- Monitoring bodies providing an independent review of involuntary admissions;
- The establishment of a mental health fund to ensure sustainable financing for mental health care, including capacity-building for those working in mental health.

In Egypt, neuropsychiatric disorders are estimated to contribute to 15.1% of the global burden of disease (WHO, 2008).[351] Hysteria occupies a position at the top of the list of psychiatric diagnoses in Egypt. Earlier studies of psychiatric morbidity among university students in Egypt

---

[351] http://www.who.int/mental_health/evidence/atlas/profiles/egy_mh_profile. pdf, consulted on 01.07.2016

showed that anxiety states were diagnosed in 36% of the study sample.[352] The findings revealed that the most common symptoms were worrying (82%), irritability (73%), free-floating anxiety (70%), depressed mood (65%), tiredness (64%), restlessness (63%), and anergia and retardation (61%)[353]. Panic attacks were present in 30%, situational anxiety in 35%, specific phobias in 37% and avoidance in 53% of the sample.[354]

Table 8.4 Availability of Mental Health Facilities[355]

	Total number of facilities/ beds	Rate per 100,000 population	Number of facilities/beds reserved for children and adolescents only	Rate per 100,000 population
Mental health outpatient facilities	96	0.114	UN	UN
Day treatment facilities	2	0.002	UN	UN
Psychiatric beds in general hospitals	399	0.472	UN	UN
Community residential facilities	UN	UN	UN	UN
Beds/places in community residential facilities	UN	UN	UN	UN
Mental hospitals	38	0.045	UN	UN
Beds in mental hospitals	7940	9.399	UN	UN

---

[352] Okasha A., Kamel M., Sadek A. et al, Psychiatric morbidity among university students in Egypt. British Journal of Psychiatry, 131, 1977, pp.149 -154.

[353] Okasha A., Ashour A.,Psycho-demographic study of anxiety in Egypt: the PSE in its Arabic version. British Journal of Psychiatry, 139, 1981, pp.70-73.

[354] *Ibid*

[355] http://www.who.int/mental_health/evidence/atlas/profiles/egy_mh_profile. pdf, consulted on 01.07.2016

Table 8.5 Workforce and Training[356]

	Health professionals working in the mental health sector Rate per 100,000	Training of health professions in educational institutions Rate per 100,000
Psychiatrists	0.54	UN
Medical doctors, not specialized in psychiatry	0.31	UN
Nurses	2.08	UN
Psychologists	0.13	UN
Social workers	0.23	UN
Occupational therapists	UN	UN
Other health workers	UN	NA

A study investigating the demographic profile and symptoms of Egyptian patients with obsessive–compulsive disorder found that more than two-thirds of the patients were male.[357] The most commonly occurring obsessions were religion and contamination (60%) and somatic obsessions (49%), whereas the most commonly occurring compulsions were repeating rituals (68%), cleaning and washing compulsions (63%) and checking compulsions (58%).[358]The prevalence rates of depression among selected samples from an urban and a rural population in Egypt were found to be 11.4% and 19.7%, respectively.[359] Depression among Egyptian patients is manifested mainly by agitation, somatic symptoms, hypochondriasis, physiological changes such as decreased libido, anorexia, and insomnia, which is not characterized by early morning awakening. Schizophrenia is the most common chronic psychosis in Egypt and accounts for the majority of in-patients in mental hospitals. In what it concerns the children, the prevalence of scholastic underachievement in

---

[356] *Ibid*

[357] Okasha A., Khalil A., Seif El Dawla A., et al, Phenomenology of obsessive–compulsive disorder: a transcultural study. Comprehensive Psychiatry, 35, 1994, pp.191 -197.

[358] *Ibid*

[359] *Ibid*

a sample of pupils at elementary schools was 42.8%.[360] Diagnoses made in this group included attention-deficit hyperactivity disorder, depression, anxiety, speech difficulties and elimination problems, none of which had been detected by their teachers.

There are three mental hospitals in Cairo accommodating approximately 5600 patients, one in Alexandria, one in Dakahlia, one in Asyout[361] (see Table 8.4.) The Behman Hospital is the oldest and largest private psychiatric hospital in the Middle East, based in Egypt.[362]

Table 8.6 Expenditures for Medicines for Mental and Behavioral Disorders at the Country Level[363]

Type of Medicines	Expenditures at country level per year and per 100,000 population (in USD)
All the psychotherapeutic medicines	UN
Medicines used for bipolar disorders	UN
Medicines for psychotic disorders	UN
Medicines used for general anxiety	UN
Medicines used for mood disorders	UN

The number of health professionals working in the mental health sector reported above is for those who work at general secretariat of mental health which supervises and monitor the main 17 psychiatric hospital in Egypt which represents 84% of the bed capacity.[364] The total number of psychiatrists is 979, which corresponds to a rate of 1.16 per 100,000 population (see Table 8.5.) In Egypt, there are about 250 clinical

---

[360] Hassan E., Epidemiological study of scholastic underachievement among primary school children in Alexandria: prevalence and causes. Thesis, Faculty of Nursing, University of Alexandria, 1999

[361] http://scholarworks.wmich.edu/cgi/viewcontent.cgi?article=1980&context= jssw, consulted on 01.05.2016

[362] http://www.behman.com/aboutus.php, consulted on 01.07.2016

[363] http://www.who.int/mental_health/evidence/atlas/profiles/egy_mh_profile. pdf, consulted on 01.07.2016

[364] http://www.who.int/mental_health/evidence/atlas/profiles/egy_mh_profile. pdf, consulted on 01.07.2016

psychologists[365] but hundreds of general psychologists are working in fields unrelated to the mental health services. There are many social workers practicing in all psychiatric facilities, but, unfortunately, they are general social workers who have minimal graduate training in psychiatric social work. There was an attempt to educate psychiatric social workers at the Institute of Social Services in Cairo in 1960. It lasted only for two years due to a shortage of students.[366]

Mental health expenditures by the government health department/ministry are 2.29% of the total health budget. There is no data on expenditures for medicines for mental and behavioral disorders at country level (see Table 8.6.)

Egyptian Universities face economic hardships, like other sectors of Egyptian society. This affects academic output, psychology included, e.g. heavy bureaucracy, budget and administrative issues, low ratio of student/instructors. The psychology departments in Egypt are part of Faculties of Arts rather than standing as a separate discipline. Therefore, psychology finds itself between literary studies and the scientific disciplines. This, in turn, affects the impression of the field and poses serious limitations to its development. Also, in some Universities, psychology is usually practiced as part of neurology. Over the years there has been a conflict between two groups of psychologists: the first being composed of medical faculty members; and the second including the faculty members of the graduate schools. Such conflict yields a characteristic version of psychology with a split identity and a disfigured public image. Most research publications in psychology are published either in Journals of Social Studies or Egyptian Journals of psychology. Much of this literature, in my opinion, is repetitive, fragmented and non-cumulative, and does not provide normative data about local populations to be used for comparisons. Often, Egyptian researchers use exported normative data from Western countries to compare their samples. Thus, there may be a lack of reliability or validity of conclusions for Egyptian samples. Many of the Western tools of investigation, especially paper, and pencil tests, have been translated into Arabic. However, computer-based tests are still uncommon, as we (Egyptian psychologists) do not have the resources to develop an Arabic interface for such tests. Moreover, normative data for those tests are based on the Western samples, e.g. White, African-American, etc., which do

---

[365] Ghodse H., International Perspectives on Mental Health, RCPsych Publications, 2011, p.9.

[366] http://scholarworks.wmich.edu/cgi/viewcontent.cgi?article=1980&context=jssw, consulted on 01.05.2016

not necessarily fit the Egyptian or Arab populations, owing to multiple socio-cultural factors. Experimental psychology (animal psychology) does not receive much attention in the psychological institutes. Thus, there is a huge gap between preclinical and clinical psychology. The translation of Western textbooks poses an obstacle for the development of psychology in Egypt. Numerous Western textbooks have been translated into Arabic since the 1950s. Moreover, there are only two psychological associations in Egypt with limited memberships, activities and influence in the field.[367] Many subspecialties in psychology do not exist in Egypt. One such example is political psychology, which is not recognized in Egypt because its theoretical framework is not well formulated.[368] According to V. Sapiro, development of these subspecialties is important because, in the case of political psychology, it provides an understanding of human nature, emotion, and behavior in politics. Such an understanding is crucial for Egypt, where the political atmosphere is such that Egyptians were forbidden to discuss the life of their most recent president.

In what it concerns the strength of the mental health system in Egypt, it comprises:

- Available updated mental health policy and a mental health plan;
- Available essential psychotropic medicines in all mental health facilities.

And weakness:

- Mental health legislation is quite old and needs to be updated;
- Only 2% of the governmental health expenditure was directed towards mental health;
- Incomplete network of mental health facilities;
- Most of the mental health facilities are present only in or near large cities;
- The referral system to mental health professionals in primary health care is not well established;

---

[367] Ahmed R., Psychology in the Arab countries. In U.P. Gielen, L.L. Adler, & N.A. Milgram (Eds.), Psychology in International Perspective: 50 Years of the International Council of Psychologists, Swets & Zeitlinger, 1992, pp. 127- 150.

[368] Jakovljevic M., Hubris syndrome and a new perspective on political psychiatry: Need to protect prosocial behavior, public benefits and safety of our civilization. Psychiatria Danubina, 23, 2011, pp.136-138.

Currently, the mental health field in Egypt is facing numerous hardships. In the country, which in the past was a place for the first mental hospitals in the world, nowadays,very limited resources are dedicated to the psychology, as a scientific discipline. Thus said, the psychologists are experiencing a lack of the educational, training and financial support. Another big challenge is the existing stigma of mental illness, which prevents many Egyptians from addressing to the psychiatrist, and, thus, receiving essential help. Not much is currently being done to fight the stigmatization. Even though, the infrastructure of mental health facilities is one of the biggest in the region, not all those, who need treatment, can be admitted. And those, who are admitted oftentimes become mentally and physically abused.

SOMALIA

Prolonged conflict and instability have largely impacted on the mental and psychological well-being of its people. One in three Somali's has been affected by some kind of mental illness[369]. The medical reports account for severe PTSD of Somali population, suggesting that many suffered repeated trauma.The barbaric practice of enchaining a mentally ill person is still generally practiced. There are only 5 health centres in Somalia, namely, Hargeisa, Berbera, Bosaso, Garowe and Mogadishu, which provide psychological services.

Regarding the legal framework, there is no unified health policy, substance abuse policy, a national mental health programme. A national therapeutic drug policy/essential list of drugs is also absent.

In Minnesota (USA) in 1998 The Somali Mental Health Program was launched at Community University Health Care Center (CUHCC). The centre provides a variety of outpatient services for Somali refugees, including psychiatric assessments, medication management, individual and group therapy, and case management for adults and children.

---

[369] http://www.who.int/hac/crises/som/somalia_mental_health/en, consulted on 01.07.2016

Somali Mental Health Foundation

Somali Mental Health Foundation, a US-based association, funded by Somali diaspora, established Gardho Mental Health Center Head Quarters in Gardho in Puntland State of Somalia in 2011.[370]

Somaliland Mental Health Support Organisation

Somaliland Mental Health Support Organisation is another organisation based outside Somalia, namely in the UK, that aims to improve and support those people who suffer from mental health conditions in Somalia. It was launched in 2011.[371]

The number of psychiatrists per 100 000 population is 0.06 and that of social workers is 0.19.[372] Regular training of primary care professionals is not carried out in the field of mental health. The voluntary workers of GAVO have been trained about the principles of psychiatric interview, introduced to DSM-IV, given training about psychopharmacology, psychosocial rehabilitation, and hospital management. The training had lasted for 2 years and is not on a regular basis.

There are no budget allocations for mental health.

As a result of prolonged wars, the mental health domain in Somalia has been severely neglected. Even though single efforts are being made by certain psychotherapists to provide the necessary treatment, they are mostly unorganized and based on mere enthusiasm.

MAGHREB COUNTRIES

One of the Maghreb countries where psychoanalytical tradition has taken deep roots is Morocco. Moroccan analysts have created a vast professional space, which represents a connecting link between the psychoanalysis and Islam.

---

[370] http://www.somalimentalhealth.org/what-we-do/project-sites, consulted on 01.07.2016

[371] *Ibid*

[372] http://psychologyinafrica.com/profiles/2013/8/13/somalia-mental-health-profile, consulted on 01.07.2016

ALGERIA

Violence came back to Algeria between 1992 and 2000/2003. Boucebci was assassinated, the other psychiatrists and very rare psychoanalysts exiled or were staying in great discretion. An interest of some medical teams, who had to treat and accompany the victims of terrorism, have oriented towards psychoanalysis since other approaches have rapidly demonstrated their limits, like debriefing. Today the Ministry of Health does not recognize psychoanalysis. As such psychoanalysis does not exist in Algeria. If it has found its way nowadays, it`s because, as Faika Medjahed explains, "a group, which practices as psychoanalytical psychologists and family therapists, and not only as psychoanalysts."[373]

The latest legislation was enacted in 1998. An officially approved mental health policy exists and was approved, or most recently revised, in 2009. Mental health is also specifically mentioned in the general health policy.[374] The components of the current mental health policy were defined more clearly in the 4 axes of the national mental health programme established since 10 October 2001.

Code of the Family states (2003):[375]

Art.81- Any person that is *completely or partly incompetent* due to his young age or *mental defect* is legally represented by a legal guardian or one designated by will, conforming to the dispositions of the current law.

Code of the Family (2005):[376]

Art.42-The person who lacks the sense to discern due to his young age or *feebleness or mental defect* does not have the capacity to exercise his civil rights. Any child who has not attained the age of thirteen lacks the sense of discern.

Art.43-The person who has attained the age to discern, without having reached adulthood, as well as the person who has reached adulthood and suffers from mental defect, have limited capacity conforming to the prescriptions of the law.

---

[373] http://www.lemidi-dz.com/index.php?operation=voir_article&id_article=culture%40art2%402010-01-30, consulted on 01.07.2016

[374] http://www.who.int/mental_health/evidence/atlas/profiles/dza_mh_profile.pdf, consulted on 01.07.2016

[375] http://arabpsynet.com/Archives/OP/TopicJ20NumanGharaibeh2.pdf, consulted on 01.07.2016

[376] *Ibid*

Table 8.7 Availability of Mental Health Facilities

	Total number of facilities/ beds	Rate per 100,000 population	Number of facilities/ beds reserved for children and adolescents only	Rate per 100,000 population
Mental health outpatient facilities	428	1.21	UN	UN
Day treatment facilities	16	0.05	15	0.04
Psychiatric beds in general hospitals	826	2.33	12	0.03
Community residential facilities	NA	NA	NA	NA
Beds/places in community residential facilities	NA	NA	NA	NA
Mental hospitals	15	0.04	UN	UN
Beds in mental hospitals	4023	11.36	160	0.45

An epidemiological study done by the Ministry of Health (2004) showed that chronic mental disorders were diagnosed in 0.7% to 1.9% of subjects of different age groups and epilepsy in 0.2% to 0.8% of subjects in different age groups.[377] Chronic mental disorders and epilepsy were more common in those below 40 years of age and in women.

There was no rural-urban difference in prevalence of these conditions. The prevalence of posttraumatic stress disorder (PTSD) assessed using the PTSD module of the Composite International Diagnostic Interview Version 2.1 was found to be 37.4% in a community survey conducted on

---

[377] http://psychologyinafrica.com/profiles/2013/6/2/algeria-mental-health-profile, consulted on 01.07.2016

a sample of 653 subjects.[378] In Algeria, neuropsychiatric disorders are estimated to contribute to 13.1% of the global burden of disease.[379]

From the Table 8.7. we can see that the average number of psychiatric beds at the mental health outpatient facilities in Algeria is 428. Whereas, in accordance with the Table 8.8, the number of psychiatrists is 1.55 per 100,000 population.

Table 8.8 Workforce and Training[380]

	Health professionals working in the mental health sector Rate per 100,000	Training of health professions in educational institutions Rate per 100,000
Psychiatrists	1.55	0.28
Medical doctors, not specialized in psychiatry	0.42	2.26
Nurses	6.01	0.75
Psychologists	4.26	2.82
Social workers	UN	0.3
Occupational therapists	UN	0.14
Other health workers	UN	NA

Table 8.9 Expenditures for Medicines for Mental and Behavioral Disorders at the Country Level[381]

Type of Medicines	Expenditures at country level per year and per 100,000 population (in USD)
All the psychotherapeutic medicines	197,527
Medicines used for bipolar disorders	51,357
Medicines for psychotic disorders	67,159

---

[378] Mental Health Atlas 2005, World Health Organization, p.54.

[379] http://www.who.int/mental_health/neurology/chapter_2_neuro_disorders_public_h_challenges.pdf, consulted on 01.05.2016

[380] http://www.who.int/mental_health/evidence/atlas/profiles/dza_mh_profile.pdf, consulted on 01.07.2016

[381] http://www.who.int/mental_health/evidence/atlas/profiles/dza_mh_profile.pdf, consulted on 01.07.2016

| Medicines used for general anxiety | 19,753 |
| Medicines used for mood disorders | 59,258 |

The primary source of mental health financing is tax based.[382] The expenditures for medicines for mental and behavioral disorders can be consulted at the Table 8.9.

The strength of the mental health system in Algeria is:

• Existing mental health policy;
• The available range of practitioners, including psychologists.

Its weakness:

• Shortage of qualified human resources;
• Low governmental spending on mental health;
• Insufficient in-patient facilities.

For the most part, in Algeria the traditional therapies still heavily dominate over the clinical treatment. And scientific psychology does not receive sufficient support from the governmental sector. So, mentally ill people are often neglected, abandoned or/and ill-treated.

LYBIA

Decades of neglect and the 2011 conflict have left Libya's mental health system in tatters, with only 12 psychiatrists, and services highly centralized at the two psychiatric hospitals in the country's two largest cities, Tripoli and Benghazi.[383] But a new mental health programme led by the Ministry of Health and WHO, based within the National Center for Disease Control (NCDC/MOH), is set to transform Libya's institution-based approach to a community-based approach to mental health care, making mental health services available to the most remote and under-served areas of the country. "Mental health services in Libya had been extremely inadequate and couldn't meet the urgent needs of people who suffered during and after the conflict," says Dr Baderdin Najjar, Director

---

[382] Mental Health Atlas, 2005, World Health Organization, p.54.
[383] http://www.who.int/features/2013/mental_health_libya/en, consulted on 31.04.2016

of Libya's National Center for Disease Control/Ministry of Health. "This had created a huge challenge to the already worn-out health system."[384]

Table 8.10 Current Most Active Contributors
into Mental Health Field in Lybia[385]

National NGOs	International NGOs	Governmental Bodies
Lybian Association of Psychological Health	Danish Church Aid	Tripoli Psychiatric Hospital
Lybian Association of Psychological Support	International Medical Corps	Benghazi Psychiatric Hospital
Lybian Red Crescent	Hilfswerk Austria International	Tripoli Central Hospital
Office for Martyrs and Missing Statistics	International Organization for Migration	Benghazi Medical Centre Psychology Department
Office for Medical and Psychosocial Support for 17th February Injured	Mercy Corps	National Centre of Disease Control
Tawassel Org.	Medicins Sans Frontiers- Belgium Acts of Mercy Save The Children WHO	Misrata Mental Health Centre

In Libya, the mental health policy is part of the general health policy. Nearly one in every three Libyans is suffering from depression as a result of widespread human rights violations committed during the era of longtime dictator Muammar Gaddafi and the volatile and violent years that have followed his overthrow in 2011, according to a new report.[386] The freedom fighters suffer from such psychological states as: isolation, risk-taking behavior, resentment, inability to reintegrate into society etc. (see Table 8.13.) Other most frequent mental disorders of the modern Lybian population can be consulted at the Table 8.11 and Table 8.12.

---

[384] *Ibid*

[385] http://cpwg.net/wp-content/uploads/sites/2/2012/09/Libya-4Ws-MHPSS-Mapping-Report-ENG-2011.pdf, consulted on 01.07.2016

[386] http://www.middleeasteye.net/news/ticking-time-bomb-mental-health-problems-libya-1228141611#sthash.1a0Xztlw.dpuf, consulted on 01.07.2016

According with the Libya Health and Environment Report of 2010 there were 97 hospitals, 37 polyclinics, and 535 health centers functioning prior to the conflict. The availability of mental health facilities can be consulted at the Table 8.14.

Table 8.11 Mental Health Related Problems, Coping and Community Sources of Support (At Risk Group: Children)[387]

Stressors and priority MH related problems	Coping methods	Community sources of support	What more could be done to support this group?	Community attitudes
1. Aggression 2. Fear 3. Stress/ conflicts within families 4. Hyperactivity 5. Increased sexual behavior 6. Enuresis 7. Insomnia	"Children do not know what to do." Parents/ families are coping by: 1. Beating their children 2. Being overprotective 3. Waiting for services to begin	Some NGO's are trying to connect families with distressed children to clinics/ supportive centers. Otherwise, nothing is being done.	1. Community awareness raising/ educating parents 2. Encouraging parents about the dangers of TV programs and exposing children to violence 3. More funding/ support to existing centers that help children	Most people understand that children have been affected by the conflict. When children have special needs, including mental health problems, the community feels pity for them. A child with any disability is seen as a "burden on a family, especially girls."

---

[387] http://internationalmedicalcorps.org/document.doc?id=239, consulted on 01.05.2016

Table 8.12 Mental Health Related Problems, Coping and
Community Sources of Support (At Risk Group: Women)[388]

Stressors and priority MH related problems	Coping methods	Community sources of support	What more could be done to support this group?	Community attitudes
1. Loss of security and routine 2. Fear 2. Loss of loved ones 3. Hopelessness 4. Financial fears 6. Unemployment 7. Weakened social Connections 10. Symptoms of anxiety and depression	1. Organizing charity groups 2. Working with Freedom Fighters support groups 3. Organizing bazars 4. Leaving homes to work together 5. Keeping themselves busy 6. Cleaning hospitals 7. Isolating themselves 8. Refusing to return to old routines 9. Denying/ acting like things aren't happening 10. Sewing revolutionary flags	All support being provided is financial, but no emotional psychosocial support is offered for women. Charity organizations are offering some material support, and social services are paid for internally displaced people, but there is nothing else.	1. Training local professionals to help women would help more than approaching women directly. 2. Teaching people the right approach to work with women. 3. More media attention regarding supportive services for women 4. More groups/ organizations for women (including women's centers)	People are not as judgmental as they were before, but still women with mental health problems are afraid that the community will judge them.

---

388 *Ibid*

Table 8.13 Mental Health Related Problems, Coping
and Community Sources of Support (At Risk Group:
Freedom Fighters (generally age 16-30))[389]

Stressors and priority MH related problems	Coping methods	Community sources of support	What more could be done to support this group?	Community attitudes
1. Isolation 2. Risk taking behavior 3. Resentment 4. Inability to reintegrate into society 5. Feeling a sense of authority (acting as if they are the law, there are no repercussions and that they have no responsibilities, resulting in chaos and instability in society)	1. Isolate themselves to their "brigade" and their "barracks to avoid dealing with civilians 2. Seek out any conflict and sometimes create conflict over minor issues 3. Alcohol and substance abuse 4. Surrounding themselves with their friends 5. Travel abroad for a while 6. Charity and community work to help rebuild Libya	1. Charities raise money to help injured but funds are paying for hospital stays and food rather than psychological treatment (which new government has said it will pay for, but is not currently) 2. Organizations are gathering information regarding the wounded and missing, 3. Charities are organizing local blood donation centers	1. The Temporary Government should treat those with physical injuries with transparency so people can follow the progress. 2. The NTC should reassure them that they will not be oppressed by a Gadaffi like regime. 3. Give them information regarding their future as combatants and the strategy for the future so they can ultimately lay down their weapons.	The community initially loved the FF and rejoiced at their presence, however recently it has become negative due to: 1. Community members don't want to praise them for fear of feeding their entitlement to power, status or money. So,

389   http://internationalmedicalcorps.org/document.doc?id=239, consulted on 01.05.2016

	7. Talking about what happened with family and friends.	4. Local youth organization arrange gatherings at Martyr Square for youth where professionals give lectures about Libya's political future and information about possible future roles for the FFs in the community 5. Community members visit the injured to provide support, they provide them with basic personal items (clothes toiletries), some charities gathering money to pay their medical treatment. 6. Many organizations who talk about helping but none focus on helping freedom fighters reintegrate into society	4. Government must pay them a salary and give them a feeling of importance and respect. 5. Arrange job opportunities for them as a way to integrate them into society and keep them busy. 6. The government must create a database of all injured so follow up can take place and money is directly allocate to those in need	community members are belittling them and dismissing their efforts. 2. Some FFs looted and are squatting in people's houses; this has resulted in an attitude change towards all FFs even those who are upholding the law

Table 8.14 Availability of Mental Health Facilities[390]

Name	Average number of patients per day (past month)	Number of beds:	Staffing
Tripoli Al Razi Psychiatric Hospital	150-250 in OPD	60 (m and f) for acute,120 (m and f) for chronic, 40 (m) for forensic cases	20 psychiatrists; 6 psychologists (none studied clinical psychotherapy); 12 social workers
Benghazi Psychiatric Hospital	50 in OPD	300 (full capacity 400)	17 psychiatrists; 40 psychologists; 20 social workers
Tripoli Central Hospital Psychiatric Office	3-4 (clinic is open 4 days a week in the mornings)	NA	2 psychiatrists; 1 psychologist; 0 social worker
Benghazi Medical Center Psychiatric Clinic	5 Number of inpatients: 300 (full capacity 400)	NA	2 psychiatrists; 0 psychologist; 0 social worker
Misrata Psychiatric Office	30	NA	2 psychiatrists; 2 psychologists; 0 social worker
Misrata Amal Alghad Private Clinic	10-13; 150 psychiatric patients per week	NA	1 psychiatrist; 10 psychologists; 3-4 social workers

Office for Medical and Psychosocial Support for Freedom Fighters

In Benghazi, the Office for Medical and Psychosocial Support for Freedom Fighters has been operating and is employing 15 psychologists: 1 psychologist was trained by Tawassel Organization in treatment of trauma/ PTSD) and 10 social workers.[391] Benghazi Rehabilitation Center is employing 5 psychologists and 5 social workers.

---

[390] http://internationalmedicalcorps.org/document.doc?id=239, consulted on 01.05.2016

[391] http://internationalmedicalcorps.org/document.doc?id=239, consulted on 01.05.2016

Zintan Hospital

In the Nafuza mountains, Zintan Hospital has received visits from two psychologists for six days a week and Yefrin Hospital from one psychologist for two days a week while both have received visits from a psychiatrist every two weeks. The two psychologists who provided the services were from Tunisia and received some training and their salary from MSF-Ch. After the departure of MSF, IMC has taken over funding for one of the Tunisian psychologist and is in the process of identifying national psychologists for further training. NGOs play an active role in the mental health field of Libya, among them there are Lybian Association of Psychological Support, Lybian Red Crescent, and others (see Table 8.10.)

Mental Health Professionals' Association of Libya

Mental Health Professionals' Association of Libya (MH PAL)[392] was established during the recent war of liberation in Libya and it represents an effort to bring together mental health professionals of Libyan background under one virtual roof. The hope is that these professionals will use the organization as a means through which to share ideas and expertise on all aspects, mental health and well-being relevant to Libya, both at home and abroad.

Educational opportunities for psychologists typically are limited to BA level degrees, which typically focus on general or educational psychology but do not provide any clinical training in mental health (see Table 8.15, Table 8.16 and Table 8.17). Focus groups discussions with psychologists revealed that they are using old texts in Libyan universities, and feel unprepared to work directly with beneficiaries/clients once they obtain their degree. From IMCs conversations with psychologists from over eight health facilities, not one of them had on-the-job training. Some of them reported that they have asked senior psychologists for guidance, but most of them work independently following graduation, with no supervision or support. The exceptions seem to be in the Psychiatric Hospitals, where "the best" psychologists go for training. Furthermore, from our conversations with psychologists, only 5 were identified in all of Libya who have skills in clinical interventions (the only intervention mentioned typically was CBT). When asked how the treatment process develops, psychologists generally explained that they typically do some type of assessment (based on their own judgment) and then intervene in an ad-hoc manner by "listening

---

[392] http://mhpal.weebly.com, consulted on 01.07.2016

and giving advice." There typically is no follow-up or referral, unless the person is identified as someone needing psychotropic medications. They expressed the need for practical training to improve their skills including working with people with disabilities due to the war.[393] In Misrata MSF has provided some training and supervision for psychologists since August 2011.[394] Several psychologists have been working under supervision of MSF in 2 hospitals (Anoor Hospital (2 psychologists), Ras Atuba Hospital (2)), 2 Medical Centers (Ras Atuba Medical Center (1), Health Center Askerat (1)), 6 Polyclinics (Almahjub poly clinic (3), Red crescent poly clinic (2), Red crescent poly clinic (private, 2),Asafwa private clinic (1), Red crescent "Arwesat" private clinic (1), Qasar Ahmed clinic (2)) and Altadhamon Physical Rehabilitation Center (1).[395]

The proportion of health budget to GDP is 2.9%[396]. In Lybia the per capita total expenditure on health is 239 US dollars, and the per capita government expenditure on health is 134 US dollars[397].

Table 8.15 MHPSS Degrees Offered in Libya[398]

University	City	MD	Psychology	Social Work
University of Garyonis	Benghazi		√	√
Al Arab Medical University	Benghazi	√		
Nasser University	Tripoli		√	√
Tripoli University (prev. Alfatha)	Tripoli	√	√	√
Omar Mukhtar University	Albayda		√	√
Misrata University	Misrata	√	√	√
Sabha University	Sabha	√	√	√

---

[393] http://internationalmedicalcorps.org/document.doc?id=239, consulted on 01.05.2016

[394] *Ibid*

[395] http://internationalmedicalcorps.org/document.doc?id=239, consulted on 01.05.2016

[396] Mental Health Atlas 2005, World Health Organization, p. 287.

[397] *Ibid*

[398] http://internationalmedicalcorps.org/document.doc?id=239, consulted on 01.05.2016

AlTahadi University	Sirte	√	√	√
Alzawya University	Alzawya	√	√	√
Almargib University	Khoms	√	√	√
Open University (16 branches)	Across Libya		√	√

Table 8.16 Overview of Preparation of Psychologist[399]

Total years of study	Institution and Department	Degree Obtained	Place of Intern-ship	Duration of Intern-ship	Further Education and training	Career options	Most popular career path	Main Universities offering degree	Private Sector
4 years	University (National Vocational diploma prior to 19865), Dept. of Education and Psychology	BA Psychology	Hospitals, Polyclinics, Schools, Orphanages, Residential Homes, Nurseries, Social Service department.	1 year with prospect of employment	Masters from several Libyan Universities, Training in workplace (work specific), Scholarship for PhD abroad	Work within schools, hospitals or place of internship.	Working in schools, hospitals	Benghazi university syllabus includes clinical psychology with clinical training.	Psychologist are becoming more and more available in private sector health care

399   *Ibid*

Table 8.17 Sample Libyan Curricula of Psychologist[400]

First year	Second year	Third year	Fourth year
Introduction to Psychology	Childhood and adolescence mental health	Research Design Psychology	Psychology of Geriatrics
Principles of counseling and guidance	Psychology and physiology	Contact	Psychopathology
The basics of scientific research	Schools of Psychology	Psychological tests Theories of learning	Field Exercises Graduation Project Psychology of Special groups
Descriptive statistics	Educational Psychology	Think of a mass Applications of psychological	Cognitive Psychology
Introduction to Sociology	Social Psychology Mental Health Terminology	Psychopathology Professional Psychology	Clinical Psychology Experimental Psychology
Arabic Language	Research Methodology	Environmental Psychology	Forensic Psychology
History of the Arab Islamic civilization	Constructive Recommendation	Psychology of language	Psychology
Islamic culture	Measurement and Evaluation Behavioral problems	Theories of Guidance and Counseling	

The strength of the mental health system in Lybia is:

- Available mental health policy;
- Available educational opportunities for mental health workers, even though, limited.

Its weakness:

- Insufficiency of qualified human resources;
- Limited (or none) management or maintenance treatment for mental disorders;
- No supervision for mental cases.

As we can see, the war has led to the destruction of the mental health sector, which prior to the revolutionary events, was counting around 100

---

[400] http://internationalmedicalcorps.org/document.doc?id=239, consulted on 01.05.2016

functioning hospitals, and as much mental health centers. At present times, Lybian mental care sector is heavily dependent on international aid and outsourcing of foreign doctors. Psychological education, training, and funding come as a part of humanitarian assistance from different NGOs. The Lybian population is massively suffering from PTSD, while the local hospitals lack sufficient resources, as well as qualified workforce, to provide the adequate therapies.

MOROCCO

Morocco is undergoing the following reforms: decentralization, integration of mental health into primary health care, reduction of the number of beds in mental hospitals, and an increase in the services available to patients at the community level.[401] Education levels in Morocco: 70% of women and 43% of men are illiterate,[402] which influences their choice of recourse to mental health treatments.The National Mental Health Program, launched in 1974 and revised in 1994, was not properly implemented. The conference Contribution of the North African Psychopathology, held at the Institute of the Arab World in April 1990, and an international symposium on the theme Psychotherapies of North African Patients in April 1992 in Casablanca, gave a kick to the creation of the Moroccan Association for Psychotherapy. The main issue discussed during this colloquium was the definition of the concept of cultural specificity that does not deny the universality of psychic mechanisms. The symposium was attended by North African as well as European therapists. The other associations, in particular, the Moroccan Association for Psychotherapy and the Moroccan Association of Psychiatrists in Private Practice, have helped to sensitize practitioners to the notion of "psychotherapy". Numerous meetings were held in the context of these associations, or as part of Cooperation and Cultural Action of the Embassy of France and French institutes. They brought together practitioners from various backgrounds, mostly French and Moroccan. This awareness stage lasted during one decade (1990-2000) before other associations would appear in the Moroccan analytical space. Psychoanalytic training steadily was growing in demand.

---

[401] WHO-AIMS Report on Mental Health System in Morocco, 2006, p. 25.

[402] http://www.humanityinaction.org/knowledgebase/314-mektab-and-sabr-cultural-and-societal-factors-affecting-mental-health-treatment-for-moroccan-adolescents, consulted on 01.05.2016

Moroccan Association of Psychotherapy

Moroccan Association of Psychotherapy (L'Association Marocaine de Psychothérapie) was created in 1992. Its objectives include: enabling knowledge about different psychotherapies, assisting Moroccan educational institutions to fulfill better their role in teaching psychotherapies and supporting the training of psychotherapists. This association has largely fulfilled its first two goals. The other associations were created either in the continuity of the MAP`s work, either independently. MAP brought together psychoanalysts, cognitive-behavioral and systemic therapists, as well as the therapists, who conduct researches on traditional therapies. Each discipline was governed by its own group of specialists. This separation allowed reducing criticism that sometimes was expressed concerning the integration of different disciplines. Some years later, other associations were established, such as Moroccan Association for Cognitive and Therapies (MACT), created in 1999, Moroccan Association for Research and Systemic Family Therapy, created in 2000, as well as others.

Moroccan Psychoanalytic Association

Moroccan Psychoanalytic Association (La Société Psychanalytique Marocaine) was established in 2001.[403] Among its member-founders, there are Jalil Bennani, Leila Cherkaoui, Abdeslam Dachmi, Khalid El Alj, Mohamed Jamai, Ahmed Farid Merini, Abdellah Ouardini, Hachim Tyal. During long years, a group, composed of practitioners psychiatrists and psychologists. Moroccan Psychoanalytic Association has assigned as its objective to assure the training of psychoanalysts in Morocco, promotion, and development of psychoanalysis, with respect to the professional ethics. MPA organized several psychoanalytic meetings with renowned speakers, which were open to the public, including French institutions of Rabat and Casablanca. It also held closed seminars designated for practitioners only. Creation of the MPA was preceded by the organization of inaugural days for this transmission of psychoanalysis in Morocco entitled The New Psychoanalytic Meetings in Rabat. These were public lectures and seminars for professionals. These events were organized with the support of the Cultural Service of the Embassy of France. The first psychoanalytic society in the North African country and the second in an Arab country, after Lebanon, MPA`s activity was made possible only after the 2000s. And there are several reasons for that. First of all, before that time the

---

[403]   http://www.spm-maroc.ma/, consulted on 31.04.2016

analytical practice was marginal and only a few psychoanalysts were capable of creating an institution. Secondly, psychoanalysis can exist only in a context of freedom, and the Moroccan society was not ready yet for this practice. Finally, this foundation meant great responsibility. It was not enough to proclaim the existence of an association but continue working on its consistency. It was necessary to have a platform for meetings, reflections, theories, and training. It was necessary that the time comes for the foundation to mature, which would ensure its duration. Such analysts as Guyomard, Fethi Benslama, Monique David Menard, Serge Tisseron, Pascale Hassoun and Chawki Azouri have also contributed with their support to the organization. Moustafa Safouan was rendering his helping hand, notably, in inviting certain analysts, such as, Elie Doumit, who responded favourably to the initiative. The Association has united the representatives from different schools and these practitioners interact constructively with each other. That was the main ambition. Since the day of its creation MPA has remained faithful to fulfillment and consolidation of its primary objective of psychoanalytic training of the members practitioners. In addition, regular lectures were opened to the public. Among its main speakers, there were: Patrick Guyomard, Jean Cournut, Jean- Pierre Winter, Elie Doumit, Guy Rosolato Roland Gori. Among other organized seminars and working groups there can be mentioned:

- Elie Doumit's seminar The Lacanian Spawning;
- Jalil Bennani's seminar on the theme of identification;
- Farid Merini's research group on the Matter of the Father;
- Abdellah Ouardini`s reading group The Work of Melanie Klein.

The purpose of the Moroccan Psychoanalytic Society is now to continue to expand to a greater number of practitioners.

Several NGOs also work in psychiatry and mental health, including the League for Mental Health and five patient associations.

Since many years, Institutes of Psychoanalytic Society of Paris (Instituts de la Société psychanalytique de Paris) have organized a training system, better adapted to the needs of Maghreb and Middle Eastern countries.[404] A candidate to the psychoanalytic profession should go through the personal analysis in France to organize one`s sessions of analysis several days per month. This "shuttle analysis" allows the candidate less favourable analytical conditions than the classical treatment, but it has an advantage

---

[404] Chamcham R., La psychanalyse au Maroc: questions pour demain, Casablanca : Editions La Croisée des Chemins, 2008, p.14.

---

of not forcing him/her to expatriation and separation from his/her family and culture. If training analysts evaluate positively his/her level of hearing his own unconscious, the candidate starts supervised treatment in his/her country, and writes weekly reports by fax or internet.[405]

The modern Moroccan psychoanalysts have largely contributed to the analytic research on the international level. In particular, Fethi Benslama examined what in islamicity was not taken into consideration by Freud. Also, he explores the foundation of Islam through the prism of psychoanalysis. Malek Chebel pursues the researches on the arabo-islamic imaginary, the representation of body, love, customs and seduction of Maghreb. The works connected with the exile are numerous and are not limited to the Maghreb`s authors exclusively, e.g. works of such authors as J. Hassoun, O. Douville, J. Hirt. The work, like "A Word without frontiers" (Parole sans frontières) has contributed to the prosperous debate concerning the role of migration in the psychopathologic and psychoanalytic research. The significant questions motivate the researches about Maghreb, highlighting its very particular place, its relation to the foreign languages, without excluding the issues of identification. The psychoanalytic practice has become widely popular in Morocco. And there are more and more young people who come.[406] The age gap of the patients is between 3 and 80. Children between 3-10 years are most frequently referred to a psychologist by a school. Those who go to a psychoanalyst are well-off people. That is to say, a minority capable of paying the honorarium of session. According to Jalil Bennani, "this is a choice, based on personal motivation...". Jalil Bennani describes the tradition of the Moroccan society, where magico-religious beliefs are still present, as follows: "The North African originality lies in the coexistence of orthodox Islam and brotherly Sufism. They should not be opposed to the modernity, however, it should be seen what crossing points lead from one practice to another, which often support the desire to "try anything to heal", like some say, from dissatisfaction left by a previous practice". "...The sadness felt in certain moments when the tradition seems to have lost its vocation to be a sign, an announcement of the renewal in the style of life, announcement of cultural richness in the diversity..."[407] Psychoanalysis, through a growing demand, which is addressed to it, is a witness of the evolution of the Moroccan society. The introduction and transmission of psychoanalysis in Morocco is undeniably linked to the

---

[405]   *Ibid*

[406]   http://www.lopinion.ma/def.asp?codelangue=23&id_info=31129, consulted on 01.05.2016

[407]   *Ibid*

171

broadening of the scope of individual freedoms and tolerance of society that agrees to open up and let coexist a plurality of speech.

Mental Health Legislation "Dahir" 1-58-295 relating to the prevention of mental illnesses and protection of the patients is the latest mental health legislation. Though it is old, its articles are well formulated and were examined by WHO experts in 1998.[408] The main aim is to guarantee the proper care of the mental health establishments in treatment of the sick while protecting their rights and their property during their period of hospitalization. The Law also achieved the following: created the Central Service for Mental Health and Degenerative Diseases and the Mental Health Committee, organized mental institutions and other psychiatric services, specified different manners of patient admission and discharge, and outlined the modalities of protection of patients and their personal property.[409]

A national survey of the prevalence of mental disorders, completed in 2003 but only made public in 2007, represented a watershed for psychiatry in Morocco: 48.9% of a sample of 5600 persons representative of the general population were found to have a mental disorder, and 26.5% of respondents were depressed.[410] According to the Moroccan news website Le Matin approximately 40% of the population at the age of 15 and older suffer, or have suffered, from at least one mental disorder.[411] A WHO assisted study on the prevalence of mental disorders has been, which was conducted on representative samples (n=6000) from many regions of the country using the Mini International Neuropsychiatry Interview (MINI). Data is regularly collected from public psychiatric institutions.[412] The patients admitted in mental hospitals are primarily diagnosed with schizophrenia (70%) and affective disorders (12%).[413] Around 2% of patients spend more

---

[408] http://psychologyinafrica.com/profiles/2013/6/23/morocco-mental-health-profile, consulted on 01.05.2016

[409] http://arabpsynet.com/Archives/OP/TopicJ20NumanGharaibeh2.pdf, consulted on 01.05.2016

[410] http://www.ncbi.nlm.nih.gov/pubmed/18225431, consulted on 01.05.2016

[411] http://www.moroccoworldnews.com/2014/07/133886/health-morocco-struggles-to-cope-with-mental-illnesses, consulted on 01.07.2016

[412] http://psychologyinafrica.com/profiles/2013/6/23/morocco-mental-health-profile, consulted on 01.05.2016

[413] http://www.who.int/mental_health/evidence/morocco_who_aims_report.pdf, consulted on 01.05.2016

than 10 years in mental hospitals, whereas 70% spend less than one year.[414] In 2002 among outpatients (n=1 504 508), 34% had schizophrenia, 25.1% had mood disorders, 16.7% had neuroses and 1.8% had alcohol and drug use disorders.[415] Among inpatients (n=15 398) 65.2% had schizophrenia, 11.9% had mood disorders, 2.5% had neuroses and 5.1% had alcohol and drug use disorders (Ministry of Health, 2004). Over 20% of patients were physically restrained or secluded within the last year in both community-based psychiatric inpatient units and in mental hospitals.[416] An estimated 70% of the total admissions to mental hospitals or to community-based inpatient care facilities are involuntary.[417] 18 patients in the community-based inpatient units and 23 patients in the mental hospitals were charged for committing crimes and subsequently judged irresponsible for reason of mental illness in the past year.[418] Following inpatient treatment, these patients will undergo obligatory outpatient care as well. Only the physician can decide the time of discharge and, in case of disagreement between the physician and authorities, the case is assessed by the national commission of mental health (per Dahir 1959).

The national health system is organized in three main sectors:

I). The public sector including the Royal Armed Forces Health Service and the Ministry of Public Health. The public sector aims to implement health prevention, promotion, and treatment and rehabilitation through four networks. The primary health care network consists of:

1. the rural dispensary;
2. the community health centre;
3. the local hospital, and
4. the urban health centre.

The hospital network comprises general hospitals and specialized hospitals and is organized on three intervention levels: 1. Public health

---

[414] http://www.who.int/mental_health/evidence/morocco_who_aims_report.
pdf, consulted on 01.05.2016

[415] *Ibid*

[416] WHO-AIMS Report on Mental Health System in Morocco, 2006, p. 11,consulted on 01.05.2016

[417] http://www.who.int/mental_health/evidence/morocco_who_aims_report.
pdf, consulted on 01.05.2016

[418] *Ibid*

---

polyclinics and provincial hospitals; 2. Regional hospitals, and 3. Academic hospitals.

The rehabilitation network is in development in Morocco and presently consists of projects implemented by both government and non-governmental organizations.

II). Private sector (profit-making): composed of private clinics (cabinets) and private hospitals.

III). Private, non-profit sector represented by national fund of social security institutions and mutual fund institutions.

There are 74 outpatient mental health facilities in Morocco, of which 5% are for children and adolescents only[419] (see Table 8.18).

Recently two Psychiatric University Centres were established in Marrakesh and in Fes. There are 2,510 primary health care institutions (1,863 in rural areas and 648 in urban areas), corresponding to one establishment per 1,109 inhabitants (2004 statistics)[420]. Mental health and psychiatry are dealt with jointly by the university, public, private, and military sectors. These facilities treat 150,458 users (503 per 100,000 population)[421]. Of all users of mental health outpatient facilities, 46% are female.[422] The average number of contacts for users treated through outpatient facilities is 1.73.[423] None of outpatient facilities provide follow-up care in the community or mobile mental health teams. In terms of available treatments, the percentage of patients in outpatient facilities last year received one or more psychosocial interventions is unknown. All outpatient facilities have at least one psychotropic medicine of each therapeutic class (anti-psychotic, antidepressant, mood stabilizer, anxiolytic, and antiepileptic) available in the facility or at a near-by pharmacy all year long.[424] While there are no official day treatment facilities in Morocco, there are a number of NGO-run day centres for youth aged 17 and younger with mental retardation and their families.

[419] WHO-AIMS Report on Mental Health System in Morocco, 2006, p.10.

[420] http://www.who.int/mental_health/evidence/morocco_who_aims_report.pdf, consulted on 01.05.2016

[421] *Ibid*

[422] *Ibid*

[423] *Ibid*

[424] WHO-AIMS Report on Mental Health System in Morocco, 2006, p. 10.

Table 8.18 Availability of Mental Health Facilities[425]

	Total number of facilities/ beds	Rate per 100,000 population	Number of facilities/ beds reserved for children and adolescents only	Rate per 100,000 population
Mental health outpatient Facilities	80	0.25	UN	UN
Day treatment facilities	1	0.003	1	0.003
Psychiatric beds in general hospitals	773	2.39	UN	UN
Community residential facilities	UN	UN	UN	UN
Beds/places in community residential facilities	UN	UN	UN	UN
Mental hospitals	10	0.03	UN	UN
Beds in mental hospitals	1461	4.51	UN	UN

There are 9 mental hospitals in the country and a total of 1147 beds (3.84 per 100,000 population).[426] All of these facilities are organizationally integrated with mental health outpatient facilities. There are no beds in mental hospitals reserved for children and adolescents only. The number of beds has decreased by 11% in the last five years.[427] These facilities treat

---

[425] http://www.who.int/mental_health/evidence/morocco_who_aims_report. pdf, consulted on 01.05.2016

[426] WHO-AIMS Report on Mental Health System in Morocco, 2006, p. 11.

[427] http://www.who.int/mental_health/evidence/who_aims_report_final.pdf, consulted on 01.05.2016

9523 users (31.86 per 100,000).[428] 18% of patients are female.[429] Patients average an estimated 26 days per hospitalization. Few patients (less than 20%) in mental hospitals received one or more psychosocial interventions in the past year. All mental hospitals had at least one psychotropic medicine of each therapeutic class (antipsychotic, antidepressant, mood stabilizer, anxiolytic, and antiepileptic) available in the facility.[430] All mental hospitals, community-based psychiatric inpatient units and community residential facilities benefit from at least one yearly review/inspection of human rights protection of patients.[431] In terms of training, 11% of mental hospital staff and 7% of inpatient psychiatric units staff have had at least one day training, meeting, or other type of working session on human rights in the year of assessment.[432]

The total number of human resources working in mental health facilities or private practice is 1,464 (4.9 per 100,000 population).[433] The breakdown according to profession is as follows: 0.4 psychiatrists per 100,000 population, 0.03 psychologists, 0.007 social workers,[434] 10 occupational therapists (0.01 per 100,000 population), and 238 other health and mental health workers including auxiliary staff, non-doctor/non-physician primary health care workers, health assistants, medical assistants, professional and paraprofessional psychosocial counsellors (0.80 per 100,000 population[435] (see Table 8.19.) Despite significant progress in the last twenty years, there are still no more than 350 psychiatrists in Morocco (thirty years ago there were fewer than ten...), plus about 60 clinical psychologists, about 400 nurses specializing in psychiatry, and social workers.[436] There are about 1900 psychiatric beds in both specialized

---

[428] *Ibid*

[429] *Ibid*

[430] WHO-AIMS Report on Mental Health System in Morocco, 2006, p. 11.

[431] WHO-AIMS Report on Mental Health System in Morocco, 2006, p. 9.

[432] http://www.who.int/mental_health/evidence/who_aims_report_final.pdf, consulted on 01.05.2016

[433] *Ibid*

[434] http://psychologyinafrica.com/profiles/2013/6/23/morocco-mental-health-profile, consulted on 01.05.2016

[435] http://www.who.int/mental_health/evidence/morocco_who_aims_report.pdf, consulted on 01.05.2016

[436] http://wwww.humanityinaction.org ww.ncbi.nlm.nih.gov/pubmed/18225431, consulted on 01.05.2016

hospitals[437] and general hospital psychiatry units located in the main cities. In the teaching sector, there are currently four university psychiatry departments, with a total of five full professors, six associate professors, and five assistant professors. The number of professionals graduated in 2005 in academic and educational institutions is as follows: 663 medical doctors (2.22 per 100,000 population), 1,600 nurses (5.35 per 100,000 population), four psychiatrists (0.013 per 100,000 population), 10 psychologists with at least 1 year training in mental health care (0.03 per 100,000 population), 120 nurses with at least one year training in mental health care (0.40 per 100,000 population), and 12 social workers with at least one year training in mental health care (0.04 per 100,000 population).[438] Few (<20%) psychiatrists emigrate from the country within five years of the completion of their training.[439] The proportion of health care expenditures by the government health department directed towards mental health is 4%.[440] About half (49%) of mental health expenditures is for mental hospitals.[441] In terms of affordability of mental health services, 30% of the population has free access to essential psychotropic medicines.[442]

For those who have to pay for their medicines out of pocket, the cost of antipsychotic medication is 1.35 dollars per day, and the cost of antidepressant medication is 1.8 dollars per day, both costing roughly 2% of the daily minimum wage.[443] Only severe mental disorders are covered in social insurance schemes.[444] Information on expenditures for medicines for mental and behavioral disorders at the country level is unavailable.

---

[437] http://www.ifre.fr/c/2025, consulted on 01.07.2016

[438] WHO-AIMS Report on Mental Health System in Morocco, 2006, p. 19.

[439] http://www.who.int/mental_health/evidence/morocco_who_aims_report. pdf, consulted on 01.05.2016

[440] *Ibid*

[441] *Ibid*

[442] *Ibid*

[443] *Ibid*

[444] *Ibid*

Table 8.19 Workforce and Training[445]

	Health professionals working in the mental health sector Rate per 100,000	Training of health professions in educational institutions Rate per 100,000
Psychiatrists	0.9	0.1
Medical doctors, not specialized in psychiatry	0.01	4.45
Nurses	2.33	1.24
Psychologists	0.04	0.0
Social workers	0.01	0.0
Occupational therapists	UN	0.0
Other health workers	0.61	NA

In terms of research, there are few publications from Morocco each year on mental health. As identified on PubMed, a total of 733 health publications were produced in the country in the period 2000-2005, among which only 9 publications were on the subject of mental health.[446] Nonetheless, a majority of the psychiatrists working in mental health services in Morocco have been involved in mental health research as an investigator or coinvestigator in the last five years. Whereas, it is estimated that approximately 51-80% of nurses working in mental health services and some (21-50%) psychologists and social workers in mental health services have participated in mental health research as an investigator or co-investigator in the last five years.[447] In the last five years, mental health research in Morocco has focused on the following topics: epidemiological studies in community and clinical samples, non-epidemiological clinical/ questionnaires assessments of mental disorders, biology and genetics, services research, policy, programmes, financing/economics, psychosocial interventions/psychotherapeutic interventions and pharmacological, surgical, and electroconvulsive interventions.

---

[445] http://www.who.int/mental_health/evidence/morocco_who_aims_report. pdf, consulted on 01.05.2016

[446] WHO-AIMS Report on Mental Health System in Morocco, 2006, p. 22.

[447] http://www.who.int/mental_health/evidence/morocco_who_aims_report. pdf, consulted on 01.05.2016

The strength of the mental health system in Morocco is in:

- Availability of mental health policy;
- Availability of legislation, which covers some areas of the mental health domain;
- Accessibility of university education in mental health;
- Qualified human resources, even though, limited;
- Conduct of regular public mental health awareness programs.

The weakness is in:

- Publishing of only a few articles each year on mental health;
- Insufficiency of qualified psychological staff.

Morocco is among a few Arabic countries, where psychoanalysis took root and influenced the clinical treatment. This became possible owing to the democratic progress of the country, Moroccan openness to the world, and its tolerance towards the Western trends. Psychoanalytic debates, particularly in Morocco, have united together philosophers, sociologists, anthropologists, and theologians. Thus, creating a space for discussing new ways for the progress of modernity while respecting the traditional values. Moroccan society, which lives in between the radical contrasts: traditional healers, from one side, and modernized hospitals, from the other, has not found yet a satisfactory compromise in approaching the mental health care.

TUNISIA

Psychoanalysis reached Tunisia much later than its neighbouring country. In 2000 Khedija Besbes introduced a teaching course entitled Knowledge of Child Psychoanalysis. Whilst Ben Rajeb began to organize, under the umbrella of URPC, annual international conferences. The themes varied from ethics in psychoanalysis, fate, debt, imaginary to ritual, belief, fatherhood etc. The foreign analysts were often participating in the lectures. Rajeb managed to unite together psychologists and psychiatrists from public and private, academic and non-academic spheres around the psychoanalytic training. Other seminars, organized in the period from 2001 until 2004 by a child psychiatrist and psychoanalyst Patrick Delaroche, were held under the umbrella of URPC and, therefore, the University of Tunis. During the three-year-period, there were organized around 24 training sessions, including 15 conferences. The sessions started on the 1st of November 2001 initially in the premises of the foundation

Beit al-Hikma. Its president, Professor Abdelwahab Bouhdiba, was ensuring the closed format of the meetings, in particular, presentation of clinical cases, viewing of videotapes, psychodrama and control sessions. This "closed" group launched with 29 people, however, the number of participants has reduced to less than ten people, notably: Riadh Ben Rejeb, Faïka Bagbag, Wided Bouhouche, Rym Ghachem, Lotfi Boughanmi, Samir Jebabli, Nébil Mrad, Olfa Emna Nsiri, Khouloud Ben Mohamed, Naïma Hammami -Youssfi, Asma Labidi, and other people, who did not attend frequently. The sessions were also dedicated to the reading of psychoanalytic texts and work on basic concepts and notions. The Faculty of Human and Social Sciences of Tunis turned into a real "laboratory" of psychoanalysis and a place of consultation. Alongside these sessions, the UPC set up a "reading group" of psychoanalytical texts. Also, psychoanalytic treatment was conducted by the analyst P. Delaroche. New experience followed in the context of the scientific partnership between the URPC and the Mediterranean Group of the Psychoanalytic Association of Paris (la Société Psychanalytique de Paris, SPP). The cooperation agreement envisaged the common scientific activities, including one annual seminar of psychoanalysis, which was launched during the university year 2008-2009 at the Faculty of Humanitarian and Social Sciences of Tunis. This seminar was conducted at a pace of one session per trimester. The session included one open to the public conference and two meetings within a closed group. The closed meetings were organized primarily for clinical work intervision of practitioners. The topic of the first meeting dealt with Masculinity-Femininity. The first session took place thanks to Myriam Boubli, President of Mediterranean Group and Jean-Claude El Bez President of PSP on Friday 12, and Saturday 13 December 2008. In August 2001 the Tunisian Association of Studies in Analytic Psychology (l'Association Tunisienne d'Études en Psychologie Analytique) was established. Its founders, Radhia Ben Mabrouk and Hachmi Dhaoui, were preparing training seminars. And numerous foreign specialists, in particular, Lidia Tarantini, were attending them.

Mental Health Legislation Law No. 92-83 of 1992 on mental health and conditions of hospitalization of individuals with mental disorders was the first law in the field of mental health. The latest legislation was enacted in 2003. A national mental health programme was formulated in 1990. The goals of the programme are to promote and protect mental health and to prevent, detect and treat mental disorders. It includes as well developing human resources, protection of users' human rights, advocacy and promotion, quality improvement and monitoring system.[448] However, it neither involved users and families nor refers to financing. It no longer addressed the issue of downsizing the mental hospital because it was already done.A substance abuse policy is also present. The policy was initially formulated in 1969. The substance abuse policy was revised in 1969 and 2000.[449] Also, a national therapeutic drug policy/essential list of drugs is present. It was formulated in 1979. The national therapeutic drug policy/essential drugs list has been re-evaluated in 1993 and in 2000.

A community epidemiological study carried out on a representative sample of 5000 adults in one region reported a life time prevalence of about 9% for major depression and 0.6% of schizophrenia[450]. Women in Tunisia don't benefit from the same protection as men and suffer from a worse clinical and social outcome[451]. Given the negative social label attached to mental disorders in women and their core role in the family, they are referred to care at a later stage and quickly discontinue treatment. Women, who are underrepresented among psychiatric inpatients, usually suffer from stigmatization of insanity, which reduces their marriage prospects. Indeed, they are far more likely than men to be divorced and separated from their children, or to be rejected by their families and to end up their life in a mental hospital.

Mental health is a part of primary health care system. Actual treatment of severe mental disorders is available at the primary level. The general practitioners diagnose severe disorders and refer patients almost systematically to the second/third level care (a second level care is only available in a few regions) for treatment and monitoring. There are community care facilities for patients with mental disorders. Some NGOs provide community based care for children under the aegis of the Social Affairs Ministry.[452]The country has specific programmes for mental health for the indigenous population, elderly and children. There are services for delinquents, abandoned children, prostitutes and patients affected by HIV. There are some facilities for children and adolescents

---

[448] WHO-AIMS Report on Mental Health System in Tunisia, 2008, p. 8.

[449] http://psychologyinafrica.com/profiles/2013/4/5/tunisia-mental-health-profile, consulted on 31.04.2016

[450] Mental Health Atlas, World Health Organization, p.469.

[451] http://www.ncbi.nlm.nih.gov/pmc/articles/PMC1489820/, consulted on 01.05.2016

[452] http://psychologyinafrica.com/profiles/2013/4/5/tunisia-mental-health-profile, consulted on 31.04.2016

in the form of day care hospitals, consultancy clinics, and medico-school centres. There is also a school health programme. There is one mental hospital available in the country for a total of approximately six beds per 100,000 population[453] (see Table 8.20.) It has regular (between two to four times by year) inspections of human rights protection of patients.[454] It is organizationally integrated with mental health outpatient facilities. Four per cent of these beds is reserved for children and adolescents only. The number of beds has not changed in the last five years, but the mental hospital was downsized by half in the past twenty years (from 1018 to 560 beds).[455] The patients admitted to the mental hospital belong primarily to the groups of schizophrenia (46%) and affective disorders (31%).[456] The number of patients treated in the institution is 46 per 100,000 population.[457] The average number of days spent in the mental hospital is 27. This figure is unrepresentative because it is skewed due to a large number of long-stay patients; with the exclusion of the long-stay patients, the figure would be around three weeks. 75% of patients spend less than one year, 8% of patients spend 1-4 years, 7% of patients spend 5-10 years, and 11% of patients spend more than 10 years in the mental hospital. About half of the patients received one or more psychosocial interventions, during their stay in the last year. The mental hospital had a broad range of all psychotropic medicines of each therapeutic class (antipsychotic, antidepressant, mood stabilizer, anxiolytic, and antiepileptic medicines) available in the facility. However, many of them are not available in the primary care settings. The rate of involuntary admissions is 14% of all admissions to community-based inpatient psychiatric units and 27% of all admissions to mental hospitals. Less than 10% (5-8%) of patients were restrained or secluded at least once within the last year both in community-based psychiatric inpatient units and in the mental hospital. There are homes for the elderly and mentally challenged individuals.[458] There are 16 public outpatient mental health facilities available in the country, of

---

[453] WHO-AIMS Report on Mental Health System in Tunisia, 2008, p. 11.

[454] WHO-AIMS Report on Mental Health System in Tunisia, 2008, p. 9.

[455] http://www.who.int/mental_health/tunisia_who_aims_report.pdf, consulted on 01.05.2016

[456] *Ibid*

[457] http://www.who.int/mental_health/tunisia_who_aims_report.pdf, consulted on 01.05.2016

[458] http://psychologyinafrica.com/profiles/2013/4/5/tunisia-mental-health-profile, consulted on 31.04.2016

which 13% are for children and adolescents only.[459] These facilities treat about 1000 (995) users per 100,000 general population (only in the public sector).[460] Of all users treated in mental health outpatient facilities, 53% are estimated to be female and 8% are children or adolescents. The users treated in outpatient facilities are primarily diagnosed with schizophrenia (30%) and mood disorders (30%), followed by neurotic and somatoform disorders (25%).[461] The country does have disability benefits for persons with mental disorders. About a third of people who receive social welfare benefits do so for a mental disability.[462]

Table 8.20 Beds in Mental Health Facilities
and Other Residential Facilities[463]

Type of Facility	Percentage
Mental hospitals	46%
Community based psychiatric inpatient unit	29%
Other facilities	19%
Forensic units	6%

The total number of human resources working in mental health facilities or private practice per 100,000 population is 8.2.[464] The breakdown according to profession is as follows: 1.5 psychiatrist, 0.2 other medical doctors (not specialized in psychiatry), 3.7 nurses, 0.3 psychologists, 0.2 social workers, 0.1 occupational therapists, 2.2 health or mental health workers[465] (including

[459] http://www.who.int/mental_health/tunisia_who_aims_report.pdf, consulted on 01.05.2016

[460] *Ibid*

[461] WHO-AIMS Report on Mental Health System in Tunisia, 2008, p. 10.

[462] *Ibid*, p. 6.

[463] WHO-AIMS Report on Mental Health System in Tunisia, 2008, p. 13.

[464] *Ibid, p. 19.*

[465] Mental Health Atlas 2005, World Health Organization, p.470.

auxiliary staff, non-doctor/non-physician primary health care workers, health assistants, medical assistants, professional and paraprofessional psychosocial counsellors). As for medical doctors, we included only those who work full-time in mental health facilities, however, all of the primary care physicians also provide mental health care. The number of professionals graduated last year in academic and educational institutions per 100,000 is as follows: 2 medical doctors (not specialized in psychiatry), 0.1 psychiatrists and 3 nurses.[466] The number of psychiatrists per 100 000 population is 1.6. The number of psychologists per 100 000 population 0.6[467] (see Table 8.21.) 15% of psychiatrists emigrate to other countries (mainly France) within five years of the completion of their training.[468] Regular training of primary care professionals is carried out in the field of mental health. Though training has been provided to some primary care personnel, a system of follow-up has not been developed yet. A manual for training of physicians has been prepared. The country also suffers from a crucial shortage of mental health professionals, especially the psychosocial workers (e.g. psychologists, social workers).[469]

Table 8.21 Workforce[470]

	Health professionals working in the mental health sector Rate per 100,000
Psychiatrists	1.5
Medical doctors, not specialized in psychiatry	0.2
Nurses	3.7
Psychologists	0.3
Social workers	0.2
Occupational therapists	0.4
Other health workers	2.2

[466] WHO-AIMS Report on Mental Health System in Tunisia, 2008, p. 22.

[467] http://psychologyinafrica.com/profiles/2013/4/5/tunisia-mental-health-profile, consulted on 31.04.2016

[468] http://www.who.int/mental_health/tunisia_who_aims_report.pdf, consulted on 01.05.2016

[469] WHO-AIMS Report on Mental Health System in Tunisia, 2008, p. 6.

[470] http://www.who.int/mental_health/tunisia_who_aims_report.pdf, consulted on 01.05.2016

There are no budget allocations for mental health. Details about expenditure on mental health are not available. The primary sources of mental health financing in descending order are tax based, out of pocket expenditure by the patient or family, private insurances and social insurance. The country has disability benefits for persons with mental disorders. Mental health patients are provided financial, treatment and transportation benefits. Over 30,000 USD dollars allocated by the WHO every two years to help to implement the NMHP and the allocations provided to the mental hospital and 50,000 USD dollars from the National Budget for the Mental Health National Programme.[471] Consequently, we can only estimate that an approximate 1% of health care expenditures are devoted to mental health. Of all the expenditures spent on mental health, 50% are probably devoted to the single mental hospital which comprises more than half the country psychiatric beds.Information on expenditures for medicines for mental and behavioral disorders in Tunisia is unavailable.

The Tunisian system of mental health has got its strong and weak points. The strengths of the Tunisian mental health system are:[472]

- A strong political will to develop a comprehensive mental health system affordable to all;
- The existence of a mental health policy, plan and legislation and their periodical updating;
- A dense primary care network accessible to 90% of the population;
- Strong family involvement and support;
- The existence of mechanisms to protect the human rights of patients;
- The availability of essential medicines in all facilities;
- The ongoing process of training on mental health for primary care staff;
- The policy of sectorization (catchment areas) which allows closer mental health services to the community;
- The development of more outpatient care in place of inpatient care;
- The equal distribution of psychiatrists between public and private sectors.

---

[471] WHO-AIMS Report on Mental Health System in Tunisia, 2008, p. 8.

[472] WHO-AIMS Report on Mental Health System in Tunisia, 2008, p. 28.

And its weaknesses:[473]

- The lack of mental health services in the face of an increasing demand for care;
- The imbalance between the mental hospital and the community mental health facilities: the mental; hospital remains the main provider of inpatient and outpatient care, given the limited number of ambulatory facilities;
- The poor extent of community care;
- The absence of community residential facilities;
- Limited child and adolescent mental health services;
- The shortage of human resources, especially psychosocial workers;
- The imbalance between drug treatment and psychosocial interventions (i.e., patients have limited access to psychosocial interventions);
- The imbalanced access to care between serious and minor mental illnesses;
- The meager financing of mental health services;
- The mediocre involvement of NGO's;
- Unsatisfactory involvement of other relevant sectors;
- The lack of interaction between mental health providers and primary care staff;
- The strong social stigma attached to mental disorders and psychiatric care;
- The absence of an effective mental health information system at all levels;
- The large volume of "gray research" that is not more widely published.

Tunisia is currently undergoing the stage of historical transformations, which paroxysmal manifestation started with the immolation of Bouazizi. It was accumulating with the social dissatisfaction, which burst out in its first and primitive origins. Tunisian revolution, by causing a rupture (thus, inciting a breach in the Other), has turned the hidden content into the manifest one. The toppling over of 50 years of dictatorship embodies a passage of the Tunisian object of enjoyment of the Other into a free and desiring subject. Once a denied subject was disconnected from the "One" total and totalitarian. The anguishing emptiness, which followed in the form of depression, paranoia, phobia, as well as other symptoms, prompted

---

[473] *Ibid*

the emergence of the defense, which sometimes was searched for in a figure of God, and sometimes in one's own liberation from it.Surprisingly, this bipolarity coexisted in Tunisia long before, however, certainly, it did not dare to come out of silence. The revolution unleashed the reticence of the gay community, who are now claiming their place in the Tunisian society. They have launched a gay newspaper and radio. Also, a publication of a book A Virgin? New Sexuality of Tunisian Women has raised up the taboo topic of the surgical restoration of a hymen, and, thus, sexual contacts before marriage, which are prohibited by Islam. This work was another attempt to display the modern realities of a Tunisian woman.

MASHRIQ COUNTRIES

Psychoanalytic tradition in Mashriq region has not developed, except Lebanon and, to a lesser extent, Syria. Lebanon has been devotedly following the tradition of the French psychoanalytic thought since its independence. And it is still continuing owing to the abundant support of the French analysts coming to provide the seminars, supervision, control groups and others.

IRAQ

Iraq is a Middle Eastern country of 30 million largely Muslim population who have lived through extremely difficult conditions for many years, including physical privations, political repression, and prolonged conflict. During 1980s-2003 the country was still plunged into wars and UN sanctions were active. This period is characterized by the sharp decline in health services. Many psychiatrists fled Iraq, and all plans for mental health strategies were blocked by regime in power.[474] In 2003 (pre invasion period), in particular, a few weeks before the war in 2003, ex-regime released convicted forensic prisoners into the streets. Immediately in post-invasion time, in 2003 violence, looting, and destruction of health infrastructure were regularly taking place, which undermined health services. Al-Rashid Hospital, the 1200 bed chronic care psychiatric facility, was hit particularly hard. Many international NGOs entered the scene out of goodwill to assist with humanitarian needs. In 2004-The first Iraqi Interim Health Minister and the CPA declared mental health

---

[474] http://www.ourmediaourselves.com/archives/93pdf/Sharma_2011_Int_Iraq.pdf, consulted on 01.07.2016

a key priority area[475], and this led to specific appointments and the setting up of committees to take things forward. An Iraqi expatriate psychiatrist was appointed to the new position of National Advisor in Mental Health in February 2004. International collaboration, inauguration of a National Mental Health Council and formulation of a comprehensive National Strategy followed. By October 2004, a Mental Health Act was submitted and approved by the Cabinet. Mental health was on the map as a public health priority, although it still needed to be integrated into policy. This was a considerable achievement given the absence of overall policy in the health sector at this time. With the high turnover of Health Ministers from 2004 to 2007, significant efforts were required to keep mental health on the agenda. Implementation of the Mental Health Act stalled, and mental health policy efforts fragmented, with the challenge of convincing each new Health Minister that it was a priority.

2007 - a psychiatrist was appointed Minister of Health and there were positive indications that the mental health system would be strengthened. Reliance on external support and funding became increasingly critical for the sustainability of mental health services. There were also efforts to put specific areas of mental health on the agenda. According to Al-Obaidi, child and adolescent mental health, with an emphasis on preventive and family and school-based services, was promoted.

2009 - 2011 The Iraq Ministry of Health has put primary care as the central plank of health care provision to the population, with emphases on competence, leadership, guidelines, standards and effective referral systems. Mental health is one of the core priorities, alongside maternal care, malnutrition, and non-communicable diseases.

In 2005 Iraq passed mental health legislation focusing on the rights of consumers, patients` families, and caregivers (e.g. access to care, determination of capacity, guardianship, voluntary and involuntary hospitalizations, law enforcement, and mechanisms for implementing legislation).[476]

According to the World Health Organization, mental health disorders are the fourth leading cause of ill health in Iraqis over the age of 5 years.[477] There is little doubt that years of political and social repression, punctuated

---

[475] http://www.ourmediaourselves.com/archives/93pdf/Sharma_2011_Int_Iraq.pdf, consulted on 01.07.2016

[476] Shi L., The Nation's Health, Jones & Bartlett Publishers, 2011, p.755.

[477] http://www.doctorswithoutborders.org/news-stories/special-report/healing-iraqis-challenges-providing-mental-health-care-iraq, consulted on 01.07.2016

by wars and followed by a post-war period characterized by interrupted and insufficient basic services, have taken their toll on the Iraqi people. Few people in Iraq have remained untouched by the trauma associated with years of unrest and instability. In 2004 Al-Jawadi found that 37.4% of children had mental health disorders (10.5% PTSD, 6% enuresis, and concluded the importance of mental health education.[478] Among primary healthcare patients in Al-Nasiriyah City in 2005 prevalence rates of anxiety and depression were 8.4% and 10.2% respectively.[479] The Association of Psychologists of Iraq (API) surveyed over 1,000 children across Iraq during a four-month period and concluded that "92% of the children examined were found to have learning impediments, largely attributable to the current climate of fear and insecurity."[480] We observe that, even if PTSD remains present, other disorders are more dominant, in particular, specific phobias and major depressive disorders.[481] The diagnoses of admissions to community-based psychiatric inpatient units were primarily from the following two diagnostic groups: schizophrenia (69%) and other diagnosis, such as epilepsy, organic mental disorders (15%).[482]

In Iraq has a dual system of work: the health staff is allowed to work in the national services in the morning and in private practice in the evening, 2% of psychiatrists work only for government administered mental health facilities, 5% work only private, and while 92% work for both the sectors.[483] Mental health services in Iraq have historically been highly centralized in urban areas and hospital based, with 1 psychiatrist per 300,000 before 2003 falling to 1 per million until recently.[484] General primary health care services are relatively sparsely distributed, with 1 primary care centre

---

[478] Al -Jawadi A., Prevalence of childhood and early adolescent mental disorders among children attending primary health care centres in Mosul, Iraq: a cross-sectional study, BMC Public Health, 2007,№ 7, p.274.

[479] Sharma S., et al., Mental Health Policy in Iraq since 2003, a Post-Invasion Analysis, p. 3.

[480] Ibid, p. 4.

[481] http://applications.emro.who.int/dsaf/EMRPUB_2009_EN_1367.pdf, consulted on 01.05.2016

[482] Mental Health System, WHO AIMS Report, 2006, p.11.

[483] Ibid, p.16.

[484] World Health Organisation. AIMS Country Report on Iraq, WR Iraq. Iraq; 2007

(40 healthcare workers including 4 general practitioners) to 35,000 population[485] (see Table 8.22.)

A mental health programme in northern Iraq emphasized the need to meet the needs of those affected by the Anfal, particularly women, also through community and decentralized facilities (WHO-EMRO 2009).[486] In 2009 Doctors Without Borders/Médecins Sans Frontières (MSF), in collaboration with the Iraqi Ministry of Health (IMoH), launched a program aimed at opening up access to psychological counseling, and at catalyzing the integration of mental health care as a crucial component of the Iraqi health system. The project focused on nonpharmaceutical approaches to address the anxiety and depressive disorders, which research shows are the most common of the mental health disorders experienced by the Iraqi population, and which are considered highly amenable to psychological counseling approaches.

Table 8.22 Beds in Mental Health Facilities
and Other Residential Facilities[487]

Type of facility	Percentage
Mental hospitals	74%
Forensic unit	13%
Other residential facilities	7%
Inpatient units	6%

Over the past four years, MSF and the IMoH have introduced psychological counseling services in two hospitals in Baghdad and one

---

[485]   http://www.ncbi.nlm.nih.gov/pmc/articles/PMC2964529, consulted on 01.05.2016

[486]   Sharma S., et al., Mental Health Policy in Iraq since 2003, a Post-Invasion Analysis, p. 10.

[487]   Mental Health System, WHO AIMS Report, 2006, p.12.

in Fallujah.[488] In Iraq, an estimated 18.6% of the population suffers from mental illness, that is 5.9 million people.[489] Al-Rashad Hospital, on the outskirts of Baghdad, houses 1,300 patients suffering from different types of psychological illnesses, mainly schizophrenia and depression.[490] The hospital is dealing with a lack of medical cadres, with only 11 doctors, as noted by the media manager of Baghdad's Rusafa Health Department, Qassem Abdel Hadi Dayekh. Despite the growing numbers of psychological illnesses in Iraq, there are only three psychiatric hospitals, Al-Rashad and Ibn Rushd in Baghdad, and Suz Hospital in Sulaimaniyah, according to Dayekh.[491] The International Red Cross restored services in Al-Rashad Hospital, which was looted and damaged following the invasion.[492] In 2006 there were working 16 psychologists (5% of mental health force) in mental health facilities in Iraq in contrast to 47 psychologists in 2010.[493] The distribution of workforce in the mental health sector can be consulted at the Table 8.23. The first mental health budget was for 2.5 million US dollars, or 0.32% of the total health budget drawn up by the CPA.[494] Funds were put into mental health training, psychiatric units in hospitals, and site visits. After 2003 health services were theoretically free at the point of use, as user fees were eliminated in line with the Coalition Provisional Authority's (Cpas) initial policy of free care.[495] However, in the absence of other income generating measures or increased budgets, this reduced the flexible income available to support salaries and for local purchasing, and user fees were informally reintroduced. In accordance to WHO`s data, by 2004 nearly half of total health expenditure came from out-of pocket expenditure, and there was no social insurance.

---

[488] http://www.doctorswithoutborders.org/news-stories/special-report/healing-iraqis-challenges-providing-mental-health-care-iraq, consulted on 01.05.2016

[489] http://www.epic-usa.org/mental-illness, consulted on 01.05.2016

[490] http://www.al-monitor.com/pulse/originals/2014/05/iraq-increase-mental-illnesses-social-stigma.html#ixzz42aJVwv7B, consulted on 01.05.2016

[491] http://www.al-monitor.com/pulse/originals/2014/05/iraq-increase-mental-illnesses-social-stigma.html#ixzz42aJrLU6R, consulted on 01.05.2016

[492] Sharma S., et al., Mental Health Policy in Iraq since 2003, a Post-Invasion Analysis, p. 11.

[493] *Ibid, p. 8.*

[494] *Ibid, p. 10.*

[495] *Ibid, p. 5.*

Table 8.23 Workforce[496]

	Health professionals working in the mental health sector Rate per 100,000
Psychiatrists	0.3
Medical doctors, not specialized in psychiatry	0.02
Nurses	0.5
Psychologists	0.06
Social workers	0.09
Other health workers	0.47

The sources of Ministry of Health state that post-2003 medications were also theoretically free when available and supplied through the national health system by two state-run pharmaceutical companies: Kimadia and Samara Drug Industries. However, they were frequently unavailable and illegally diverted from the public to the private sector and the black market. Equipment was also in short supply or outdated: some ECT machines were over 20 years old.[497] Information on expenditures for medicines for mental and behavioral disorders at the country level is unavailable.

The strengths of the Iraqi mental system are as follows:

- Available mental health policy;
- Public education and awareness campaigns are regularly conducted by governmental agencies;

Its weaknesses:

- No sufficient training for psychologists;

---

[496] http://applications.emro.who.int/dsaf/EMRPUB_2009_EN_1367.pdf, consulted on 01.05.2016

[497] Sharma S., et al., Mental Health Policy in Iraq since 2003, a Post-Invasion Analysis, p. 5.

- Not enough support for researches in psychology domain;
- No sufficient equipment and psychiatric medicine.

Despite the destructing war, which the country was going through from 2003 until 2011, the mental health sector is actively functioning. The mental health domain receives active governmental support in terms of reformation, promotion and funding. Besides that, more and more psychiatrists and psychologists are graduating every year in Iraq, which enables the local mental care sector with quality staff.

JORDAN

In 2008 WHO partnered with Jordan's Ministry of Health and the Jordanian Nursing Council, under the Royal Patronage and support of HRH Princess Muna Al Hussein, on a reform of the mental health system, based on evidence and best practices.[498] The first national mental health policy was supported by a large number of stakeholders, including the National Steering Committee, which elaborated its implementation plan. In April 2014 the 2nd Regional meeting took place in Amman, Jordan regarding launch of the clinical field studies under auspices of WHO.

The Mental Health Law makes part of the Public Health Act No. 54 from 2002. The Chapter 4 article 15 of this law permits the designation of a section (a ward) in a general hospital for the treatment of persons with mental illness or addiction provided that there is at least one psychiatrist on staff to direct the unit.[499] Article 16 stipulates that patients may be admitted voluntarily or involuntarily. The involuntary admission may take place exclusively in the following circumstances:

1. If the condition of the person with mental illness or addiction requires a treatment that can only be administered in a hospital setting.
2. If the person with mental illness or addiction is causing destruction to property.
3. If a court issues an order for involuntary treatment based on a psychiatric opinion.

---

[498] http://www.emro.who.int/jor/jordan-news/mental-health-in-jordan.html, consulted on 01.05.2016

[499] http://arabpsynet.com/Archives/OP/TopicJ20NumanGharaibeh2.pdf, consulted on 01.05.2016

Article 17 gives the Minister of Health the discretion to refer the person who was involuntarily committed to a committee of specialists in the field to ensure that the person, in fact, meets the criteria for involuntary admission (and if not, for the person to be discharged or not admitted) except for point 4 in article 16 (Risk of serious harm to self or another).[500]

One study suggested a prevalence of depression of greater than 30% in 493 randomly selected participants.[501] At CMH hospital 70% of patients with acute admissions are males. The diagnostic distribution is as follows: organic mental disorders (2.9 %), substance use disorders (1.4 %), psychotic disorders (74 %), mood disorders (20 %) and others (1.4%). The stay in chronic wards is as follows: more than 10 years (10 %), 5-10 years (7 %), 1-4 years (5 %), and less than one year (78 %).[502]

Jordan has one of the most modern healthcare infrastructures in the Middle East.[503] Jordan's health system comprise three major sectors: public, private and donor (see Table 8.24.) The public sector works on two major public programs, which are totally administered by the Ministry of Health (MOH) and Royal Medical Services (RMS). The smaller public programs are organized on the basis of the universities, such as: Jordan University Hospital (JUH) in Amman and King Abdullah Hospital (KAH) in Irbid. The private sector, which is currently a leader in offering services in the mental health field, includes 60 hospitals and many private clinics. Over 1.6 million Palestinian refugees in Jordan get access to primary care through the United Nations Relief Works Agency (UNRWA).[504] Whilst the MOH is the major institution sponsor and provider of health care services in Jordan, each of the health care sub-sectors receives financing from extra sources. Ministry of Health is the main and only responsible institution for the health matters of the Kingdom, including:

a) Maintainance of public health by offering preventive, treatment and health control services.

---

[500] *Ibid*

[501] Laeth S.et al., Barriers to the Diagnosis and Treatment of Depression in Jordan. A Nationwide Qualitative Study, Journal of the American Board of family Medicine, March 1, 2005 vol. 18 no. 2, pp.125-131.

[502] http://www.hcst.gov.jo/userfiles/file/Health.pdf, consulted on 01.05.2016

[503] *Ibid*

[504] http://icai.independent.gov.uk/wp-content/uploads/ICAI-UNRWA-report-FINAL-110913.pdf, consulted on 01.05.2016

---

b) Organization and supervision of health services offered by the public and private sectors.

c) Provision of health insurance for the public within available means.

d) Establishment and control over the management of health educational and training institutes and centers according to relevant provisions of the legislations enacted. The MOH provides primary, secondary and tertiary health care services. Primary Health Care services are mainly delivered through an extensive primary health care network. MOH owns and operates 30 hospitals in 11 governorates, with 4333 hospital beds accounting for 38.7 percent of total hospital beds in Jordan.[505] There is one community residential facility for long stay homeless patients (MOH) with a capacity of 150 beds (0.37 per 100 000 population) and over 93% of the residents suffer from chronic psychotic disorders mainly schizophrenia and the vast majority are on antipsychotic medications with no psychosocial interventions. In addition to its general public health functions[506], the MOH has a dual financing function. First, it is responsible for administering the Civil Health Insurance Plan (CHIP) which covers civil servants and their dependents. Individual certified as poor, the disabled, children below the age of six years, and blood donors are also formally covered under the CHIP, which covers about 34 percent of the population. There are 64 outpatient mental health facilities available in the country including the private sector, of which one is for children and adolescents only.[507] In 2010 In Irbid of about 1 million population, 700 people were seen in one week at the outpatient facilities including the main psychiatric clinics in Princess Besma Hospital (MOH), Prince Rashid Hospital (RMS), King Abdullah University hospital, Al Ramtha Clinic (MOH) and three private clinics (303 users per 100,000 general population).[508] Of all users treated in mental health outpatient facilities, 39% were females and 2.6% were children or adolescents (below the age of 16 years). A national

---

[505] http://apps.who.int/medicinedocs/documents/s17239e/s17239e.pdf, consulted on 01.05.2016

[506] http://www.hcst.gov.jo/userfiles/file/Health.pdf, consulted on 01.05.2016

[507] National ReportonMental Health System and Services in Jordan. The Higher Council for Science and Technology, 2010, p. 28.

[508] http://www.hcst.gov.jo/userfiles/file/Health.pdf, consulted on 01.05.2016

mental health authority (MOH) exists which provides advice to the government on mental health policies and legislation.[509] This authority was expected to be endorsed by the Minister of Health in 2009 to coordinate all aspects of mental health with other health sectors including the private one.

Table 8.24 Availability of Mental Health Facilities[510]

Name	Percentage
Ministry of Health	58%
Private	28%
Royal Medical Services	11%
University	3%

The Royal Medical Services

The Royal Medical Services (RMS) accounts for 35% of population coverage,[511] and it mainly provides secondary and tertiary care services. It owns 11 hospitals (7 general and 4 specialist), 2131 beds, which constitutes 19% of all hospital beds in Jordan. It employs 8.4% of all practicing physicians. RMS also delivers health services to military and security personnel on the basis of the military insurance. The Military Health Insurance system currently covers 1,500,000 people of whom less than 10% are active military and police personnel.

Jordan University Hospital

Jordan University Hospital (JUH), which is affiliated with Jordan University and its medical school, has over 522 beds. It is one of the most specialized and high-tech medical centers in the public sector, along with

---

[509] National Report on Mental Health System and Services in Jordan. The Higher Council for Science and Technology, 2010, p.27.

[510] http://apps.who.int/medicinedocs/documents/s17239e/s17239e.pdf, consulted on 01.05.2016

[511] Jordan National Health Accounts, Technical Report No. 49, 2000, p.33.

King Hussein Medical Center and King Abdullah Hospital. It owns 4.7 % of the total number of hospital beds in Jordan and registered 3.4 % of the admissions in 2008. JUH has an occupancy rate of 68 % and employs 2% of physicians.

King Abdullah Hospital

King Abdullah Hospital (KAH) is affiliated with Jordan University of Science and Technology (JUST). The total bed capacity of the hospital is 650 beds and the operating (opened beds) are 504 beds. It has 4.5% of the total number of hospital beds in Jordan and fixed3.8% of the admissions in 2008. The hospital serves as a teaching hospital to the Faculty of Medicine at JUST and as a referral hospital for all public sectors in the Northern Region.

The United Nations Relief and Work Agency (UNRWA) for Palestine Refugees

The United Nations Relief and Work Agency (UNRWA) for Palestine Refugees works on the basic health programs, accessible to refugees, which make up about 600,000 of the population. The UNRWA`s programmes comprise preventive, curative, and family planning services. Currently, UNRWA controls 25 health centers and MCH centers. For in-patient services, they cooperate with MOH, RMS, and some private hospitals.

The Institute for Family Health

The Institute for Family Health (IFH) is a regional model providing comprehensive family healthcare services and training for professionals and caretakers in the fields of family healthcare, child protection, and rehabilitation for survivors of gender-based violence and torture.[512] The IFH provides integrated healthcare including medical and reproductive health services, psychological, social and legal counseling, and services for children with disabilities. IFH also leads national gender-based violence initiatives, conducts human rights awareness programs, and implements capacity building for community-based organizations and other national

---

[512] http://www.nooralhusseinfoundation.org/index.php?pager=end&task=
view&type=content&pageid=35, consulted on 01.07.2016

and international organizations.[513] IFH operates a multidisciplinary women's health and counseling center, a child development unit, and Jordan's first specialized rehabilitation center for trauma victims serving local community members and refugees from neighboring areas of conflict.[514] IFH was established in 1986 with support from Save the Children (Sweden) as a national model for primary healthcare services for mothers and children. The institute was the first health center in Jordan to provide comprehensive training for medical professionals, which initially focused on early detection and intervention for children with disabilities.Since 2002 IFH has expanded its services to address gaps in family health needs, providing comprehensive counseling services to all family members with a special focus on adolescent females and women through IFH's Women's Health Counseling Center. In response to the emerging need to address mental health issues, IFH established Jordan's first Trauma Center in 2008. The center provides specialized rehabilitation services to individuals suffering from psychological disorders, survivors of gender-based violence and torture, and other war-related trauma. IFH's Trauma Center is the first national rehabilitation center providing basic and advanced psychosocial counseling services in Jordan and focusing on behavioral and psychological disorders as well as treatment for those suffering from war-related trauma, torture, and organized violence. IFH is providing mental health and psychosocial counseling services based on internationally-recognized intervention approaches adapted within the context of the MENA region and targets vulnerable groups through individual, family, and group counseling services.[515] In what it concerns mental hospitals, there is one that belongs to the MOH with a capacity of 260 beds of which 150 beds for acute male and female patients (4.6 beds per 100 000 population).[516] And another one, Al-Rashid Mental Hospital is a private hospital with a capacity of 70 beds (1.25 per 100 000 population). The length of stay in the acute wards ranges from few days up to 3 months (average is 3 weeks). In the last couple of years Ministries of health, information, educations, WHO, Jordan Association of Psychiatrists and the Jordanian Society of Psychology have all promoted public education

---

[513] http://www.irct.org/media-and-resources/irct-news/show-news.aspx?PID= 13767&Action=1&NewsId=3923, consulted on 01.07.2016

[514] *Ibid*

[515] http://www.nooralhusseinfoundation.org/index.php?pager=end&task= view&type=content&pageid=35, consulted on 01.07.2016

[516] National Report on Mental Health System and Services in Jordan, The Higher Council for Science and Technology, 2010, p. 30.

and awareness campaigns. These campaigns have targeted the general population, children, adolescents, trauma survivors and women[517].When service users were asked if they ever wanted talking therapy during their stay in hospital, 68.1% said that they did. When service users were then asked if they had had the talking therapy in hospital, 16.8% said they did have talking therapy. There was a gap of 51.3% between those who wanted the talking therapy in hospital and those who said they had talking therapy[518]. When service users who did have talking therapy in hospital were asked if they found it helpful, 55.0% said they definitely did and 5% said they did not.[519]

There are 1.2 psychiatrists and 6.9 psychologists per 100,000 population[520] (see Table 8.25.) In terms of staffing in mental health facilities, there are 0.17 psychiatrists per bed in community-based psychiatric inpatient units, in comparison to 0.04 psychiatrists per bed in mental hospitals.[521] The distribution of human resources between urban and rural areas is unequal. The density of psychiatrists, as well as the mental health staff in or around the capital, is two times greater than the density of same staff in the entire country. Regarding the training programs of all medical doctors, 6% of the curriculum is devoted to mental health.[522]The total number of human resources working in mental health facilities (MOH, RMS, AlRashid hospital and University hospitals) per 100,000 population is 6.52.[523]The breakdown according to profession is as follows: 70 psychiatrists (1.2 per 100,000 population), two medical doctors, not specialized in psychiatry (0.04 per 100,000), 261 nurses (4.66 per 100,000), 400 psychologists registered in the country (7.14 per 100,000), but only 11 are known to provide service in the four sectors.[524]The majority (62%) of physician-based primary health care doctors make on average at least one referral per month to a mental health professional. In terms of

---

[517]   National Report on Mental Health System and Services in Jordan, The Higher Council for Science and Technology, 2010, p. 35.

[518]   *Ibid, p. 47.*

[519]   http://www.hcst.gov.jo/userfiles/file/Health.pdf, consulted on 01.07.2016

[520]   *Ibid*

[521]   *Ibid*

[522]   National ReportonMental Health System and Services in Jordan. The Higher Council for Science and Technology, 2010, p.6.

[523]   http://www.hcst.gov.jo/userfiles/file/Health.pdf, consulted on 01.07.2016

[524]   National Report on Mental Health System and Services in Jordan. The Higher Council for Science and Technology, 2010, p. 33.

professional interaction between primary health care staff and other care providers, a few (less than 30%) primary care doctors have interacted with a mental health professional at least once a month in the last year.[525]

The availability of psychotropic drugs in mental health facilities can be consulted at the Table 8.26. The WHO-AIMS Report for Jordan, 2007 showed that total health expenditure as percent of GDP is 10.6 % and what is devoted to mental health is not known.[526]

Table 8.25 Workforce[527]

Health professionals working in the mental health sector	Rate per 100,000
Psychiatrists	1,09
Medical doctors, not specialized in psychiatry	0,54
Nurses	3,95
Psychologists	0,27
Social workers	0,30
Occupational therapists	0,09

Table 8.26 Availability of Psychotropic Drugs in Mental Health Facilities[528]

Type of mental health facility	Percentage
Outpatient facilities	84%
Mental hospitals	75%

Jordan's mental health field is among the most advanced in the Arab world owing to its strong sides, which are:[529]

[525] *Ibid*

[526] *Ibid, p.14.*

[527] http://apps.who.int/medicinedocs/documents/s17239e/s17239e.pdf, consulted on 01.05.2016

[528] http://apps.who.int/medicinedocs/documents/s17239e/s17239e.pdf, consulted on 01.05.2016

[529] National Report on Mental Health System and Services in Jordan. The Higher Council for Science and Technology, 2010, p.73.

- High coverage of the urban and rural population by the mental health system;
- The predominance of outpatient care compared with inpatient care. However, this could be regarded as a lack of sufficient inpatient facilities;
- Promoting equity of access for the whole population;
- Availability of essential psychotropic medications in all facilities;
- The majority of the population have a free of charge service.

However, the weak sides, on which Jordan is purposefully working, also exist. And they as follows:

- Lack of a national program on mental health;
- Lack of an information system (central) that works well even in rural areas;
- Lack of practical mechanisms to protect the human rights of patients (e.g. legislation, review/inspection boards);
- Only a small proportion of all health resources are spent on mental health;
- Training provided to mental health and primary care staff is not enough;
- Consumers' associations are not available in the country;
- Lack of proper integration of mental health services in primary health care;
- Lack of general hospital inpatient units;
- Shortages of psychiatric nurses, psychiatric social workers, and clinical psychologists.

In Jordan the mental health system is weaker in comparison to other health sectors. Moreover, it experiences a shortage of human resources. Since a long time Jordan has shifted to a community-based approach in the mental health field, which makes its services more available to the population. Also Jordan has been selected as one of six countries in the world to implement the Mental Health Gap Action Program, which aimed to reduce the number of people, who needed psychological treatment and did not receive it. Also, Jordan is actively collaborating with WHO to fight the stigma of mental illness. Therefore, Jordan is seen as a progressive and proactive country in terms of developing and sustaining the mental health sector.

LEBANON

Lebanon has a developed history of the psychoanalytic practice. It continues to host numerous analytical conferences, seminars and workshops on the international level. Also, it is a place for various analytical associations, in particular:

The Lebanese Society of Psychoanalysis

The Lebanese Society of Psychoanalysis (La Société Libanaise de Psychanalyse). Among its main objectives LSP proclaims:[530]

- Promote psychoanalysis as the scientific practice and independent discipline in the context of the humanitarian studies.
- Train analysts and candidates to the practice of psychoanalysis, in particular: personal analysis, supervision, technical and theoretical learning;
- Ensure that members of LSP have all necessary means for the development of their training;
- Reflecting on the format of clinical psychoanalysis based on its structural, social, religious and family specificities of the Lebanese culture;
- Organize exchanges with foreign psychoanalytic societies on the issues of training, education and transmission of psychoanalysis;
- Promote meetings of psychoanalysts in Lebanon without political or religious discrimination;
- Organize and develop a profession of psychoanalyst on associative, administrative and legal bases;
- Defend practice of members of LSP legally, if necessary;
- Preserve independence of psychoanalytic practice vis-a-vis any power, and independence of LSP vis-a-vis any attempt of influence, disregarding its origin;

LSP consists uniquely of psychoanalysts-associate members; psychoanalysts-affiliated members; members practitioners; interested auditors; honorary members and benefactors[531].

---

[530] http://www.slp-web.org, consulted on 01.07.2016

[531] http://www.slp-web.org/les-membres, consulted on 01.07.2016

The Lebanese School of Psychoanalysis

Lebanese School of Psychoanalysis and Psychotherapy (Ecole libanaise de psychanalyse et psychotherapie)[532] pursues the following goals:

- Train future analysts and psychotherapists to exercise their practices and ensure the continuation of their training;
- Advance education that progressively addresses the clinical, theoretical and institutional aspects of psychoanalysis and psychotherapy;
- Open a free clinic where different analysts and psychotherapists could offer some of their time to provide their services. This center could also turn into a place of confrontation of different clinical perspectives. It could partner with international NGOs for projects in the social psychology field;
- Arrange for those psychotherapists and psychoanalysts, who wish, clinical internships in psychiatric and psychotherapeutic institutional services of the Hospital Mount Lebanon;
- Organize meetings with emphasis on clinical teaching, particularly, psychosis.

The Lebanese Association of the Development of Psychoanalysis

The Lebanese Association of the Development of Psychoanalysis (L'Association Libanaise pour le Développement de la Psychanalyse, ALDeP) was attached to the International Psychoanalytic Association (IPA) and European Association of Psychoanalysis (la Fédération Européenne de Psychanalyse, EPF) in capacity of Study Group starting from January 2010. Founded by five Lebanese psychoanalysts, members of IPA, it was officially recognized by a State on the 26th of March 2009. Its official journal starts from the 2nd April 2009. Its objectives include transmission and development of psychoanalysis as a scientific discipline and therapeutic method, in compliance with Freudian texts and his successors. The ALDEP also considers that it is not in the interest of modern psychoanalysis to stay aside from an international psychoanalytic movement that brings together associations as scientifically rich as diverse in their complementarity. The ALDeP`s members believe that staying aside from this movement would lead to a risk of isolation and impoverishment

---

[532] http://mlh.com.lb/departments/psychiatry/ecole-libanaise-de-psychanalyse-et-de-psychotherapie, consulted on 31.04.2016

of psychoanalytic discourse, which has not ceased enriching since Freud`s time. Thus, one of the main goals of opening ALDEP was joining this movement in their work on implementation of procedures for membership in the International Psychoanalytical Association (IPA), founded by Freud in 1910; this association was acknowledged for its plurality of the training models (French model, Eitingon model, and Urugayan model) highlighting theoretical and practical diversity. Since January 2010 ALDeP was attached to IPA in the capacity of Study Group. ALDeP is placed in the continuation of evolution of psychoanalytic thought of Lebanon. The main changes evolved mainly around the Lebanese Society of Psychoanalysis (the first one founded in the Arab Middle East in 1980), from which there emerged groups and associations.

Arab Regional Center for Research, Training & Policy Making in Mental Health

Arab Regional Center for Research, Training&Policy Making in Mental Health was established at the American University of Beirut in October 2010.[533] It proclaimed its main mission as development of research, training, and policymaking capacities necessary to enhance mental health academia and care in the Arab region. It works on the following tasks: establish a database of research from the region, a network of professionals to encourage collaborative work, exchange expertise, and knowledge, and support professionals in conducting research in mental health through capacity building. The organization also aims at:

- working on ICD revision process;
- provision of training in the ICD-11 changes;
- training of IRB reviews, research protocols;
- conducting field studies;
- protection of professional ethics;
- establishment of a database of regional studies;
- creation of a network of regional professionals.

The first attempt of classification of mental & behavioral disorders in Arab countries took place in a form of a regional conference in Beirut in June 2011. The event gathered over 20 professionals from 10 countries of the region, who were elaborating together the recommendations to WHO

---

[533] https://www.aub.edu.lb/fm/shbpp/ethics/Documents/Brigitte-Khoury-mental-health-research-arab-region.pdf, consulted on 01.07.2016

and its International Advisory Group for the revision of ICD-10 Mental & Behavioral Disorders based on the experience of the Arab region. The participants also agreed to enhance further collaboration. An estimated 17% of Lebanon's population suffers from mental health problems, yet almost 90% have no access to treatment[534]. 49% of the population sampled had experienced a war-related distressing event of some type and the survey was compiled before war 2006.[535]

Mental health policy is absent. Details about the mental health legislation are not available.

Lebanon has a predominantly private mental health system, which relies heavily on the private sector and NGOs to provide mental health services[536] (see Table 8.27.) International Medical Corps has been a leader in mental health programming since first arriving in Lebanon in 2006 when child-friendly spaces were established to provide war-traumatized children with a secure place to play. There are 3 dedicated mental hospitals in Lebanon. The largest inpatient psychiatric hospital has over 1200 beds providing acute and long-term care for patients of all ages with mental disorders, including psychiatric illnesses and mental retardation. The hospital is over-crowded and standards of care are suboptimal.[537] In rural areas, mental healthcare is provided by family physicians, internists or specialists, and while some physicians charge specialists fees, others may charge fees as low as LL 15 000 (10 US dollars) per visit.[538]

---

[534] http://odihpn.org/magazine/addressing-mental-health-needs-in-lebanon, consulted on 01.07.2016

[535] *Ibid*

[536] *Ibid*

[537] http://applications.emro.who.int/emhj/1506/15_6_2009_1596_1612.pdf, consulted on 01.07.2016

[538] *Ibid*

Table 8.27 Availability of Mental Health Facilities[539]

Residential facility	Number	Number of beds
Residential facilities specifically for people with substance abuse (including alcohol) problems (e.g. detoxification inpatient facilities)	5	90
Residential facilities specifically for people (of any age) with mental retardation	3	120
Residential facilities specifically for youth aged 17 years and younger with mental retardation	3	65
Residential facilities specifically for people with dementia	2	60
Residential facilities that formally are not mental health facilities but where, nevertheless, the majority of the people residing in the facilities have diagnosable mental disorders (e.g. mental retardation, substance abuse, dementia, epilepsy, psychosis)	2	15

The country ranks high in the Middle East based on the number of mental health professionals, with 60 psychiatrists and 100 clinical psychologists for every four million Lebanese, and 274 general practitioners per 100,000[540] (see Table 8.28.) Although its mental health expertise is internationally renowned, like many countries in the Arab world Lebanon does not have a national policy on mental health, and very little long-time planning is being done at the ministerial level. Budget allocations from the health sector for mental health average just 5%, lower than most European states but higher than the global average of 3,2%.[541] The cost of training a psychologist for a Bachelor's degree is estimated at a range of LL 6.15 million (4000 US dollars) in public universities to LL 94.05 million (61 000 US dollars) in private universities.[542]

---

[539] http://www.moph.gov.lb/Publications/Documents/WHO_AIMS_Lebanon2015.pdf, consulted on 31.04.2016

[540] https://internationalmedicalcorps.org/sslpage.aspx?pid=2178, consulted on 01.07.2016

[541] http://odihpn.org/magazine/addressing-mental-health-needs-in-lebanon, consulted on 01.07.2016

[542] http://applications.emro.who.int/emhj/1506/15_6_2009_1596_1612.pdf, consulted on 01.07.2016

There are no budget allocations for mental health. Details about expenditure on mental health are not available. Availability of psychotropic drugs in mental health facilities is is shown in the Table 8.29. The primary sources of mental health financing in descending order are tax based, out of pocket expenditure by the patient or family and social insurance. The Ministry of Health has contracts with the private sector and needy patients receive free treatment.[543]

The strong points of the Lebanese mental health system are:

- Existing mental health legislation;
- Available mental health policy;
- Accessible medicines at mental health facilities;
- Extensive network of mental health facilities;
- Provision of training for primary health care physicians in mental health;
- Accessibility of education in mental health field.

Its weak points refer to the following issues:

- Researches in the field of mental health are not supported on the national level;
- The number of mental health professionals working in community care is not sufficient.

Table 8.28 Workforce[544]

Mental health professionals	Health professionals working in the mental health sector Rate per 100,000
Psychiatrists	1,26
Medical doctors, not specialized in psychiatry	0,87
Nurses	3,26
Psychologists	3,42
Social workers	1,38
Occupational therapists	1,06
Other health workers	4,02

543   Mental Health Atlas 2005, World Health Organization, p.281.

544   http://www.moph.gov.lb/Publications/Documents/WHO_AIMS_ Lebanon2015.pdf, consulted on 31.04.2016

Table 8.29 Availability of Psychotropic Drugs
in Mental Health Facilities[545]

Name of mental health facility	Percentage
Mental Health Outpatient Facility	100%
Community-Based Psychiatric Inpatient Unit	100%
Mental Hospital	80%

As shown above, psychoanalysis reached Lebanon many decades ago and proved itself as an efficient treatment method in the Islamic context. Devastated by war, the Lebanese people are still reliving memories of the traumatic events. Unfortunately, the majority of them do not even have a proper access to the mental health treatment. This occurred for the main reason of financial non-affordability of the private hospital's services, which constitute 90% of the national mental health sector. Mental disorders are common in Lebanon, with a prevalence equivalent to that in Western Europe. However, the number of individuals with mental disorders who are not receiving treatment is considerably higher in Lebanon than in Western countries.[546] Lebanon has got lots of qualified mental health specialists, such as psychiatrists, clinical psychologists, psychoanalysts, social workers, psychiatric nurses and others. However, the mental health system does not receive sufficient funding and governmental support.

PALESTINE

Previously the health affairs of the population of the Palestinian Authority were fully run by the United Nations Relief and Work Agency for Palestine Refugees in the Near East (UNRWA). At present, there is also the Ministry of Health of the Palestinian Authority. Concern over the mental health of Palestinian refugees extends back for many years. In addition to the usual psychiatric morbidity, this population has been subjected to the harsh realities of refugee life and political pressures of severe proportion for decades.

Actual in-patient psychiatric services are composed of a 320-bed facility in the West Bank (established back in 1960) and a 34-bed unit in Gaza (established

---

[545] http://www.moph.gov.lb/Publications/Documents/WHO_AIMS_Lebanon2015.pdf, consulted on 31.04.2016

[546] http://www.thelancet.com/journals/lancet/article/PIIS0140-6736(06)68427-4/abstract, consulted on 01.07.2016

in 1979). The Gaza Community Mental Health Centre was founded to address a range of mental health needs of the population. It is an active centre for mental health that also advocates human rights and tries to provide for the promotion of mental health, diagnostic, treatment, and rehabilitation. Human resources for mental health in Palestine include 18 psychiatrists, 40 clinical psychologists, 17 trained social workers and 72 psychiatric nurses.[547]

Psychoanalytic Work Group for Peace in Palestine/Israel

Psychoanalytic Work Group for Peace in Palestine/Israel was formed by Nadia Ramzy, Faculty Member of the St. Louis Psychoanalytic Institute and co-editor of the International Journal of Applied Psychoanalytic Studies. In 2004, Ramzy, long interested in the psychosocial dynamics of the "intractable conflict" between Palestinians and Israeli Jews, gathered together Toronto-based Palestinian psychoanalyst George Awad, Israeli psychologist Carlo Strenger, and several Jewish American, Arab-American and Arab-Canadian psychoanalysts, to form a work group in hopes of helping North American psychoanalytic colleagues to better understand the Palestinian as well as the Israeli perspective on this conflict that is at the heart of intensifying global tensions.[548] The group gathers twice a year for weekend-long meetings and participates in discussion groups on the application of psychoanalysis to social issues and prejudice at American Psychoanalytic Association meetings. Periodic conference calls continue the work in between the meetings. The goal of the organization is to engage other psychoanalysts through public events to listen to one another and express diverse perspectives and concerns, modeling empathic speaking and listening, and motivating others to become actively engaged in social action projects designed to facilitate peace and justice in the Middle East. Among the guests there have been invited: psychiatrist Joel Kovel, Israeli filmmakers Udi Aloni, Carlo Strenger, and psychoanalyst and holocaust survivor Henri Parens. The group is composed of Muslims, Christians, and Jews of Arab and Euro-American ethnicity. By openly discussing the psycho-political micro-dynamics, they believe to be able to understand better the obstacles, which lay on the way to working for peace among the traumatized Israelis and Palestinians, the U.S and other regional powers. According to the participants, the group experience provides

---

[547] http://applications.emro.who.int/emhj/0703/emhj_2001_7_3_336_347. pdf?ua=, consulted on 01.07.2016

[548] http://www.apadivisions.org/division-39/publications/newsletters/activist/ 2011/10/peace-in-palestine.aspx, consulted on 01.07.2016

an opportunity to engage "close up and personal" with individuals who represent some of the rich diversity of the major players in the conflict.

Strong points of the mental health system in Palestine comprise:

- Existing officially approved mental health plan;
- Relatively good distribution of mental health centers;
- Technical assistance and financial support of WHO and other international NGOs.

Its weak points:

- Absence of needed mental health infrastructure;
- Financial resources distributed to the mental health sector are relatively small;
- The existing outpatient facilities do not fulfill the criteria for community mental health services.
- No sufficient training for mental health staff.

It is difficult to talk about the mental health field in Palestine, since, as such, it does not exist. The numerous international medical delegations, which render assistance in the context of the humanitarian aid, is, probably, the sole source of psychological intervention for Palestinians.

SYRIA

The psychoanalytical practice in Syria has been mainly limited to the activity of the Psychoanalytical School of Damascus.

Psychoanalytic School of Damascus

Rafah Nashed, a Syrian psychoanalyst, who received her education abroad, was at the roots of training the first generation of Syrian psychoanalysts. During the first two months, the group was working on the Freud`s texts once per week at the small hospital at the outskirts of Damascus. Later, on the demand of the participants, the training was extended, on the basis of which, in 2000 the Psychoanalytic School of Damascus was established. Three analysts from this group commenced their own active practice after. The graduates of this group used to organize meetings two times per month. The first French psychoanalyst, who accepted participation in professional exchange was Françoise Myret, who arrived from Lyon for one seminar about the children as per Françoise

Dolto.[549] During the war period in Syria Rafah Nashed was imprisoned by the governing regime. She was among 1,180 people detained for their alleged involvement in anti-government activities. On the 15th of November 2011, Dr Nashed was released.

The latest legislation concerning the organization of the admission and discharge of patients in government psychiatric hospitals was enacted in 1965. A mental health policy is present, which was initially formulated in 2001. A national mental health programme was also formulated in 2001.

Officials from the International Medical Corps, who have done extensive work with refugees in Syria and along its borders, said in an interview that was based on a nearly 6,000-person caseload sampling from Syrians, that 31% have severe emotional disorders.[550] Within this categorization, 20 % have depressive disorders like anxiety and 6% suffer from bipolar disorders.[551] Schizophrenia, at 10%, was the most common form of psychotic illness across the region.[552]

In Syria there were only two public psychiatric hospitals. One is located in a rural area outside Damascus but now operates with limited capacity because of security concerns. The second one, in Aleppo, has closed its doors. With 51 beds and about 30 consultations per day, Ibn Rushd covers only a tiny fraction of the need in Syria. Only people from the capital can reach the hospital. People in the rest of the country, especially those living in areas hardest hit areas by conflict, are practically left without mental health services.

National Centre for Mental Health (NCMH)

National Centre for Mental Health (NCMH) was set up as a result of the disastrous but inevitable rise in mental health issues amongst Syrian children, due to the conflict. The centre offers psychosocial treatment to children and their parents. Special needs section includes rehab sessions for children with syndromes such as Asperger's, autism, PTSD, and

---

[549]   Rafah N., Histoire de la psychanalyse en Syrie, Topique 1/2010 (№ 110), pp. 117-127.

[550]   http://kristof.blogs.nytimes.com/2014/08/01/syrias-mental-health-crisis/?_r=0, consulted on 01.07.2016

[551]   http://applications.emro.who.int/emhj/1506/15_6_2009_1596_1612.pdf, consulted on 01.07.2016

[552]   http://kristof.blogs.nytimes.com/2014/08/01/syrias-mental-health-crisis/?_r=0, consulted on 01.07.2016

depression. The special needs section had 700 visits in 2014.[553] Each year these numbers double. There is a separate clinic for adults where they are assessed and assigned to relevant therapy. Services for adults are also conducted outside of the clinic at medical points located in Reyhanli. The special needs service is also offered for children in schools via the outreach projects. This has already covered 3 schools, reaching over 5,000 children.[554] Teachers and volunteers are trained to deal with children with special needs. Psychologists are also trained to meet the increasing need, and in turn, can train others. NCMH also has a newly established female rehab section which helps women who have been raped and sexually abused. The research section of the NCMH conducts valuable research to assess the situation on the ground in Syria and the needs of the people.[555] Even before the conflict, mental health care was in short supply in Syria, whose 21 million people were served by only 70 psychiatrists.[556]

There are 0.5 psychiatrists per 100 000 population, and no psychologist registered.[557]

Details about expenditure and sources of financing of mental health field are not available.

The main strength of the mental health system in Syria is:

• Extended ancient tradition of treating mental illnesses;

Its weaknesses:

• The mental health infrastructure is destroyed because of war;
• The mental health professionals have fled the country.

Despite the fact that Syria was a homeplace for the first mental hospitals in the world, the current state of its mental health infrastructure suffers from total destruction. Moreover, the mental health experts had to leave the country as soon as the war erupted. There were undertaken attempts

---

[553] https://www.syriarelief.org.uk/programmes/medical-aid/national-centre-for-mental-health, consulted on 01.07.2016

[554] *Ibid*

[555] https://www.syriarelief.org.uk/programmes/medical-aid/national-centre-for-mental-health, consulted on 01.07.2016

[556] http://www.emro.who.int/syr/syria-news/mental-health-care-in-syria-another-casualty-of-war.html, consulted on 01.07.2016

[557] Mental Health 2005, World Health Organization, p.451.

to introduce the psychoanalysis in the country, however, they failed due to the politico-social conditions.

GULF COOPERATION COUNTRIES

The psychoanalysis has not been practiced in GCC until the recent years. However, even nowadays it is not largely favoured. The local graduates, having returned from their studies in the West, have brought in the clinical methods, which include psychoanalytic techniques of free associations and dream interpretation. They are becoming frequently applied alongside with other therapies.

BAHRAIN

The Kingdom of Bahrain's mental health policy was formulated in 1993 and includes the following components:[558]

1. Developing community mental health services;
2. Downsizing large mental hospitals;
3. Developing a mental health component in primary health care;
4. Human resources;
5. Involvement of users and families;
6. Advocacy and promotion;
7. Human rights protection of users;
8. Equity of access to mental health services across different groups;
9. Financing;
10. Quality improvement;
11. Monitoring systems.

The mental health plan was formulated in 1997. This plan contains the same components as the mental health policy but it also includes reforming mental hospitals to provide more comprehensive care. In addition, a budget, timeframe, and specific goals are identified. In addition, a list of essential medicines is present. These medicines include 1. Antipsychotics, 2. Anxiolytics, 3. Antidepressants, 4. Mood stabilizers and 5. Antiepileptic drugs.

The patients admitted to the mental hospitals belong primarily to the following two diagnostic groups: schizophrenia, schizotypal and delusional disorders (39%), followed by mood (affective) disorders and

---

[558] Mental Health System in Kingdom of Bahrain, 2010, p.8.

mental and behavioural disorders due to psychoactive substance use (both 20%).[559] There is one psychiatric hospital with a capacity of 289 beds.[560] The number of beds has increased by 6% in the last five years.[561] The hospital is organizationally integrated with mental health outpatient facilities. Six percent of the beds in the mental hospital are reserved for children and adolescents only. Based on admissions, the number of patients in the mental hospital is 107 per 100,000 population. The average number of days spent mental hospitals is 74.7 days.[562] The mental hospital has at least one (2-5 of each group) psychotropic medicine of each therapeutic class (anti-psychotic, antidepressant, mood stabilizer, anxiolytic and antiepileptic medicines) available in the facility. In terms of affordability of mental health services, 100% of the population has free access to essential psychotropic medicines.[563] A monthly social welfare aid (50 Bahraini dinars) through the Ministry of Social Development is given to those with disabilities, including mental retardation and autism, according to specific criteria. 43% of people who receive social welfare benefits (in the form of a disability grant) do so for a mental disability, mental retardation or autism.[564] Distribution of beds in mental health facilities can be consulted at the Table 8.30.

Table 8.30 Beds in Mental Health Facilities and Other Residential Facilities[565]

Name of mental health facility	Percentage
Mental hospitals	93%
Other residential facilities	7%
Forensic unit	0%

[559] Mental health system in Kingdom of Bahrain, 2010, p.10.

[560] http://www.moh.gov.bh/pdf/mohnewsletter/healthmatters-english.pdf, consulted on 01.07.2016

[561] http://www.who.int/mental_health/evidence/mh_aims_report_bahrain_jan_2011_en.pdf, consulted on 01.07.2016

[562] *Ibid*

[563] *Ibid*

[564] Mental health system in Kingdom of Bahrain, 2010, p.16.

[565] http://www.who.int/mental_health/evidence/mh_aims_report_bahrain_jan_2011_en.pdf, consulted on 01.07.2016

National Centre for Mental Health

Based on the Royal College of Surgeons Ireland (RCSI) 5 year training program, 7-8% of this training for undergraduate medical doctors is devoted to mental health.[566]Seven mental health clinics have been opened in the health centers and patients are referred to them according to the Table 8.31.

Table 8.31 Mental Health Clinics of Bahrain

Mental Clinic	Covered Health Center
Bank of Bahrain and Kuwait -Hidd Health Center Clinic	Bank of Bahrain and Kuwait health center. Muharraq health center. National bank of Bahrain health center-Arad. National bank of Bahrain health center-Dair. Shaikh Salman health center.
Naim Health Center Clinic	Naim health center
Shaikh Sabah Health Center Clinic	Shaikh Sabah health center. Hoora health center. Ibn Sinna health center.
Jidhafs Health Center Clinic	Jidhafs health center. Budia health center. Bilad AlQadeem health center
Isa Town Health Center Clinic	Isa Town health center. A'Ali health center Yousif Engineer health center
Hamad Town Health Center Clinic	Hamad Town health center. Mohammed Jassin Kanoo health center. Kuwait health center. Zallaq health center. Budia clinic
Ahmed Ali Kanoo Health Center Clinic	Ahmed Ali Kanoo health center Hamad Kanoo health center East Riffa health center Sitra health center Jaw Askar clinic

The clinics provide the services for all people referred by the doctors working in the primary health care centers and aged 18 years or older. Children below 18 years of age and patients with substance abuse problems

---

[566] Mental health system in Kingdom of Bahrain, 2010, p.12

are referred to the child and adolescent and al-Moayed units respectively in the psychiatric hospital. Certain diagnoses and emergency cases are referred directly to the psychiatric hospital.[567]

King Hamad University Hospital

King Hamad University Hospital`s[568] mental health department is a comprehensive center for maintenance of physical and mental health that offers full range of services in culturally diverse environment. It aims at providing inclusive services, including those in the mental health area.The mental health unit aspires to excel in providing out-patient, consultation liaison to all medical services in King Hamad Hospital. As per goals, it strives to:

- provide the high level of care with the major focus on positive outcome and patient`s satisfaction;
- provide the supportive environment to talk openly about concerns and feelings;
- offer psychometric testing to help diagnose illness;
- work with local community and network in order to offer patient all resources available through the kingdom.

The philosophy of the hospital maintains that successful treatment occurs in an environment which is safe and which meets the psychological and physical needs of patients. The staff attempts to include the patient`s family into the process of rehabilitation, believing it to be the most effective way to successful recovery. Treatment includes comprehensive assessments of the psychological, emotional, and social needs of patients who are experiencing psychosis, anxiety, depression, behavioral aberrations, organic mental symptoms, or substance abuse disorders. Psychology department provides services to individuals of all ages and may work with single individual or with groups or family. The head of the unit is a psychiatrist who provides the following services:

Psychologists liaise with physicians and other health professionals about their finding and both parties determine the treatment of the patient thereafter. The social workers of the hospital ensure the assessment of patients and families, help obtain information about patient and caregiver's psychosocial functioning

---

[567] http://www.moh.gov.bh/EN/MOHServices/Services/OurPrimaryServices/ Curative/MentalHealth.aspx, consulted on 01.07.2016

[568] http://www.amh.org.bh/our-services/psychiatry-mental-health, consulted on 01.07.2016

environment, which would aid in the development of intervention and treatment strategies and help to identify the emotional, social and environmental strength, provide education to patient and their families around issues related to adaption to patient`s diagnosis, illness, treatment and or life situation. In addition, the social worker participates in discharge planing,coordinates follow-up services for patients, makes referral and ensures that all related clinical procedures are carried out in line with hospital policies and procedures.

The Bahrain Institute for Special Education

The Bahrain Institute for Special Education BISE[569] established in 2002 and is a non-profit making organization exists to make a positive difference for individuals with special needs especially children with learning difficulties such as dyslexia and attention deficit hyperactivity disorder by disseminating current and accurate information and advice, and by providing independent, specialist consultancy, evaluation and educational services. The Bahrain Institute for Special Education is a facility, which works to advance the development and education of individuals with learning difficulties and other special needs children.[570] The Bahrain Institute for Special Education competes for the recognition of its leadership in Bahrain in the sphere of providing quality services in diagnozing and treating the individuals with special needs. The Institute publishes information and practical guides, organizes conferences and workshops, and provides advisory and consultancy services for families and professionals concerned with the care and development of individuals with special needs.[571] The institution aims to provide individuals with special needs with the skills, which will help them to live a normal life. The integration of a child with special needs into the normal life is BISE`s priority. It also updates its members and associates of relevant information pertaining to special education through its newsletter and website.

American Mission Hospital

American Mission Hospital is also in charge of providing psychiatry/ mental health services in Bahrain[572].

---

[569] http://www.bised.org/portal/english/page.php?id=1, consulted on 01.07.2016

[570] http://www.bised.org/portal/english/page.php?id=1, consulted on 01.07.2016

[571] http://www.bised.org/portal/english/page.php?id=1, consulted on 01.07.2016

[572] http://www.amh.org.bh/our-services/psychiatry-mental-health, consulted on 31.04.2016

Over 3.7% of health care expenditure by the government health department is directed towards the sole mental health hospital which is the main provider of mental health services in the Kingdom.[573] Hussein A. Gezairy, WHO Regional Director for the Eastern Mediterranean Region, said that "Bahrain is among the countries of the region that have developed national mental health programs based on integrating mental health within primary health care."[574] In practice, it has led to 1. Advanced access to mental health services and treatment of co-morbid physical conditions;

2. Improved prevention and detection of mental disorders; 3. Amelioration of financial accessibility of psychological services.

The total number of psychiatrists working in mental health facilities or private practice is 58 giving a rate of 5.6 per 100,000 population[575] (see Table 8.32.) 83% of psychiatrists work only for government administered mental health facilities, 14% work only in private practice, while 3% work for both sectors.[576]Twenty-two psychosocial staff (psychologists, social workers, and occupational therapists) work in the mental hospital.[577] Two physiotherapists also work in the mental hospital.

According to WHO`s statistics, 3.7% of health care expenditure by the government health department is directed towards the sole mental health hospital which is the main provider of mental health services in the kingdom. In terms of affordability of mental health services, 100% of the population has free access to essential psychotropic medicines.[578] A monthly social welfare aid (50 BD) through the Ministry of Social Development is given to those with disabilities, including mental retardation and autism, according to specific criteria. Over 43% of people who receive social welfare benefits (in the form of a disability grant) do so for a mental disability, mental retardation or autism.[579]

---

[573] Mental health system in Kingdom of Bahrain, 2010, p. 8
[574] http://www.albawaba.com/news/who-praises-bahrains-mental-health-program, consulted on 01.07.2016
[575] Mental health system in Kingdom of Bahrain, 2010, p. 14
[576] *Ibid*
[577] *Ibid*
[578] Mental health system in Kingdom of Bahrain, 2010, p. 14.
[579] Mental health system in Kingdom of Bahrain, 2010, p. 16.

Table 8.32 Staff Working in the Mental Health Hospitals[580]

Mental health professionals	Number
Psychiatrists	49
Medical doctors, not specialized in psychiatry	0
Nurses	199
Psychologists	22
Social workers	2

Although the exact proportion of released publications on mental health in the last five years is unknown, the researches have mainly focused on epidemiological studies in community and clinical samples, non-epidemiological clinical/questionnaire assessments of mental disorders, services research, psychosocial/psychotherapeutic interventions, in addition to pharmacological, surgical and electroconvulsive interventions. Information on expenditure on drugs in mental health facilities is unavailable.

The strengths of the mental health system in Bahrain are:

- Well-established mental health system;
- Available mental health policy and plan;
- Mental health, as a part of the primary health care strategy.

Its weaknesses are:

- Limited availability of community based mental health services;
- No Mental Health Act, nor human rights inspections of the hospital;
- Insufficient mental health professionals.

The mental health field in Bahrain receives the essential support and funding from the government, which enable the construction of the well-equipped mental hospitals and treatment centers. However, a shortage of qualified human resources still makes the mental treatment difficult to access.

---

[580] http://www.who.int/mental_health/evidence/mh_aims_report_bahrain_jan_2011_en.pdf, consulted on 01.07.2016

KUWAIT

In 1970 John Racy in an article entitled "Psychiatry in the Arab East" stated:"there is an acute need for professional staff in all categories; but if choices must be made or a list of priorities established, the order would be social workers first and foremost, nursing personnel second and psychiatrists last". It was also clear that there is a blurring of the social work role and that of the occupational therapist. In what it concerns Kuwait, there was one trained occupational therapist on the team but none in the hospital.The significant clinical areas of the hospital were: out-patients and casualty (which was open 24 hours a day), admission units, a long-stay/rehabilitation area and an addiction unit. Liaison occurred with the Kuwait Prison Service and a closed male ward served as a forensic unit. A specialised unit, the Al Reggae Centre, which had been set up after the Gulf War to treat patients suffering from post-traumatic stress disorder, was off site.

An officially approved mental health policy exists and was approved or most recently revised in 2005. Mental health is specifically mentioned in the general health policy. A mental health plan exists and was approved or most recently revised in 2010. The mental health plan components include:

- Timelines for the implementation of the mental health plan;
- Shift of services and resources from mental hospitals to community mental health facilities;
- Integration of mental health services into primary care.

Mental health legislation as such does not exist. Legal provisions concerning mental health are also covered in other laws (e.g. welfare, disability, general health legislation, etc.). A lawyer, Stephen Poitras from the WHO, who visited the country to further the course of formalising mental health legislation, disclosed: "I came to appreciate that working with unwritten rules of procedure, rather than formal legislation, does allow for flexibility in the management of the patient which has benefits for the clinician, when working with patients and their families. The family exerts considerable control over the individual family members in the Arabian culture. I was able to write a paper on this issue, comparing the practices in the UK and Kuwait". If mental health legislation is to be accomplished in Kuwait it will require the support of the public and law-givers and this will take time.In September 1997, the Islamic Organisation for Medical Science in association with WHO organized a conference in Kuwait Inter-Country Consultation on Mental Health Legislation in

Different Law Traditions including Islamic Law. The conference work was based upon the WHO Guidelines for the Promotion of Human Rights of Persons with Mental Disorders.[581]

There has been an increase in mental disease in Kuwait, primarily depression. Out of the mere four million people that populate the country, 200,000 have been diagnosed with depression. There was a major leap from 2010 to 2011 and rates increased by a whopping 40 percent.[582]The suicide rate for males is 2.5 per 100, 000 population and for females is 1.4 per 100, 000 population.[583] Based on WHO`s statistics from 2008, in Kuwait, neuropsychiatric disorders are estimated to contribute to 20.2% of the global burden of disease. Dubbed Taqabbal, the campaign, which aimed at understanding the mental illness, and elimination of the social stigma associated with it, was launched at various Kuwaiti public places in 2014. During the campaign, lectures were given to both public and private high schools and universities by specialists in the field of mental health and included the broadcasting of a documentary film regarding the pain of living with mental illness in an ignorant society. Among the speakers, there were invited: Dr Mohammad Al-Suwaidan, Dr Mariam Al-Awadhi, Dr Naif Al-Mutawa and Dr Adel Al- Zayed. The organizers also held a walkathon on the Arabian Gulf Street to raise mental health awareness among the public. Participants were taking part in the walkathon to support the cause and enjoy the workout.

During the walkathon, individuals were introduced to different mental health illnesses through various mediums.[584] The availability of mental health facilities can be checked at the Table 8.33.

---

[581] http://pb.rcpsych.org/content/24/3/111, consulted on 01.07.2016

[582] http://www.borgenmagazine.com/mental-illness-kuwait-rise/, consulted on 01.07.2016

[583] http://chartsbin.com/view/prm, consulted on 01.07.2016

[584] http://news.kuwaittimes.net/one-every-five-people-kuwait-mentally-ill/, consulted on 31.04.2016

Table 8.33 Availability of Mental Health Facilities[585]

	Total number of facilities/ beds	Rate per 100,000 population	Number of facilities/ beds reserved for children and adolescents only	Rate per 100,000 population
Mental health outpatient Facilities	25	0.82	6	0.2
Day treatment facilities	1	0.03		
Psychiatric beds in general hospitals	0	0.00	0	0.00
Community residential facilities	UN	UN	UN	UN
Beds/places in community residential facilities	UN	UN	UN	UN
Mental hospitals	1	0,03	UN	UN
Beds in mental hospitals	1000	32.78	UN	UN

There are 2,62 psychiatrists and 2,29 psychologists per 100,000 population[586](see Table 8.34.) The majority of primary health care doctors have received official in-service training on mental health within the last five years.

The first premises in which formal psychological services were delivered for psychiatric patients in Kuwait were constructed in 1940. In spite of shortage of specialized staff and inadequate medical and psychiatric provisions, the premises were considered fairly adequate for the range of available services. The special section was designated for female patients.

---

[585] http://www.who.int/mental_health/evidence/atlas/profiles/kwt_mh_profile.pdf, consulted on 01.07.2016

[586] *Ibid*

As a result of the government interest on this important aspect of health, the mental health services center was designated as the Mental & Psychological Illness Hospital. In 1959 it was renamed as it is currently known Psychological Medicine Hospital. The hospital became equipped, organized and managed in accordance with modern systems to regulate patient's admission and other activities. Services delivered by the Psychological Medicine Hospital were expanded to include the formal teaching of male and female paramedical students of the diploma schools available at the time. The first psychiatric clinic was opened at the school health department in 1965, followed by establishing psychiatric clinics in the general hospitals of the health regions. These clinics were established as subsidiaries of the Psychological Medicine Hospital, and that is the way they have been run till date. New programs were added to the package of services offered by the Hospital in accordance with the natural development undergone by the Kuwait community as well as new treatment approaches.

Table 8.34 Workforce and Training[587]

	Health professionals working in the mental health sector Rate per 100,000	Training of health professions in educational institutions Rate per 100,000
Psychiatrists	2.62	0.13
Medical doctors, not specialized in psychiatry	UN	3.28
Nurses	13.77	3.93
Psychologists	2.29	1.31
Social workers	0.66	2.29
Occupational therapists	0.13	0.66
Other health workers	UN	NA

Kuwait Psychological Medicine Hospital

Services provided by Kuwait Psychological Medicine Hospital include treatment for adults, child, adolescent, geriatric and forensic patients.[588] A separate service for addiction and substance abuse is also available. The

---

[587] http://www.who.int/mental_health/evidence/atlas/profiles/kwt_mh_profile.pdf, consulted on 01.07.2016

[588] http://www.psychiatrykuwait.com/hospitalHistory.html, consulted on 01.07.2016

psychiatric services are provided through inpatient hospital and outpatient clinics management program.The hospital also serves as a training and educational site for psychology students. The Department is extensively involved in many teaching programmes in Kuwait, among them:

- Undergraduate medical student teaching and clinical training;
- Psychology student teaching and clinical training;
- Undergraduate occupational therapy student teaching and clinical training and others.

In October 1996, an expatriate team commenced working at the Kuwait Hospital for Psychological Medicine on a three-year government contract to develop quality improvements in the mental health service in Kuwait.[589] The team comprised of administrative, medical and nursing staff, including nurse trainers and an occupational therapist and social worker. The Kuwait Hospital for Psychological Medicine, which has approximately 450 beds, serves the whole population of Kuwait, comprising 800 000 Kuwaitis and 1.2 million expatriates. Each of the five medical teams serves one of the five regions into which Kuwait is divided. The service offered was reminiscent of the mental health services in the UK before the development of the present community-style approach. There was a lack of trained nursing personnel and only 7% of the 280 nursing staff had had a formal training in psychiatric nursing. In addition, the social work staff, only numbering eight, was a serious deficiency. The monthly meeting of the Medical Council was central to the management of the medical department. It was with the agreement of the Medical Council that four committees were formed, responsible to the Council, building on the existing strengths of the department:

- the Education Committee responsible for the educational activities of the Medical Department;
- the Drugs and Therapeutics Committee dealing with all relevant matters involving this area of work;
- the Quality Assurance Standing Committee which had been already in existence with an audit Sub-Committee;
- the Research and Ethics Committee to approve protocols of research proposals and consider any ethical matters arising in the work of the hospital.

---

[589]   http://pb.rcpsych.org/content/24/3/111, consulted on 01.07.2016

Al Seef Hospital

The Psychology Department at Al Seef Hospital is the first private hospital in the State of Kuwait to offer mental health treatment services.[590] The hospital cares for providing quality mental health treatment in a safe, confidential, and therapeutic manner. The highly qualified and experienced mental health professionals collaborate with the patients to destigmatize and normalize the notion of seeking mental health treatment. The hospital specializes across a full-range of mental health treatment for children and adults. These include a wide range of mental health conditions related to mood (depression and anxiety), situational stressors and life changes (dealing with pregnancy, marriage, divorce, relational problems and medical illnesses), children and adolescent related issues (behavioral problems, attention difficulties, and mood disturbances), and body image issues (eating disorders). The mental health department also works closely with other departments within the hospital to synergise treatment and provide the patients with holistic and comprehensive care for their overall wellbeing.

The hospital offers the following psychological services:

- Psychological consultations to patients admitted to other medical services at Al Seef Hospital (including radiology, internal medicine, family medicine, surgery, obstetrics, and gynecology), who experience significant mental illness symptoms, enabling them to better understand and manage their health towards recovery. The consultation service provides a range of services, including psychological evaluation, collaboration with medical specialists, and arrangement for follow-up.
- Individual psychotherapy. The psychotherapists conduct one-on-one personalised sessions – approximately 60 minutes each - for individuals to assess and help them understand their respective behavioral problems, their medical and personal background, and identify solutions to help them improve their level of functioning and relationships.
- Group psychotherapy. The group psychoeducational sessions (approximately 60 minutes, and 3-10 patients per group) focus on specific coping strategies and topics such as anger management, frustration tolerance, social skills, and parenting. These topics are explored by all group members and solutions are solicited.

---

[590] http://www.alseef-hospital.com/our_medical/Psychology.html#, consulted on 31.04.2016

- Family therapy sessions (approximately 60 minutes) are highly effective and beneficial for a family experiencing distress, difficulties, and friction amongst familial members. Family members learn to appropriately interact with one another in order to improve the communication and overall functioning of the family as a unit.
- Couples psychotherapy and premarital counseling. This modality is not only helpful to couples who experience tension and conflict in their relationship, but it is also helpful for couples who would like to gain increased insight into one another. Premarital counseling is valuable for couples who plan to marry and would like to develop skills in order to navigate their way through marriage successfully.
- School consultations. The clinicians of Al Seef Hospital often visit children's schools to observe a patient in his/her natural academic environment. Such a service can be beneficial in order to gather information related to a child's functioning in the school setting and to consult with teaching personnel, provided there was written consent from the minor's guardians.
- Psychological testing is useful in gaining a better understanding of an individual's personality structure, psychopathology, cognitive capabilities and more. They are often used in a variety of settings to determine whether students require special education programs, in clinical settings to learn more about the mental illness present in clients, and in the workplace, to better understand employees' personalities and work styles.[591]

Al Raggae Center

Of particular note was the Al Raggae Center in 1992, which was specialized in treating the epidemic of Post Traumatic Stress Disorder (PTSD) that was consequent on the brutality of the Iraqi invasion.[592] Psychological services provided by the centre involve IQ assessment; cognitive functions assessment; memory assessment; personality assessment; psychotherapy; counseling; social work services; family therapy; group work etc. The research unit of the Centre is devoted to clarifying the roots, diagnosis and treatment of psychiatric illnesses. Rapid exchange of information between research and clinical specialties enhances immediate contributions to the

---

[591] http://www.alseef-hospital.com/our_medical/Psychology.html#, consulted on 31.04.2016

[592] http://www.psychiatrykuwait.com/hospitalHistory.html, consulted on 01.07.2016

mental health of patients and the public at large. Regarding the hospital inpatient program, there are two distinct wards; the acute wards are where all patients are initially placed usually. These wards are located in the main hospital. If the staff determines that the patient is not a danger to self or others, the individual may be moved to subacute wards. This type of ward is not as restrictive as the acute unit. These subacute wards try to make life as normal as possible for the patients and many activities are provided. Subacute wards are located in the new hospital. In most cases the patient can be back to family, in others the patient is transferred to a medium or long term environment according to the patient's level of functioning.[593]

Kuwait Centre for Mental Health

Kuwait Centre for Mental Health.[594] As a result of the government interest in the health domain, the mental health services center was designated as the Mental & Psychological Illness Hospital. In 1959 it was renamed into Psychological Medicine Hospital. The hospital became equipped, organized and managed in accordance with modern systems to regulate patient's admission and other activities. However, it also has its weaknesses, such as: infrastructure (the building is unable to accommodate the large number of patients and the increase of population); shortage of beds; shortage in staff (laboratory technologists, filling staff, specialized nurses, ward clerks, public relations, security, pharmacist, social workers, psychologists, psychiatrists); no HIS (Hospital Information System), internet access, no information technology department; shortage of isolation rooms; unstable administration; no day care facility; no community outreach service; scattered buildings; poor communication with other medical services; transfer of highly skilled medical staff to other governmental hospital, or migration; liability to assault from visitors, and patients, with no security service; legal issues and unreliable involvement of the press; no mental health act.[595]

Mubarak Hospital Mental Health[596].

The Mental Health Unit at Mubarak Al-Kabeer Hospital in Kuwait is the country's first mental health service that is based completely at a general hospital. It is based at Mubarak Al-Kabeer Hospital, Kuwait's largest

---

[593] http://www.psychiatrykuwait.com/hospitalHistory.html, consulted on 01.07.2016

[594] http://kcmh.jimdo.com/introduction/, consulted on 01.07.2016

[595] *Ibid*

[596] http://www.mkhpsych.com/about, consulted on 01.07.2016

academic hospital, which covers a catchment area of 1.2 million residents. Prior to the establishment of the unit, all publicly-funded psychiatry and mental health services in the country where based at the Kuwait Center for Mental Health – Kuwait's National Mental Health Hospital, or were satellite clinics of this central psychiatric hospital. In 2015, the Mubarak Mental Health Unit was established by a Ministerial Resolution and Dr. Mohammad Alsuwaidan was appointed as the founding head of this newly established program. The aim was to augment the clinical services provided at the Kuwait Center for Mental Health by providing additional services closer to the community and primary care levels of mental health care.Under Dr. Alsuwaidan's leadership, Mubarak Hospital Mental Health is taking an active role in medical student/resident, professional, inter-professional and community education about mental health, helping to train family doctors to provide mental health services at the primary care level and introducing advanced, cutting-edge and high-quality clinical services in psychiatry.[597]

FSRI

FSRI is registered in the U.S. as a non-profit organization and is designed to provide the highest quality care for the entire Kuwait community.[598] As the only registered non-profit mental health care provider in Kuwait, the Psychology Department at FSRI is fully committed to helping all individual and families residing in Kuwait. The Psychology Department is a full-service department and offers an incredibly broad range of services, including individual therapy for children, adolescents and adults to address a range of concerns including behavioral issues, academic difficulties, low mood, anxiety/worry, family difficulties, eating concerns and many other. The department also offers marriage/couples counseling and family counseling. The other psychological programs offer group therapy including Relationships Group, a Substance Abuse Group, a Meditation Group, and others. FSRI also has a unique program in collaboration with Yale University which enables Kuwaiti psychologists to offer telehealth medication consultations with doctors at Yale University. All clinicians are licensed or are supervised by licensed clinicians and all treatment full adheres to the Code of Ethics put forth by the American Psychological Association (APA) and the Middle East Psychological

---

[597] http://www.mkhpsych.com/about, consulted on 01.07.2016

[598] http://www.fsrikuwait.org/psychologicalServicesDept.html, consulted on 31.04.2016

Association (MEPA). The clinic also specializes in educational psychology and psychological assessments for children, adolescents, and adults. Using the latest testing instruments, the psychologists do not just identify areas of weakness but are instead focused on individuals' strengths. All assessments are also focused on interventions and determining concrete recommendations to reach the solution. The FSRI psychologists test for the following concerns:

- Intelligence and cognitive assessments (WISC-IV);
- Academic ability (WIAT-III);
- Attention and concentration difficulties (ADHD);
- Learning disabilities including reading, writing, and math disabilities;
- Developmental disabilities including Autism and Asperger's;
- Dementia and geriatric concerns;
- Specific diagnostic concerns including depression, anxiety, social anxiety, eating disorders, bipolar disorder, addictions, OCD, schizophrenia, childhood anxiety/depression, personality disorders, forgiveness, anger, and marital satisfaction and many others.

Psychology Department is headed by Dr. Nick Scull, the President and Founder of the Middle East Psychological Association, with psychologists and counselors rigorously adhering to the standards of treatment and confidentiality as defined in the American Psychological Association. Experienced and specialized medical team, mostly educated and trained in Canada.[599]

Kuwait Center for Autism

Kuwait Center for Autism was established in 1994 by Dr. Samira Al-Saad, a mother of a girl with autism[600]. The main mission of the center is to spread autism awareness and ensure an accurate educational program to children with autism for improving their educational, societal and conceptional abilities taking into consideration the individual differences and in the meantime supporting their vocational talents and the possibilities of integration with society. The Educational Training Program is presented on scientific and educational basis that suits the autistic child abilities and

---

[599] *Ibid*

[600] http://in-car.ca/linkfiles/Kuwai_Center_for_Autisim.pdf, consulted on 01.07.2016

to evaluate the child and determine the level of his/her abilities to join him/her, in the class that fits his/her age and abilities. An individual educational plan is set to assess the improvement of the student all through the year.

1. The Early Intervention Program is an intensive rehabilitation program for children from age 3 to train the basic skills such as work behavior, work skills, enhancing communication programs and behavior modification plans and helping families by designing a self-help program.

2. The Friends Club Program is an entertainment program to enable the autistic child to spend the weekend with his brothers and other children in a pleasant atmosphere of fun and entertainment and structure under the supervision of specialized persons.

3. The Summer Camp is arranged during summer holidays and so far 8 summer camps have been arranged giving the children the chance to have a mixture of entertainment, training and amusement in a structured environment. This camp is open to all students of autism and Down syndrome from different schools and establishment in and outside Kuwait.

4. The Swimming Club Program is an afternoon program setup every year during summer holiday for children with autism and special needs and their brothers and friends under the supervision of trainers. It is an essential step to join autistic children with normal and external society in such clubs teaching them many interaction and communication skills.

5. The Youth House Program aims to train youths suffering from autism and pervasive developmental disorder (PDD) concerning self-help skills, in addition to communication and social interaction through several activities and programs specially planned to achieve these goals.

6. The Occupational Program is composed for people with special needs to find a suitable job to secure a better life for them. This program began at the center by employing one young man with autism and another young lady with Down syndrome.

7. The Evaluation&Diagnosis Unitaids to fulfill the devotion of family needs, studying the main difficulties of their children with the cooperation of genetic centres for medical tests and then perform the academic and psychological evaluation. Finally, the parent gets a detailed psychological report with the needed recommendations.

8. The Consultation and Training are contributed by specialists in the field of autism invited from different countries of the world, for continuous information on the latest developments in the field of autism.

9. Widen the scope of employing adults with special needs. Assist in establishing specialized programs for children with Autism in many Gulf countries (Jeddah, Riyadh, Jubail, Bahrain, Qatar, and Sharjah) & in Arab countries (Egypt, Jordan, Lebanon).

Such efforts include training, curriculum development, educational manuals and other services. Conferences and workshops are held for families, teachers and workers in the field of autism and special needs, also all those who have relationship and interest in autism in and outside Kuwait. The 1st International Conference in the region was in 2000 & the 2nd in 2003[601]. Publication series are introduced since the establishment of the center to spread understanding and awareness of autism by composing or translating specialized books into Arabic language to overcome the clear shortage of such books (more than 50), audio or video in the Arabic library. Silent Scream Magazine (1997), the first scientific specialized magazine in the Middle East concerned in autism syndrome. It speaks for those who are suffering autism and other difficulties, as many translations, research stories, interventions and the updated information in science and researches in this field.[602] Gulf Autism Union established (2002) to bring together the professionals and institutions in the field of autism in the Gulf region which is soon to be converted to the Arab Autism Union. To maintain the ISO 9001:2000 certificate acquired (in 2005 & 2008) to ensure the quality of service provided and also to improve the efficiency & productivity of the different services provided. Autism Accreditation Status was awarded (2010) to the center by National Autistic Society-Accreditation, UK for Quality Autism Provision.[603] Medical Unit, to provide fast and professional care to the students of the center in case of accidents & emergency. Research Unit, with a Study Hall & Research Hall to continue old researches currently being done with Harvard University, Faculty of Medicine & Kuwait University & start or cooperate with more researches to identify the causes of autism. The Center has so far published many research articles in scientific journals and international conferences and will continue to do so. Training Center, to train the parents, teachers, and other workers in

---

[601] http://in-car.ca/linkfiles/Kuwai_Center_for_Autisim.pdf, consulted on 01.07.2016

[602] *Ibid*

[603] *Ibid*

this field through workshops conducted by international professionals and therapists in the autism field[604]. Autism Diploma courses for teachers and professionals were also conducted at the centre in cooperation with the University of London. Among the academic papers on autism, published in Kuwait, there are:

- "The Identification of Training and Educational Needs for Autistic Children from Parents' Perspective in Kuwait and Saudi Arabia", An Article published by Educational Journal Kuwait University No. 45 - 1997 "Special needs and the 21st century in Arab World", a research paper presented to the 7th National Conference on Autism - Cairo/1998.
- "The identification of training and educational needs for children with special needs", a research paper presented to 2nd International Congress on Rehabilitation - Dubai, UAE/1998.

The Organization has won the international prizes, including:

- Princess Haya Award for Special Education for 2011 for best practices in educating and rehabilitating special needs individuals according to international standards and distinguished quality programmes, creating a competitive and qualified environment that is capable of advancing and sustaining future services.
- Prince Salman Bin Abdul Aziz of Riyadh (Saudi Arabia) award for 2010 was awarded for establishing programs for Autism in GCC region.
- Chaillot Prize 2009 finalist awarded by the Delegation of the European Commission to organizations which promotes the rights of vulnerable groups or which promotes general awareness of human rights as an appreciation for their positive developments in the area of human rights promotion in the GCC region.
- Jan Amos Comenius Medal for 2008 awarded by the UNESCO & the Ministry of National Education, Youth and Sport of the Czech Republic to acknowledge the significant contribution to the development of education in the autism field.
- Jaber Prize for Quality Management 2008 on best establishment run by a Lady (Kuwait) with level of quality provided and recognized as a model to be followed by other organizations.

---

[604] *Ibid*

- Corporate Social Responsibility (CSR) Award Kuwait 2007 in conducting awareness campaigns in Kuwait by non-profit organizations
- Philip Morris Award 2003 for Charitable Organizations in recognition of its effort towards supporting children with autism in Kuwait to make a difference in their lives.
- U. A. M. Women Society (U.A.E.) in 2003, the prize in the field of social services.

The Kuwait Association for Learning Differences

The Kuwait Association for Learning Differences (KALD) is a social welfare association that collaboratively works towards helping students with learning differences in private schools in Kuwait. Kald was established in 2007 and is funded by Masharea Al Khair/ Kuwait Project Company. Its Board of Trustees comprises of educators, specialists and parents who volunteer to offer their time and effort to serve students with Learning Difficulties. Members of KALD has chosen "Learning Differences" instead of "Learning Difficulties" because they believe that the targeted students are intelligent people and the only difference between them and other students is that they have their own way of learning.[605]

Kuwait Dyslexia Association

Kuwait Dyslexia Association began its journey in the field of specific learning disabilities in 1999[606]. KDA organizes and provides training courses for teachers, remedial intervention programs for children, and in English and Arabic assessments. It also develops dyslexic friendly software and publishes magazines.

Social Development Office Council of Ministers

Social Development office Council of Ministers was established in response to Iraq, military invasion on (22nd of August 1990) and auspices of his Highness Sheik Jaber Al-Ahmad Al-Sabah to promote national, mental, health and welfare of the state of Kuwait and to support the

---

[605] http://www.kaldkuwait.com/Files/Others/KALD_Directory_English.pdf, consulted on 01.07.2016

[606] *Ibid*

psychological rehabilitation of society. The aim starts to move psychological and educational variables in Kuwait City[607].

Kuwait Counseling Center

Kuwait Counseling Center provides comprehensive assessments, therapy, and training services to children, adolescents, adults, couples, families, and groups to resolve special needs; interpersonal, academic, nutritional, and/or stress of life problems.[608] The Center operates under the strict code of ethics of the American Psychological Association and the American Counseling Association AND complies with the standards of privacy and confidentiality published by HIPAA. The staff consists of trained and licensed therapists. In a comfortable and supportive atmosphere, they offer a confidential and personalized approach tailored to each client individual needs.

Kaizen Centre

Kaizen is a private center that provides comprehensive human services in the form of therapy, assessments, workshops and training. The services are available to individuals, families, groups, organizations, and institutions.[609] Kaizen staffs are bilingual and comprised of licensed clinical psychologists and qualified professionals.

Fatma Clinic

Fatma Clinic was established by the well-known Dr. Fatma Al Awadhi. Dr. Fatma is a Consultant Developmental Pediatrician, and she provides medical consultation, assessments and diagnosis for children with special needs.[610] She is also licensed by several programs from around the world to provide specific cognitive trainings and programs. Individualized training programs are provided for children according to their needs. Assessments include the medical history and clinical exams, developmental assessment, assessment of intellectual ability, behavior and social interaction and other specific assessment for each child as needed.

---

[607] http://www.kaldkuwait.com/Files/Others/KALD_Directory_English.pdf, consulted on 01.07.2016

[608] *Ibid*

[609] *Ibid*

[610] *Ibid*

Al-Razi Counseling and Assessment Center

Al-Razi Counseling and Assessment Center was established by Dr. Kazem Abal in 1994 making it the oldest and most highly recommended psychology clinic in Kuwait.[611] Al-Razi Center is known for its innovative treatment programs and has become the standard of the industry in Kuwait due to its outstanding reputation for accurate diagnosis and effective treatment of the full range of psychological, emotional, social and educational disorders for children and adults. Dr. Kazem Abal, who has a doctorate in educational psychology and Dr. Vincenza Tiberia, also an educational psychologist and the first licensed clinical psychologist in Kuwait are among the most experienced staff members providing services there. Al-Razi Center is also the first psychological assessment center in Kuwait providing all types of testing services for children and adults including IQ testing, Psychoeducational Test Batteries, Neuropsychological Assessment and Personality Testing to name a few.

Al-Dana Center For Psychological Social And Educational Consultation

The center plays a pivotal role in the field of mental health and psychological counseling along with the dissemination of cultural psychological and personal development, potential of the individual and the discovery and development capabilities.[612] It also has the latest therapeutic methods for different kinds of mental disorders and to keep pace with the circumstances of the times and challenges.

Tatweer Int. Counseling, Research & Training Center

TCRC Tatweer Int. Counseling, Research & Training Center is a full-service center specialized in counseling, social and family therapy, and educational assessment & support provided for children.[613] Assessment is provided to complete the treatment for the client to get a full diagnosis of their issues. Research service is offered within the area of psychology, social, and education. The centre applies behavior analysis, behavioral counseling, evaluation, diagnosis sessions, behavioral assessment, early intervention & treatment to help to treat children and adults developmental disabilities.

---

[611] *Ibid*

[612] http://www.kaldkuwait.com/Files/Others/KALD_Directory_English.pdf, consulted on 01.07.2016

[613] *Ibid*

The Guidance Centre For Social And Psychological Consultation & Training

The Guidance Centre For Social And Psychological Consultation &Training was established in 2009 and aims to provide psychological counseling services for all social and community groups of different ages and for all psychological marital work and children's disorders.

Behavior & Family Consulting Center

Behavior & Family Consulting Center was established in 1994. The center offers consulting that helps the patients understand themselves, discover their abilities. The centre also offers consulting to help family members understand the family life, overcome the difficulties encountered, develop the skills of interaction, communication and problem-solving to achieve efficiency and stability of the family, and cope with their marital life and family relations.

In Kuwait, the total expenditure on health as a percentage of gross domestic product is 3.31% and the per capita government expenditure on health is 748.0 US dollars (WHO, 2006).[614] Information on expenditure on drugs is unavailable.

The strengths of the mental health system are as follows:

• The healthcare system is one of the best in the world;
• Availability of the mental health policy;
• Extensive network of delivering mental health care;
• Sufficient funding.

Its weaknesses comprise:

• Insufficient professional workforce.

Kuwait ranks high in depression rates, probably, hitting the highest statistics in the region. There is no legal coverage for mental health domain in Kuwait, which makes the service-providers and service-consumers more vulnerable in front of the law. Despite the constantly increasing abundancy in mental centers, the qualified mental health workers severely lack.

---

[614] http://www.who.int/mental_health/evidence/atlas/profiles/kwt_mh_ profile.pdf,consulted on 01.05.2016

OMAN

Psychiatry in Oman is generally based on the Anglo-American model. The first steps towards instituting a system in Oman of biomedical care for psychiatric patients were undertaken in the mid-1970s in a missionary hospital, Al-Rahma Hospital. An Indian psychiatrist dispensed outpatient services, which later developed into the provision of custodial care. Parallel services evolved in the late 1970s in the southern part of the country. The first specialised psychiatric hospital, Ibn Sina, was opened in 1983. At the beginning, it had two wards, one for male and the another for female patients. It also provided outpatient services. The one hospital catered for the needs of the whole population (then nearly 1.5 million). In the early 1990s, a psychiatric teaching service was initiated within the teaching hospital of Sultan Qaboos University[615].

The last revision of the mental health plan was in 2005[616] and includes the following components:

1) Developing community mental health services;
2) Developing a mental health component in primary health care;
3) Human resources;
4) Involvement of users and families;
5) Advocacy and promotion;
6) Human rights protection of users;
7) Equity of access to mental health services across different groups;
8) Financing;
9) Quality improvement;
10) Monitoring system.[617]

An officially approved mental health policy exists and was approved, or most recently revised, in 2009. Mental health is specifically mentioned in the general health policy. Other components of mental health plan include:[618]

---

[615] https://www.researchgate.net/publication/259640865_Psychiatry_in_the_Sultanate_of_Oman, consulted on 01.07.2016

[616] http://arabpsynet.com/Archives/OP/TopicJ20NumanGharaibeh2.pdf, consulted on 01.07.2016

[617] *Ibid*

[618] http://www.who.int/mental_health/evidence/atlas/profiles/omn_mh_profile.pdf, consulted on 01.05.2016

- Timelines for the implementation of the mental health plan;
- Funding allocation for the implementation of half or more of the items in the mental health plan;
- Integration of mental health services into primary care.

Dedicated mental health legislation does not exist. However, legal provisions concerning mental health are covered in other laws (e.g. welfare, disability, general health legislation etc.).

Doctors at Sultan Qaboos University (SQU) Hospital revealed in 2009 that they diagnosed 2,200 women with depression, an increase of more than 20 percent on the previous year.[619] In May 2014, a study conducted on students by the Department of Behavioural Medicine at SQU showed that 27% had depression of varying grades.[620] Another study investigating the rate of depression among secondary school students in Oman found that 17% of the respondents showed symptoms.[621] Some maladjustment indicators of youth are becoming increasingly common. Firstly, the incidence of deliberate self-harm increased from 1.9 cases per 100 000 in 1993 to 12.8 per 100 000 by 1998 among female adolescents.[622] Secondly, there has been an increase in the numbers of addicts seeking rehabilitation, drug overdoses, and drug-related deaths; there has also been a rise in drug shipments confiscated by law enforcement officers[623]. The popular mind-altering substance in Oman appears to be cannabis, although the extent of its use is hard to quantify. Finally, there is evidence that the traditional admiration of a plumpish figure is eroding, and that eating disorders are becoming increasingly common in young Omanis.[624] One study found that only 5.2% of anxiety disorder cases are actually treated.[625] Females were

---

[619] https://www.y-oman.com/2015/03/changing-minds-fighting-depression/, consulted on 01.07.2016

[620] https://www.y-oman.com/2015/03/changing-minds-fighting-depression/, consulted on 01.07.2016

[621] Afifi M., Positive health practices and depressive symptoms among high school adolescents in Oman, Singapore Med J 2006; 47(11), pp.960-967.

[622] https://www.researchgate.net/publication/259640865_Psychiatry_in_the_Sultanate_of_Oman, consulted on 31.04.2016

[623] Ghodse H., International Perspectives on Mental Health, RCPsych Publications, 2011, p.168.

[624] https://www.researchgate.net/publication/259640865_Psychiatry_in_the_Sultanate_of_Oman, consulted on 31.04.2016

[625] http://www.ncbi.nlm.nih.gov/pubmed/19781054, consulted on 31.04.2016

13.5 times more likely to seek assistance than males were, highlighting the Arab males fear of expressing his emotions in public.[626] Unfortunately, this behaviour leads to other, more physical dangers. For instance, experts have linked reckless driving on Oman's roads to anxiety and other psychological distress. There are definite advances being made especially when it comes to treatment for conditions such as anxiety disorder.

Most services are dispensed within general tertiary hospitals, but there are two specialised centres, both in the capital city. Apart from the teaching hospital, the multidisciplinary infrastructures often essential for psychiatric services have remained rudimentary, due to a lack of suitable staff. There are substandard facilities for occupational therapy and psychiatric rehabilitation remains basic[627] (see Table 8.35.) The country's only psychiatric facility is Al Masarrah Hospital in the capital, Muscat[628]. The WHO-AIMS Report also states that there are 26 outpatient mental health facilities throughout the country.[629] It was opened in 2013 by Oman's minister for social development, Sheikh Mohammed bin Sayed al-Kalbani.[630]The hospital contains over ten wards for men, women and children, as well as secure units used to treat criminals and addicts. It also has a day care centre, a multi-purpose sports hall, swimming pool and open-air sports facilities. The 60,000 m2 facility has been built to international standards and has taken four years to complete. It also receives patients who are referred from other hospitals around the country.There are also two community-based psychiatric inpatient units offering their services to Omani locals. Day treatment facilities and community residential facilities are non-existent.There are also campaigns run by local healthcare facilities aimed at promoting wider awareness about this topic. One which is called Not Alone involves individuals talking about their battle with various mental health conditions in a public environment.

---

626 http://www.caminorecovery.com/treatment-for-anxiety-oman, consulted on 31.04.2016

627 https://www.researchgate.net/publication/259640865_Psychiatry_in_the_Sultanate_of_Oman, consulted on 31.04.2016

628 http://www.caminorecovery.com/treatment-for-anxiety-oman, consulted on 31.04.2016

629 http://www.who.int/mental_health/who_aims_oman_report.pdf, consulted on 01.07.2016

630 http://www.constructionweekonline.com/article-21907-new-127m-mental-health-hospital-opens-in-oman, consulted on 01.07.2016

Al-Harub Medical Centre

Al-Harub Medical Centre (AHMC) is one of the leading healthcare facilities specialized in offering alternative and mainstream medicinal services in Oman. They are a centrally located in Muscat providing mental health, educational, chiropractic, physical integrated therapy, and others[631]. There are fewer than 15 registered mental health professionals for a population of nearly 3 million people scattered over 300 000 km2 (see Table 8.36.) Most psychiatrists have been recruited from abroad, although some have been naturalised. The duration of general medical training in students at Sultan Qaboos University is 7 years (4 years pre-clinical, 3 years clinical). Graduates then spend 1 year on internship, rotating between three out of four specialties (internal medicine, general surgery, child health, obstetric and gynecology)[632]. Behavioural science, which encompasses diverse disciplines, including sociology, anthropology, and psychology, is taught in the second and third years of the pre-clinical course, in order for Omani trainees to appreciate the social and cultural aspects of illness and well-being. In their sixth year, clinical students spend 8 weeks on a clinical clerkship in psychiatry, which is their first exposure to psychiatry. The 8-week programme includes supplementary lectures on various aspects of clinical psychiatry and allied fields, patient case presentation, case histories and clinical interview.[633]

Table 8.35 Availability of Mental Health Facilities[634]

	Total number of facilities/ beds	Rate per 100,000 population	Number of facilities/ beds reserved for children and adolescents only	Rate per 100,000 population
Mental health outpatient facilities	26	0.89	2	0.07

---

[631] http://www.alharubmedical.com/pge.php?id=20, consulted on 01.07.2016

[632] http://www.rcpsych.ac.uk/pdf/IPv3n4.pdf, consulted on 31.04.2016

[633] https://www.researchgate.net/publication/259640865_Psychiatry_in_the_Sultanate_of_Oman, consulted on 31.04.2016

[634] Mental Health Atlas 2011, WHO, Department of Mental Health and Substance Abuse

Day treatment facilities	0	0.00	NA	NA
Psychiatric beds in general hospitals	12	0.41	0	0.00
Community residential facilities	0	0.00	NA	NA
Beds/places in community residential facilities	0	0.00	NA	NA
Mental hospitals	1	0.03	0	0.00
Beds in mental hospitals	64	2.20	0	0.00

Table 8.36 Workforce and Training[635]

	Health professionals working in the mental health sector Rate per 100,000	Training of health professions in educational institutions Rate per 100,000
Psychiatrists	2.31	0.10
Medical doctors, not specialized in psychiatry	0.41	1.17
Nurses	6.57	24.72
Psychologists	0.17	0.34
Social workers	0.07	0.93
Occupational therapists	0.10	0.03
Other health workers	UN (information unavailable)	NA

[635] Mental Health Atlas 2011, WHO, Department of Mental Health and Substance Abuse

Table 8.37 Expenditures for Medicines for Mental and
Behavioral Disorders at the Country Level[636]

Type of Medicines	Expenditures at country level per year and per 100,000 population (in USD)
All the psychotherapeutic medicines (N03AG01, N05A, N05B, N05C, N06A)	187,837
Medicines used for bipolar disorders (N03AG01, N05A, N05B, N05C, N06A)	7,608
Medicines for psychotic disordersN05A (excluding N05AN)	55,086
Medicines used for general anxiety (N05B &N05C)	2,435
Medicines used for mood disorders (N06A)	22,708

In 2016 to promote mental health, the Whispers of Serenity Clinic organised a movie night at the clinic on Thursday in Muscat.[637] "This event (movie night) is a first of many to come, which is planned to be held on a monthly basis.[638] The movie Call Me Crazy had five stories, with each character portraying a mental disorder. The first story talked about schizophrenia and the second about bipolar disorder. The third story was interlinked with the first to show the impact of mental health illness on the family as a whole. The fourth story talked about depression and the last one dealt with post-traumatic stress disorder. The You Are Not Alon campaign, promoted by Whispers of Serenity Clinic, has featured prominent figures and personalities from different backgrounds, who have offered to engage in the awareness programme and to show the public and every patient that: "You are not alone, we are here to help you." Recently, Al Said, the clinic's manager, was awarded the Golden Recognition Award by the Arab Women Council for her efforts in social responsibility and for the Not Alone initiative to raise awareness about mental health in the Arab region.She was also awarded an Honorary Doctorate for youth volunteer projects, as well as the Middle East award for contributions to society

---

[636]   *Ibid*

[637]   http://timesofoman.com/article/77848/Oman/Health/Whispers-of-Serenity-Clinic-organises-movie-night-to-raise-mental-health-awareness, consulted on 01.07.2016

[638]   *Ibid*

from the GR8! Women Achievers Awards, held both in the United Arab Emirates in May and January, respectively last year. To fight stigma against mental illness, campaigners have launched a drive in the schools and colleges of Salalah city in the southern Dhofar province. "The campaign aims to raise public awareness about mental health and fight the tendency of ostracising those afflicted with mental illness," Dr Hamed Al Sinawi, Senior Consultant Psychiatrist at the Sultan Qaboos University Hospital (SQUH) told the Times of Oman[639].The survey, campaigners said, was an initial step in Your Mental Health campaign that aims to raise public awareness about mental health and fight stigma against mental illness. They said 612 individuals from all over Oman participated in the electronic survey including 59% females.Of the total number of participants, 41% were from Muscat and the rest were from other provinces.They fell in the age bracket of 15 years to 65 years with about 46% aged 15-30 years.Those who worked in the health sector represented 25% of the total respondents while the remaining worked in different sectors, for example, educational, industrial, governmental and students.Campaigners said the study revealed that one out of three respondents knew someone with symptoms indicative of mental illness and the overall score that measures the perception towards mental illness was "favourable". However, the age group of 15-30 years had "less positive" attitude towards mental illness and people with mental disorders compared to the older age groups.[640]

The total number of human resources working in mental health facilities or private practice per 100,000 population is 14.18[641]. In terms of staffing in mental health facilities, there are 0.27 psychiatrists per bed in community-based psychiatric inpatient units, in comparison to 0.34 psychiatrists per bed in the mental hospital.[642] As for nurses, there are 0.69 nurses per bed in community-based psychiatric inpatient units, in comparison to 1.84 per bed in the mental hospital. The density of psychiatrists in or around the largest city (Muscat) is 2.42 times greater than the density of psychiatrists in the entire country.[643] There are only 67 psychiatrists, 11 assistant psychiatrists, 183 nurses, 12 psychologists and

---

[639] Oman health: Campaign to fight stigma of mental illness launched, *Times of Oman*, from 3rd January, 2016

[640] *Ibid*

[641] Mental health system in Oman, WHO AIMS Report, p.6.

[642] *Ibid*

[643] *Ibid*

8 social workers working in or for mental health facilities in Oman.[644] In 2006, 85 general medical doctors, 493 nurses, 1 psychiatrist and 21 nurses specialized in mental health care, and 1 occupational therapist with at least 1 year training in mental health care graduated from various institutions in or outside Oman.[645] Around 9% of the training for medical doctors is devoted to mental health, in comparison to 7% for nurses.[646] Over 6% of primary care doctors and 3% of nurses received at least 2 days of refresher training in mental health in 2006.[647]

The expenditures for medicines for mental and behavioral disorders at the country level can be consulted at the Table 8.37.

The strength of the Omani mental health system is:

- Available mental health policy;
- Mental health services, including, essential psychotropic medicine, are free to the entire Omani population.

Its weaknesses:

- No available comprehensive mental health legislation that protects and promotes the human rights of people with mental disorders;
- Insufficiency of human resources working in the mental health;
- Oftentimes no treatment solutions are available for certain diseases;
- No available refresher training system for working professionals.

The mental health in Oman is principally based on the classical tradition, and all innovations should pass through the rigorous examination of the Ministry of Health. This also concerns the psychoanalysis, which till nowadays has not been introduced in the country. Omanis, who suffer from mental and psychosomatic disorders, continue to seek treatment abroad since the local mental health system cannot offer the effective solutions.

QATAR

The National Mental Health Strategy was launched on the 9th of December 2013. It sets out Qatar's vision to provide the best possible mental health services for our citizens while changing attitudes towards mental

---

[644] *Ibid*

[645] Mental health system in Oman, WHO AIMS Report, p.6.

[646] *Ibid*

[647] *Ibid*

illness[648]. The vision for Mental Health in Qatar comprises: "Good mental health and wellbeing for the people of Qatar, supported by integrated mental health services with access to the right care, at the right time and in the right place." Qatar's first National Mental Health Strategy is a critical part of the National Health Strategy (2011-16) and demonstrates progress in transforming the health sector and developing integrated health services. The National Mental Health Strategy contributes to the human development pillar of the Qatar National Vision 2030, which recognizes that a healthy mind is as important as a healthy body. The National Mental Health Strategy outlines a 5-year plan to design and build a comprehensive and integrated mental health system, including education, services, leadership and research. The strategy includes a new model of care that will change the way mental health services are delivered in Qatar, giving people a range of choices on how and where they receive care when they need it. Qatar's public and private health service providers are united behind this integrated plan.[649] The Supreme Council of Health, Hamad Medical Corporation and Primary Health Care Corporation are the key healthcare partners in the delivery of the strategy. The Strategy includes 10 pledges which describe the benefits for Qatari people as the system delivers wide changes for mental health.[650] A key outcome of implementing the Mental Health Strategy is to increase the number of people who have access to the care they need. This is planned to be achieved by reducing stigma, offering treatment in a range of settings, building a mental health trained workforce, improving facilities and increasing financial investment over the next five years.[651] The Supreme Council of Health has set a clear vision to create a high-quality mental health system for Qatar and will take a leading role in monitoring the successful implementation of the strategy.

2013 Qatar National Mental Health Strategy is in place.[652] Action plan (2014-2015) for mental health promotion and prevention included:

- Developed baseline indicators to measure improvements in attitudes and awareness of mental health;

---

[648] http://www.moph.qa/health-strategies/national-mental-health-strategy, consulted on 01.05.2016

[649] *Ibid*

[650] https://www.moph.gov.qa/health-strategies/national-mental-health-strategy,consulted on 01.05.2016

[651] *Ibid*

[652] http://nhsq.info/app/media/1166, consulted on 01.05.2016

- Mental health service level performance measures developed;
- Priority mental health research programs identified;
- Access to assessment and treatment for mild mental illness assured by a trained
  Primary Care health professional;
- First specialist community mental health service hub created;
  2015-2016-Mental Health Law enacted and implemented by December 2015 included:
- Four Primary Care Mental Health Teams;
- Second specialist community mental health service hub;
- Mechanisms in place to facilitate service user and family participation in mental health policy, planning and promotion;
- Integrated care pathways implemented and audited for priority conditions;
  2016-2017-Regulatory and Quality Standards for mental health include:
- Third specialist community mental health service hub operational by March 2017;
- At least two functioning national, multi-sectoral promotion and prevention programs in mental health by March 2017 (Aligned to WHO Mental Health Global Action Plan);
- Inter-disciplinary teams established across all mental health services by March 2017;
- Mental health training available to all health professionals by March 2017
  2017-2018-20% of people with mental illness will receive their treatment in primary care settings by April 2018;
- Fourth specialist community mental health service hub operational by April 2018;
- Service coverage for people with severe mental disorders will increase by 20% by April 2018 (Aligned to WHO Mental Health Global Action Plan);
- Minimum of 12.5 psychiatric beds per 100,000 population by April 2018 (NHS / General Secretariat of Development Planning);
- 50% of Psychiatric Inpatient Beds co-located with general hospital settings by April 2018;
- The increase in investment in mental health as a proportion of the total health budget by April 2018.

The National Mental Health Strategy, which has a theme of "Changing Minds, Changing Lives", also contains a 10-point pledge, which includes[653]:

- Raising public awareness about mental health and reducing the stigma associated with mental illness;
- Providing more information about mental health in healthcare centers;
- Educating healthcare professionals so that they can pick up on problems at an early stage;
- Developing specialist services that meet the differing needs of individuals and groups;
- Ensuring mental health research evidence translates into improvements in clinical practice and patient outcomes.

The strategy document also assesses the total cost of mental health disorders in Qatar – putting it at an estimated QR1.7 bn (467 million US dollars) per year. It also states that three out of six of the "most burdensome diseases" in the country and three of five of the top causes of disability are mental disorders.

Dedicated mental health legislation does not exist. However, legal provisions concerning mental health are covered in other laws (e.g. welfare, disability, general health legislation etc).

Subjective well-being was measured in a series of questions relating to energy, money and satisfaction with various aspects of their life[654]. Satisfaction was again coded into two categories of satisfied and dissatisfied, with satisfaction being assumed if the respondent had stated that they were very satisfied or satisfied with the different spheres of well-being that were asked. Over 95% of the respondents stated that they had enough energy for everyday life, while only 81.3% stated that they had enough money to meet everyday needs. Age had the strongest relationship to energy, with younger age groups having a higher percentage of respondents with enough energy compared to the older ages.

---

[653] http://dohanews.co/qatar-launches-strategy-to-combat-rising-mental-health-woes, consulted on 01.05.2016

[654] http://www.biomedcentral.com/content/supplementary/1478-7954-12-18-S1.pdf, consulted on 01.05.2016

Table 8.38 Availability of Mental Health Facilities

	Total number of facilities/ beds	Rate per 100,000 population	Number of facilities/ beds reserved for children and adolescents only	Rate per 100,000 population
Mental health outpatient facilities	16	1.06	3	0.20
Day treatment facilities	2	0.13	0	0.00
Psychiatric beds in general hospitals	0	0.00	NA	NA
Community residential facilities	1	0.07	0	0.00
Beds/places in community residential facilities	15	0.99	0	0.00
Mental hospitals	1	0.07	0	0.00
Beds in mental hospitals	60	3.98	0	0.00

A lower proportion of females than males stated they had enough energy (93.7% and 97.2% respectively),[655] while more non-Qataris felt that they did have enough energy compared with Qatari nationals (96.5% and 93.5% respectively).[656] Feeling that there was enough money did not vary greatly between gender or nationality status. The percentage of respondents in Al Rayyan who felt they did not have enough money was lower than in Doha, with figures of 77.3% and 81.7% respectively. There was no large variation in the responses to having enough money to meet needs by wealth quintile, indicating that this variable may not measure wealth that accurately.[657]

---

[655] http://www.biomedcentral.com/content/supplementary/1478-7954-12-18-S1.pdf, consulted on 01.05.2016

[656] *Ibid*

[657] *Ibid*

The statistics for existing mental health facilities can be found at the Table 7.38.

Sidra

Sidra represents the vision of Her Highness Sheikha Moza bint Nasser, who is also its Chairperson.[658] Mental health services for children also belong to Sidra's competency. As a hospital and research center focusing on the health of women and children, addressing the mental health care needs of pregnant women and that of children, will be a part of the overall service of care.

Hamad Medical Corporation's Psychiatry Department

Hamad Medical Corporation's (HMC) Psychiatry Department recently hosted the first Annual Symposium of Community Mental Health Services in Qatar, which brought together mental health experts from the region and key stakeholders in Qatar's mental health community.[659] The Symposium was attended by staff from HMC, Primary Health Care Corporation, patients and their families and caregivers, social service workers and other community-based organizations. The Department has a capacity of 76 inpatient beds and an average of 1700 outpatient contacts per month. HMC offers special expertise in general adult psychiatry, child psychiatry, geriatric psychiatry, substance abuse (addictions), liaison psychiatry, community psychiatry, and psychotherapy.[660] The department adopts a multidisciplinary approach to mental health provision. The team consists of psychiatrists, nurses, psychologists, psychotherapists, social workers, and occupational therapists, all following a comprehensive biopsychosocial model of care, provided at the level of inpatients, outpatients, day patients, and community services.[661] The department works closely with HGH Emergency Department as a primary source of input to the service. There are also close links through consult-liaison service or clinics with the Pediatric and Dermatology department, Rehabilitation department at Rumaillah, Al-Amal hospital, Kidney Transplant unit, the Women's

---

[658] http://www.sidra.org/introduction, consulted on 01.05.2016

[659] https://www.hamad.qa/EN/news/2015/June/Pages/HMC-holds-1st-Annual-Symposium-of-Community-Mental-Health-Services-in-Qatar.aspx, consulted on 01.05.2016

[660] http://site.hmc.org.qa/ips/aboutus.htm, consulted on 01.05.2016

[661] *Ibid*

Hospital, in addition to the Psychiatry service at Al-Khor hospital. The Faculty and residents are actively involved with research and scholarly activities. The department won a number of research awards, including the Medical Director's Research Award grant in 2011, and a number of grants awarded by Qatar Foundation's National Priorities Research Program. Clinical Services at Psychiatry Department. The corporation is divided into the following units:

- Outpatient unit: This is the main primary mental health service in Qatar and is the point of entry into the services for the majority of patients. The average number of the patients contact the outpatient service is 1700 per month. Five attending physicians are assigned for supervised clinical teaching for residents during working hours, in addition to other service clinics run by attending physician. The clinic has its own records and pharmacy. Treatment modalities in the clinic include pharmacotherapy, psychotherapy, and behavioral therapy. Social and psychological services are also available in the clinic.[662]

- Inpatient units: there are five inpatient units, two male units, two female units and one male high-care unit. Currently, the total number of beds is 76. The patients are usually admitted through the outpatient service, accident and emergency department of HGH, and community services. Each unit has a treating team consists of two attending psychiatrists (one consultant and one specialist), a senior resident and one or two junior residents. All teams operate under the graded responsibility concept with junior residents supervised by senior residents.

- Community care services: This service started in 1993 and at present is undergoing major development. A Community Team provides Day Programs, Residential care, Home Based Outreach and Crisis Intervention.[663] The community team consists of two attending psychiatrists (one consultant and one specialist) and an adequate number of community nurses.

- Extended care facility: The Extended Psychiatric Care Facility is located within the complex of the Extended Care Facilities of Rumailah Hospital. It consists of 3 villas, each housing 5 male patients with the long-standing psychiatric illness who are unable to live alone in the community and who have no relatives who

---

[662] http://site.hmc.org.qa/ips/aboutus.htm, consulted on 01.05.2016

[663] *Ibid*

---

can take them in.[664] The villas are staffed primarily with nursing staff members who work in 3 shifts. Patients are encouraged to do their Activities of Daily Living (ADLs) independently and be responsible for their own medication. Daily activities and outings are organized and supervised by the staff and a psychiatric consultant makes rounds weekly. Medical care is provided in the complex where the villas are located in the form of a fully-staffed medical clinic.

- Day patients: Day patients' service is part of the community service and under the care and responsibility of the community team. Patients attend on different days of the week, to be engaged in several therapeutic activities with special emphasis on psychosocial rehabilitation[665].
- Consultation-liaison psychiatry: A 24 hour Consultation-liaison service to other facilities of the Hamad Medical Corporation (HMC) is available. The Consultation-liaison team provides cover for HGH. The consultation-liaison team consists of two attending psychiatrists (consultant and specialist) and one resident under rotation.
- Emergency psychiatry services: The Emergency psychiatry service is an interdisciplinary clinical learning assignment in the context of a hospital medical/surgical emergency room (HGH). The emergency psychiatric service is under the clinical duties of the consultation-liaison psychiatry team during the morning working hours. After the morning working hours the emergency service is covered by the senior residents in-house on call, second on call (specialist) and the consultant on call for that day.
- Geriatric psychiatric services are based at the Psychiatry Department of HMC. Currently, the Geropsychiatry team consist of two full-time attending psychiatrists (consultant and specialist), two community mental health nurses (key workers). The team provides a variety of hospital-based and community-based services to address the mental health needs of elderly people through assessment, counseling, education, therapy, and liaison with geriatric medicine homecare services at Rumailah Hospital and geriatric inpatients units at Skilled nursing facility units, Hamad Medical City.

---

[664] *Ibid*

[665] *Ibid*

- Child psychiatry service: the team of professionals' works intensively with the referring clinician and the patient's family to ensure the high expectations for treatment when dealing with children. Child psychiatrists provide treatment and consultation in the following clinical setting: Outpatient Child & Adolescent Clinic at Psychiatry Dept., Outpatient Child Clinic and Inpatient Units at Pediatric Department of HGH, Child Rehabilitation Unit at Rumailah hospital, Pediatric Emergency Center.
- Drug dependence service: This is mainly an outpatient service for patients with substance abuse and drug dependence. Patients who need admission are admitted to an inpatient unit[666]. The treating team conducts a bio-psychosocial model plan of treatment for the patient and their families.
- Psychological service: The psychology unit is based at the psychiatry department and provides psychological services for patients of all ages by qualified, professional psychologists. Psychologists are active members of inpatient multidisciplinary teams. Their main duties are to provide psychological assessment for children with developmental and psychiatric disorders, psychodynamic assessment for patients with marital issues and dysfunctional relationships, administer cognitive and psychometric assessment and provide psycho-education for patients and families[667].
- Psychotherapy service: The Psychotherapy unit is integrated into the Department of Psychiatry. It consists of a group of mental health clinicians (MD, PhD, and Masters levels) who are trained in the practice of various forms of psychotherapy. They work with individuals of all ages, with couples, families and groups. A variety of psychotherapy approaches is practiced: supportive, psychodynamically-oriented, cognitive behavioral therapy, psychotherapy combined with medication management, and play therapy.[668] The clinicians of the Psychotherapy unit are also actively involved in the psychotherapy curriculum of the residency training program offering extensive didactic teaching and supervision to the Residents throughout their years of training. In what it concerns the Residency training program, the department offers four-year general psychiatry- training program. The program has been fully and consistently accredited by the Arab Board of Medical

---

[666] http://site.hmc.org.qa/ips/aboutus.htm, consulted on 01.05.2016
[667] *Ibid*
[668] *Ibid*

Specialization since 1993. It prepares the residents for the Arab Board examination leading to certification in psychiatry - the basis for future independent practice.

Naufar Healthcare and Rehabilitation Centre Qatar

Naufar Healthcare and Rehabilitation Centre Qatar is a state-of-the-art healthcare facility for treatment and rehabilitation for substance abuse. Naufar has a vision to be an internationally recognized centre of excellence for providing specialized healthcare and social care, teaching and training, and research in the field of substance abuse.

The project includes community/outreach services, residential programs, assessment services, and prevention/awareness/research/education programs. A 50,000 square meter facility, which includes 249 beds, which will include male adult units, a male dual diagnosis unit, a male secure unit, a male adolescent unit, a female unit, five VIP villas, and a halfway house. Program durations will typically range from three months to six months (except the acute dual diagnosis unit, which will be up to three months).[669]

Child Development Centre

Child Development Centre was established in 2013, CDC provides a network of internationally qualified and licensed professionals who offer child-centered and evidence-based early detection and intervention for children with developmental delays. The aim of Child Development Center is to create a leading, comprehensive, multi-disciplinary therapy and support center for children with mild to moderate special needs. Based on the reason for referral and needs of the client, the Clinical Director will develop an individually tailored battery of tests that provide a high quality and comprehensive assessment.[670] A full psychological evaluation typically includes an in-depth clinical interview in addition to tests of ability/intelligence, academic achievement tests, personality tests, behavior rating scales, and various scales assessing psychopathology. Information from this evaluation provides a broad view of psychological functioning, which consists of intellectual and academic strengths and weaknesses, personality patterns, and various psychological diagnoses including autism spectrum

---

[669] http://www.adr-medical-recruitment.co.uk/vacancies/qatar--naufar-healthcare-and-rehabilitation-centre, consulted on 01.05.2016

[670] *Ibid*

disorder. For educational psychological reports, the WIAT-II (UK), and Stanford Binet-5 are administered in creating a comprehensive assessment for the child. Annual Autism Conferences provide an opportunity for important dialogue about identifying the needs of children on the autism spectrum and their families in Qatar.[671]

There are 1,66 psychiatrists and 1,26 psychologist working in the Qatari mental health sector per 100,000 population[672] (see Table 8.39).

Table 8.39 Workforce and Training

	Health professionals working in the mental health sector Rate per 100,000	Training of health professions in educational institutions Rate per 100,000
Psychiatrists	1.66	0.13
Medical doctors, not specialized in psychiatry	0.20	UN
Nurses	10.94	1.59
Psychologists	1.26	0.00
Social workers	0.46	0.00
Occupational therapists	0.40	0.00
Other health workers	UN	NA

The global average for a government mental health budget is 2.8% of total spending. Although Qatar's total expenditure on mental health has yet to be released, the 2011 Mental Health Atlas submission states that Hamad Medical Corporation Psychiatric Services represent 1.95% of the country's health budget. This figure does not include primary health care services or private clinics.[673] Information on expenditures for medicines for mental and behavioral disorders in Qatar is unavailable.

Its strengths:

• Available mental health policy;
• Financial support from government;

[671] http://www.qatar.northwestern.edu/life/student-services/counseling-wellness, consulted on 01.05.2016

[672] http://nhsq.info/app/media/1166, consulted on 01.05.2016

[673] http://dohanews.co/qatar-launches-strategy-to-combat-rising-mental-health-woes, consulted on 01.05.2016

- Extensive mental health infrastructure.

Its weaknesses:

- Insufficient professional human resources.

Qatar considers the execution of mental health strategy to be the national priority. Currently, the construction of new on-site mental health buildings is being carried out against the background of already functioning mental care facilities. The ambitious mega-projects aim to bring the up-to-date innovations and the most knowledgeable human resources into the peninsula, thus, turning it into the health-care harbor catering for the patients` needs from the whole Middle East, and, even, the planet. More and more mental health professionals, as well as patients, choose Qatar, as a key point, where the fully-fledged medical facilities allow for proper clinical conditions and comprehensive treatment.

SAUDI ARABIA

The chronological timeline of KSA with the inclusion of major events in the mental health area starts with 1932, the year when KSA was founded by Al-Saud. In 1952 the 1st mental hospital was opened in Taif. In 1969 the 1st medical school was built in Riyadh. In 1989 primary health care centers were established. In 1997 the psychiatry training residency began. In 2007 the 1st Saudi Mental and Social Health Atlas (SAMHA-1) edited. In 2010 the 2nd Mental Health Atlas (SAMHA-2) published. In 2012 Mental Health Act was passed by the government. In 2013 Saudi National Mental Health Survey began. In 2014 and beyond the building of community mental health centers started.[674]

An officially approved mental health policy exists and most recently revised in 2008. Mental health is also specifically mentioned in the general health policy.[675] The Saudi government has recently passed a Mental Health Act (MHA) that focuses on the following areas:[676]

---

[674] Mental Health Care in Saudi Arabia: Past, Present and Future, Open Journal of Psychiatry, 2014, 4, pp.113-130.

[675] http://www.who.int/mental_health/evidence/atlas/profiles/sau_mh_profile.pdf, consulted on 01.05.2016

[676] http://www.ncbi.nlm.nih.gov/pmc/articles/PMC3743653/, consulted on 01.05.2016

---

1. Improving access to mental health care generally;
2. Ensuring the least restrictive level of care;
3. Preserving the rights of patients, family members, and other caregivers;
4. Streamlining competence, capacity, and guardianship issues, including voluntary and involuntary treatment;
5. Ensuring the accreditation of professionals and facilities;
6. Enforcing mental health laws and other legal issues;
7. Establishing mechanisms to implement these provisions.

The MHA is a strategic document because it puts governmental authority behind the mental health policy guidelines developed in 2008 that followed the 2006 Saudi Arabian Mental and Social Health Atlas. The latter sought to streamline the delivery of mental health care services to health consumers, families, and caregivers over the next 4 years. The MHA was developed after reviewing what other countries were doing globally over a period of 5 years. The MHA establishes the procedures and policies for safeguarding the rights of persons with mental illness.

While the majority of patients seen in outpatient settings have neurotic (36%) or mood disorders (35%), those admitted to inpatient mental hospitals are more likely to suffer from schizophrenia (50%), substance-abuse disorders (20%), and mood disorders (20%)[677]. In a retrospective Saudi study from the mental hospital in Taif, schizophrenia (89%) and drug addictions (61%) were the most common inpatient diagnoses, followed by mental retardation (18%), personality disorders (4%), and epilepsy (2%)[678]. The average number of outpatient visits for those with an identified psychiatric problem in KSA is 2.5 per year.[679]

---

[677] http://www.ncbi.nlm.nih.gov/pmc/articles/PMC3743653/, consulted on 01.05.2016

[678] *Ibid*

[679] *Ibid*

Table 8.40 Availability of Mental Health Facilities

	Total number of facilities/ beds	Rate per 100,000 population	Number of facilities/ beds reserved for children and adolescents only	Rate per 100,000 population
Mental health outpatient Facilities	94	0.36	19	0.07
Day treatment facilities	3	0.01	UN	UN
Psychiatric beds in general hospitals	100	0.38	UN	UN
Community residential facilities	2	0.01	0	0.00
Beds/places in community residential facilities	240	0.91	0	0.00
Mental hospitals	20	0.08	0	0.00
Beds in mental hospitals	3000	11.43	0	0.00

About one in five (19%) outpatient facilities provides follow-up care in the community, while an unknown percentage has mobile mental health teams. In terms of available treatments, 21%–50% of psychiatric outpatients in the past year received one or more psychosocial interventions.[680]

Almost all facilities (100%) have at least one psychotropic medicine available onsite from each major drug class (i.e. antipsychotics, antidepressants, mood stabilizers, anxiolytic drugs, and mood-stabilizing antiepileptics).[681] It was reported that less than 40% of those with a lifetime disorder had ever received professional treatment, and less than 20% of those with a recent disorder had been in treatment during the past

[680] http://www.ncbi.nlm.nih.gov/pmc/articles/PMC3743653/, consulted on 01.05.2016

[681] http://www.ncbi.nlm.nih.gov/pmc/articles/PMC3743653/, consulted on 01.05.2016

12 months.[682] The types of psychiatric disorder seen in outpatient and inpatient settings are similar in the US and KSA.

There are only three day-treatment facilities in KSA, which serve a variety of patients with acute and chronic mental disorders (see Table 8.40.) The goal is to minimize admissions and to optimize independent living skills and vocational rehabilitation and to provide support in the recovery process by emphasizing the development of healthy coping skills in the community. A multidisciplinary team provides comprehensive, needed services that include case management, group therapies, individual support, occupational services, leisure assessment and counseling, and medication monitoring and administration. Adequately staffed day-treatment facilities and programs need to be expanded in the Saudi setting. These are rented facilities similar to halfway houses for chronic patients whose care is managed by nursing staff, other support personnel, and on-call psychiatrists. There are five community-based psychiatric inpatient units in KSA for a total of 0.41 beds per 100,000 population, with an average length of stay of 30 days[683]. No beds are reserved for children or adolescents since inpatient admission is generally discouraged and if admission is required, it is done regardless of bed availability and only briefly. Diagnoses of admitted patients are unknown, but in general tend to be schizophrenia, bipolar disorder, and organic psychoses. About one-quarter to one-half of these patients had received at least one psychosocial intervention in the past year, and all patients had received at least one psychotropic medication in terms of antipsychotics, antidepressants, mood stabilizers, or anxiolytic drugs. Regarding patients living in halfway houses and supported housing, the primary goal of many developed nations has been to move these individuals to the independent housing, along with keeping them stable and increasing their living skills. In one UK study, two clusters of patients emerged: those with no stated goals or with the aim of staying healthy (often with lower quality of life and more psychopathology), and those with an aim to move to independent housing (with better quality of life and less psychopathology). This study suggested that besides better training of staff, more conceptual and practical efforts were needed to manage the transformation of these settings from homes for life to transitional facilities where residents receive specific interventions. Twenty-one mental hospitals

---

[682] Kessler R., McGonagle K., Zhao S., et al., Lifetime and 12-month prevalence of DSM-III-R psychiatric disorders in the United States-Results from the National Comorbidity Survey, Arch Gen Psychiatry, 1994;51, pp.8–9.

[683] http://www.ncbi.nlm.nih.gov/pmc/articles/PMC3743653/, consulted on 01.05.2016

in KSA provide twelve beds per 100,000 population, a number that has remained roughly the same between 2005 and 2010.[684] In KSA, mental hospitals treat 1.92 users per 100,000 per year.[685] The primary diagnoses of patients admitted to these facilities are schizophrenia, mood disorders, and substance use disorders, similar to psychiatric inpatients in the US. The average length of inpatient stay in KSA is 45 days, and most patients (70%) spend less than 1 year in these facilities.[686] The rest spend 1–10 or more years. Across the world, the average length of inpatient stay in mental hospitals is on the decrease compared to hospital stays for physical disorders. This has been attributed to managed care, the development of innovative community and home mental health care services, the freedom to leave against medical advice, and prospective payment systems. Hospital-at-home services can provide a safe, effective alternative to inpatient care for patients appropriate for this level of care. Furthermore, home treatment has the potential to reduce costs, reduce pressure on inpatient services, and provide care that is acceptable to patients and their families.

The total number of psychiatrists, medical physicians, nurses, psychologists, social workers, occupational therapists, and other workers in mental health facilities and private psychiatric practice in KSA is 22 per 100,000 population (see Table 8.41.) The number of psychiatrists has also been expanding in KSA. In 1977, there were only three psychiatrists to serve the entire population of KSA. By 1983, that number had increased about 10-fold, and by 2006 there were 205 psychiatrists serving a population of 23 million (0.9 per 100,000).[687] By 2010 there were over 700 psychiatrists (3.0 per 100,000), including 380 who performed primarily outpatient psychiatry and 263 who worked in mental hospitals.[688] The number of psychologists, psychiatric nurses, and psychiatric social workers has also increased over time. By profession, this breaks down to three psychiatrists, 13 nurses, two psychologists, three social workers, and one other mental health worker (auxiliary staff, occupational therapists, health assistants,

---

[684] http://www.ncbi.nlm.nih.gov/pmc/articles/PMC3743653/, consulted on 01.05.2016

[685] *Ibid*

[686] *Ibid*

[687] http://www.omicsonline.com/open-access/doctor-to-patient-ratio-and-infrastructure-gap-in-a-psychiatric-hospital-in-oil-rich-eket-nigeria-2378-5756-1000356.pdf, consulted on 01.05.2016

[688] http://www.ncbi.nlm.nih.gov/pmc/articles/PMC3743653/, consulted on 01.05.2016

medical physicians, medical assistants, professional and paraprofessional counselors). According to SAMHA-2010, the latest figures indicate 1980 nurses working in outpatient facilities and 1176 in mental hospitals. There were also 515 psychologists, social workers and occupational therapists at outpatient facilities and 611 working in mental hospitals.[689] However, most nurses caring for the mentally ill did not start out with special training in psychiatry, and psychologists and social workers often do not have post-graduate degrees. Several undergraduate and post-graduate training programs in psychology and counseling now exist at universities in KSA. These are the University of Tabuk, the King Khaled University in Abha, the King Saud University in Riyadh, the University of Dammam in the Eastern province, and the Princess Noura Bint Abdulrahman University in Riyadh. Furthermore, 13 of KSA's 21 medical schools now offer post-graduate training for allied health disciplines including nurses, psychologists, social workers and counselors. Besides a small psychiatric residency at King Saud University, specialty training in psychiatry was also almost non-existent. A second psychiatry training program existed at the Taif Mental Health Hospital in Shahar that offered a diploma in psychological medicine. According to Dubovsky, this diploma would not fulfill residency requirements for certification. Other than a few lectures on depression and organic brain syndrome, or a week-long clinical clerkship working with a psychiatrist in one of the two mental hospitals, exposure to psychotherapy or psychopharmacology was infrequent in medical school. Slightly more than two-thirds of psychosocial staff, which includes psychologists, social workers, nurses, and occupational therapists, work in government facilities. Regarding the location of employment, 380 psychiatrists are employed in outpatient facilities and 263 in mental hospitals.[690] Approximately 145 medical physicians work in mental health outpatient facilities and 165 in mental hospitals.[691] Regarding other providers, 1,980 nurses work in mental health outpatient facilities and 1,176 in mental hospitals, and 515 psychosocial allied staff work in outpatient facilities and 611 in mental hospitals.[692] In terms of the staffing of mental hospitals, there are 0.09 psychiatrists per hospital bed, 0.39 nurses, and 0.21 other mental health care staff, including psychologists and

---

[689] *Ibid*

[690] http://www.ncbi.nlm.nih.gov/pmc/articles/PMC3743653/, consulted on 01.05.2016

[691] *Ibid*

[692] Mental Health Care in Saudi Arabia: Past, Present and Future, Open Journal of Psychiatry, 2014, 4, pp. 113-130.

social workers.[693] Despite challenges in access to mental hospitals, the distribution of human mental health resources between urban and rural areas is nearly equal. The density of psychiatrists in moderate-to-large cities is only 0.19 per 100,000 lower than the density of psychiatrists in the entire country (although 80% of the population of KSA is urban).[694] Likewise, the density of nurses is only 1.16 per 100,000 lower in large cities than in the rest of the country.[695] In terms of support for the child and adolescent mental health, 15% of primary and secondary schools have either part-time or full-time school counselors, and many schools (between 51% and 80%)[696] have activities to promote mental health and prevent mental disorders. According to Dr.Stephan, school mental health education helps in reducing stigma, enhancing access to mental health services, and preventing mental disorders. They suggest a variety of strategies for expanding mental health in school. Progress began with the building in 1952 of the Taif Mental Hospital in Shahar, an hour's drive southeast from Mecca, the cradle of Islam.[697] By the early 1980's, however, there were still only two psychiatric hospitals to serve the Kingdom's population of 6 to 8 million.[698] Psychotherapy was seldom done with the chronic mentally ill who were usually medicated and housed. No electroconvulsive therapy (ECT) was performed in KSA in the mid-1980s. Although first generation antipsychotics including long-acting agents were used, they were often given at subtherapeutic levels since there were no guidelines for drug use in this part of the world. Regional studies of young persons have also reported relatively high rates of emotional symptoms. For example, Abdel-Fattah and Asal identified a systematic sample of 490 secondary school students in Taif, assessing depressive symptoms using the 21-item Beck Depression Inventory (BDI). The average age was 17 years and 38% were female[699]. One-third (33%) scored 19 or over on the BDI (moderate to severe depression) and 11% scored in the severe to very severe depression

---

[693] http://www.ncbi.nlm.nih.gov/pmc/articles/PMC3743653/, consulted on 01.05.2016

[694] *Ibid*

[695] *Ibid*

[696] *Ibid*

[697] Mental Health Care in Saudi Arabia: Past, Present and Future, Open Journal of Psychiatry, 2014, 4, pp. 113-130.

[698] http://www.ncbi.nlm.nih.gov/pmc/articles/PMC3743653/, consulted on 01.05.2016

[699] *Ibid*

range[700]. In multivariate analyses, females were about one-third more likely than males to score 19 or higher (40% vs. 29%)[701]. Birth order (last child), family history of chronic physical disease, and history of loss of a close relative were other predictors of depression. In a second study of Saudi youth, Gelban examined psychiatric symptoms in high school students ages 14 to 19, reporting results on boys and girls in separate papers[702]. In the first report on males, the 42-item Depression, Anxiety and Stress Scale (DASS) was used to assess symptoms in 1123 students attending all-boys schools in Abha. Around 59% had significant levels of either depression, anxiety or stress; 41% had significant levels of two or more of these symptoms; and 23% had significant levels of all three symptoms. Overall, 36% reported stress, 38% depression, and 49% anxiety. In the second report that focused on females and used a different methodology, the Symptom Checklist 90 (SCL-90-R) was administered to 545 students at 10 all-girls schools in Abha. The most frequent symptoms were phobic anxiety (16%), psychoticism (15%), anxiety (14%), somatization (14%), and depression (14%). Overall, 16% had one or more type of symptom, 9% had two or more symptoms, 6% had three symptoms, and 4% had all four symptoms. Greater psychiatric symptoms in males compared to females (the reverse of what is usually found) may have been due to differences in instruments used to assess psychiatric symptoms. Thus, based on these three reports on secondary school students, between 16% and 59% have significant levels of mental or emotional symptoms. Changes in KSA's mental health care system have been dramatic over the past 30 years. In order to improve the detection and treatment of mental health issues, the World Health Organization in 2000 encouraged countries to make PHC centers the point of the first contact for those with mental disorders. In situations where PHC physicians cannot handle these patients, the recommendation was to refer to psychiatrists in general hospitals (secondary level), and if psychiatrists in those settings couldn't manage patients, then they were to refer to specialty psychiatric hospitals or to teaching hospitals (tertiary level). Since most individuals first see their medical doctor for health problems, and psychiatric and medical illnesses often co-exist, the WHO viewed this system as the best way to identify and treat those with mental health problems. In KSA, which has followed the WHO recommendation, this process has worked reasonably well covering the

---

[700] *Ibid*

[701] *Ibid*

[702] http://www.ncbi.nlm.nih.gov/pmc/articles/PMC3743653/, consulted on 01.05.2016

majority of the population with mental health needs. Patients in KSA can also go directly without referral to see psychiatrists at specialty psychiatric hospitals, and some patients seek help through emergency services at either general hospitals or psychiatric hospitals without a referral. Finally, there is a private mental health care system in KSA, where patients are seen for a fee, unlike the public system which is government-funded. In addition to free-standing private psychiatric clinics, there are over 125 private general hospitals, many with private psychiatric clinics connected to them. Because of the stigma of mental illness and the ease of access to services, those who have the financial resources often prefer to consult private clinics and pay out of pocket. Private clinics offer psychotherapy, psychotropic drugs, addiction services, speech therapy, and rehabilitation services to children, adolescents, adults, and older adults. There are now at least 21 child psychiatry clinics in KSA. Limited research, however, exists on the characteristics of patients seen in these settings. The most common presenting symptoms were hyperactivity (43%), poor school performance (33%), delayed milestones (28%), anxiety (18%), attention and concentration problems (14%), and impulsivity (13%). Diagnoses were mental retardation (30%), anxiety disorder (16%), ADHD (13%), autism spectrum disorder (13%), mood disorder (4%), school refusal (4%), toileting problems (3%), and psychosis (3%).[703] At the initial interview, 86% of these children and adolescents were prescribed one or more psychotropic medication (65% one medication; 21% more than one)[704]. Polypharmacy (21%) in these clinics was considerably lower than that reported in a study of adult Saudi psychiatric patients (85%).[705] Medication alone was not the only treatment offered to children and adolescents, and psychotherapy was recommended in 55%[706]. Good results of treatment were reported, with a "stable" outcome on follow-up in 82%. Also, a shift in the types of illegal drugs used by psychiatric patients has been observed. As reviewed previously, a 1994 study of 116 patients admitted to Al-Amal Hospital in Dammam reported that 84% used heroin alone in or in combination with other drugs, 31% used alcohol, 26% used cannabis, and 10% used stimulants. A more recent review of 12,743 patients at the same Al-Amal Hospital in Dammam between 1986 and 2006 reported a change in a drug of choice. Admissions during the first decade (1986-1996) were

---

[703] Mental Health Care in Saudi Arabia: Past, Present and Future, Open Journal of Psychiatry, 2014, 4, pp.113-130.

[704] *Ibid*

[705] *Ibid*

[706] *Ibid*

for heroin (51%), alcohol (27%), cannabis (18%), sedatives (15%), amphetamines (12%) and volatile substance use (6%), which are similar to the 1994 study above[707]. In the second decade (1997-2006), however, patients were more likely to be admitted for amphetamines (48%) and cannabis (47%), but less likely for heroin (23%), sedatives (7%), or volatile substances (3%).[708] Researchers concluded that considerable shifts had occurred in the types of drugs being abused, likely reflecting changes in the pattern of use in the community.

Table 8.41 Workforce and Training

	Health professionals working in the mental health sector Rate per 100,000	Training of health professions in educational institutions Rate per 100,000
Psychiatrists	2.91	0.21
Medical doctors, not specialized in psychiatry	UN	39.97
Nurses	13.41	6.93
Psychologists	1.66	UN
Social workers	2.90	UN
Occupational therapists	UN	UN
Other health workers	UN	NA

The available finances for mental health care today are spent largely on the salaries of mental health professionals and paramedical personnel working in mental hospitals, on infrastructure development, and on the training of mental health professionals. 4% of the entire health care budget of the MOH is directed towards mental health care. Of all mental health expenditure, 78% goes to mental hospitals. Most of the population now has free access to psychotropic medications and nondrug psychological and social services (see Table 8.42.) However, mental health financing needs further support from the Saudi government. According to a WHO report, "mental health financing is a powerful tool with which policy-makers can develop and shape quality MHSs. Without adequate financing,

---

[707] Mental Health Care in Saudi Arabia: Past, Present and Future, Open Journal of Psychiatry, 2014, 4, pp.113-130.

[708] *Ibid*

mental health policies and plans remain in the realm of rhetoric and good intentions."

The psychiatric research was also strikingly underdeveloped. In the early 1980's, the medical school at King Abdulaziz University in Jeddah had just begun to study biomedical aspects of the hajj, an event where more than 2 million visitors come to Mecca during the 12th month of the Islamic calendar (Dhu al-Hijjah). No research, however, was being done on how this massive pilgrimage affected the mental health of either the visitors or the residents of KSA. In terms of academic research, only a small percentage of peer-reviewed journal publications from KSA are on mental health, although that percentage is likely to increase as more funds are now being reserved for health research in this country. This has resulted in a higher number of research publications in open-access journals, though several barriers still need to be overcome. Over 86,87% of papers published so far have primarily focused on the hospital-based epidemiology of mental disorders and health-services research. There remains a large gap in mental health research, and filling that gap needs to become a health-system priority. The Saudi MOH has begun to encourage research across all regions of KSA by allocating a budget for researchers. Further grant support is also available from the King Abdulaziz City for Science and Technology in Riyadh. In order to build capacity for psychiatric research, the MOH is also providing funds for continuing training of psychiatric nurses, social workers, psychologists, and other psychiatric staff. There is evidence accumulating that research in KSA can help to transform the understanding and treatment of mental illness, as has been the vision of the National Institute of Mental Health (NIMH) in the US. High-priority research at the NIMH that is relevant to LAMICs includes:

1. Identifying trends and gaps in mental health disparities, women's mental health, and global mental health to guide priority-setting for research funding;
2. Monitoring research efforts involving nondomestic institutions and domestic grants with foreign components;
3. Supporting capacity-building, research infrastructure development, and research mentoring in order to develop a multidisciplinary mental health research workforce.

The MOH needs to collaborate with the NIMH and other partners in order to develop a multidisciplinary research workforce in KSA.[709]

Table 8.42 Expenditures for Medicines for Mental and Behavioral Disorders at the Country Level

Type of Medicines	Expenditures at country level per year and per 100,000 population (in USD)
All the psychotherapeutic medicines	225,749
Medicines used for bipolar disorders	15,240
Medicines for psychotic disorders	191,363
Medicines used for general anxiety	1,715
Medicines used for mood disorders	17,622

The strengths of KSA`s mental health system include:

• Functioning psychiatric network;
• Psychiatric courses, which are regularly organized for GPs, along with other training courses.

Its weaknesses:

• Mental health legislative acts are not available;
• Limited community mental health care.

The first mental hospital in GCC was constructed precisely in KSA (1952). The Saudi government has been actively involved in the elaboration of national mental health policy, as well as numerous mental health acts. The Kingdom has a developed interconnected system of delivering psychiatric aid, which includes public and private hospitals, clinics for children and adolescents, as well as numerous mental health centers. The Royal Family is willingly investing into support of mental health sector, by enabling research grants and free of charge training. All Saudi nationals have a right to a free access of psychological services. However, many of them, prefer to pay to a specialist from a private clinic, and, thus, remain incognito.

---

[709] http://www.ncbi.nlm.nih.gov/pmc/articles/PMC3743653/, consulted on 01.05.2016

UNITED ARAB EMIRATES

In UAE, mental health services were established in the mid-1970s, these services were in the form of psychiatric services in some emirates (i.e. Abu Dhabi, Dubai).[710] At the same period, an undergraduate program in psychology was launched in the United Arab Emirates University. According to Fatima Al-Darmaki, an assistant professor in the counseling program in the Department of psychology and counseling of the United Arab Emirates University, in the 1980s psychological services were viewed as supportive services in the treatment of patients who were receiving psychiatric help at the hospitals. The need for the provision of psychological services in UAE society became prominent as a result of the rapid social and economic changes which have taken place within the last 30 years in addition to the external influences of other cultures. Such changes seem to impact the values, beliefs, and role expectations of individuals which may, in turn, affect the psychological health especially for those who may have not being able to adjust to these changes. Despite the ministerial endeavours to create a professional mental health infrastructure in UAE, the competent professionals are lacking. In addition, the prevailing medical treatment model of practice in UAE and the tendency of the public to seek help from religious healers seem to contribute to the underutilization of mental health services in UAE which, in turn, impinge on the importance of services delivery in the society.[711] Public trust in the mental health services and providers seem to be effected by the observed increase in malpractice by those who are not professionally competent.[712] As yet existing tradition of going to the religious healers called "Mattawa" cannot but hinder the process of the recovery of the individual. Their services were the only known method of treatment of mental health illness in UAE prior the formation of the seven emirates in 1971.[713] Mental services in the UAE, referred to as "psychiatric services", officially began in 1975 with the allocation of several beds in ward 14 of the Central Hospital in

---

[710] http://www.omicsonline.com/open-access/mental-health-services-in-the-united-arab-emirates-challenges-and-opportunities-1522-4821-1000263.php?aid=61346, consulted on 01.05.2016

[711] *Ibid*

[712] *Ibid*

[713] *Ibid*

Abu Dhabi.[714] In many cases, individuals are referred to psychiatric care through the emergency room or a general physician. A strategy to develop mental health services was initiated in 1981 with the opening of Al Amal Hospital in Dubai to provide services to the northern emirates. In 1983, a consultant psychiatrist was appointed to work in Fujairah Hospital and a specialist psychiatrist in Ras Al-Khaimah.

With the urban and demographic development, the UAE was one of the first countries in the region to develop Mental Health Act in its Decrees No.28 of 1981. This act dealt primarily with the detention of psychotic patients. Attention to mental health services began in 1985, particularly as a result of the spread of heroin in West Asia and Arab countries. In 1986 the new psychiatric hospital was planned, following Federal Law No. 6 to combat "mind affecting substances". Temporary units were opened in Abu Dhabi and Dubai.Federal Laws Associated with Mental Health in the UAE include:

- Federal Law No. 28 (1981) regarding the detention of psychotic patients.
- Federal Law No. 43 (1993) regarding the organization of correctional institutions.
- Federal Law No. 14 (1995) regarding drugs and mind influencing substances.

These laws were followed by the following periodic ministerial decrees:

- Decree No.1350 (1994) regarding the assessment of inmates with psychotic disorders and other disorders threatening their lives and those of others.
- Decree No.1444 (1997) regarding the formation of a Central Committee for Mental Health.
- Decree No. 1090 (1998) regarding the internal organization of addiction treatment facilities in the UAE.
- Decree No.1826 (1998) regarding the computerization of medical records.
- Decree No.274 (1998) regarding the formation of the Mental Health Appeals Board.

---

[714] Al-Karam C., Haque A., Mental Health and Psychological Practice in the United Arab Emirates, Palgrave Macmillan US, 2015, pp. 35-40.

The final version of proposed changes in mental health laws was submitted to the National Council in 2011 and is awaiting review and approval. The Mental Health Act of 1981 addressed the very basics of mental health services. It had twelve articles that dealt mostly with the definition of key terms as observed at that time, distinguished between voluntary and compulsory admissions, and the role of various related entities or individuals such as relatives, the police, the courts, and the medical board referred to as the "Department Board". This document clarified who could be admitted into an institution. All subsequent laws addressed mental health issues in parts, but the proposed Mental Health Law in 2011 addresses mental health services more comprehensively, and this is apparent from the first article that deals with definitions.[715] The federal government's MOH is the official body that manages health care legislation in the country.[716] However, two other semi-governmental bodies, the Health Authority Abu Dhabi (HAAD) and Dubai Health Authority (DHA) regulate their respective emirates. The practice of providing psychological services such as counseling and psychotherapy remains loosely regulated by the authorities. Several practitioners and academics have voiced their concerns and expressed a dire need for mental health legislation.[717] The lack of enforced rules of practice has enabled "bogus" psychologists and mental health workers who exploit legal loopholes to operate in the UAE's market.[718] A panel of professionals from Dubai Health Authority (DHA), Ministry of Health (MOH), Emirates Psychological Association and other institutes are currently working on regulation guidelines for the practice of psychology[719]. Despite the ongoing efforts to establish a regulatory body for the professions of psychology in the UAE, there are still a number of challenges hindering progress on this issue. According to Dr Hussein Al Maseeh, licensing procedures are going to be different from one emirate to another depending on the local authority's existing guidelines and willingness to get involved. In the UAE the licensure can be obtained with

---

[715] Al-Karam C., Haque A., Mental Health and Psychological Practice in the United Arab Emirates, Palgrave Macmillan US, 2015, p. 35-40.

[716] http://www.apa.org/international/pi/2015/06/psychology-arab.aspx, consulted on 01.05.2016

[717] Al-Shihabi R., Licensing needs for psychologists in Abu Dhabi, The UAE Psychologist. 1(2), 2011, p.4.

[718] http://www.thenational.ae/uae/health/bogus-psychologists-are-exploiting-legal-loopholes

[719] The Journal "UAE Psychologist", Mayissue, 2012

a master level education or even with the undergraduate degree and a few years of experience.The licensing source (federal versus local) will affect the scope of practice of professionals. Finally, current legislative efforts are directed toward psychiatry and clinical psychology, with no consideration of other psychological professions such as counseling or school psychology. Presently, licensure is obtained from governmental health entities such as the Abu Dhabi Health Authority (HAAD), DHA and MOH. For counselors, the Dubai Community Development Authority provides licensing. Availability of mental health facilities can be consulted at the Table 8.43.

The rate of mental health professionals per 100,000 is as follows: 0.3 psychiatrists, 0.51 psychologists, 0.25 social workers, 0.04 occupational therapists and 0.04 other health workers[720] (see Table 8.44.) The data on the number of counselors is unavailable. These numbers indicate an extreme shortage of mental health professionals and facilities in the UAE. Training psychologists in UAE is very challenging. Most of the Emiratis who provide psychological services in schools and in the community mental health agencies have minimal training in applied psychology. The only well-established public undergraduate program available is in the United Arab Emirates University (UAEU) which admits a very limited number of international students. This is due to the fact that UAEU is a federal institution funded by the government. Similarly, Zayed University (ZU), another federal institution, recently began offering a program in psychology as a major. Expatriate students seeking training in psychology have to enroll in private universities such as Middlesex University Dubai and Herio-Watt University Dubai that also offer undergraduate programs in psychology. Other universities such as New York University Abu Dhabi, American University in Sharjah offer minors in psychology or hybrid majors involving psychology. At the graduate level, only one clinical psychology masters (MSc) program exists, which was recently introduced in UAEU. It is open to both UAE nationals and non-nationals. However, the clinical program has several challenges, including finding adequate internships for students, sufficient resources (culturally relevant textbooks, bilingual faculty), and well-trained supervisors.

---

[720] http://www.who.int/mental_health/evidence/atlas/profiles/are_mh_profile. pdf, consulted on 01.05.2016

Table 8.43 Availability of Mental Health Facilities

	Total number of facilities/ beds	Rate per 100,000 population	Number of facilities/ beds reserved for children and adolescents only	Rate per 100,000 population
Mental health outpatient Facilities	3	0.06	0	0.0
Day treatment facilities	0	0.0	NA	NA
Psychiatric beds in general hospitals	25	0.53	0	0.0
Community residential facilities	0	0.0	NA	NA
Beds/places in community residential facilities	0	0.0	NA	NA
Mental hospitals	1	0.02	0	0.0
Beds in mental hospitals	80	1.7	0	0.0

The majority of psychologists currently in the UAE have undergone a Western model of training. Despite global concerns about the limited applicability of Western psychological principles to developing world populations, the psychology of the "first" and "second" worlds is still being exported to the majority worlds with little attention to the validity or appropriateness of what is being exported to ethnically diverse populations.[721] Scholars have expressed their concerns about the compatibility of Western therapeutic models with

---

[721] Moghaddam F., Taylor D., What constitutes an "appropriate psychology" for the developing world? International Journal of Psychology, 21(1-4), 1986, pp.253-267.

the UAE's culture and values.[722] To address this challenge, an indigenous movement in psychology has been initiated internationally.[723] Practitioners and researchers participating in the movement adopt psychological treatment models that were developed in a bottom-up fashion, rather than being adapted or tweaked from foreign models. Scholars in several developing countries around the world like Mexico, Philippines, Taiwan, India, and others have endorsed the indigenous psychology approach.[724] Current professionals are overwhelmed with meeting the demands of teaching or practice, which allows little time for research. Therefore, there is an ongoing reliance on Western frameworks in providing mental health care and education.[725]

Some hospitals in UAE are specialized in providing comprehensive mental health services for both inpatients and outpatients. These are located in major cities such as Abu Dhabi, Dubai, and Ras AlKhaima. Other hospitals have outpatient clinics and units for hospitalization. These facilities are well-established and their services are professionally trusted. Other mental health services are provided within the educational settings (e.g. counseling centers, school health facility, and community mental health services). The services provided by theses agencies typically involve individual therapy, group therapy and other psychological services. There are 25 beds reserved for psychiatric patients in the general hospitals, and 80 beds available in the specialized mental hospital. Recent reports indicate that there are approximately 33,000 mental patients in the country, and new admissions to public facilities are put on waiting lists that can go up to two months. The hospitals usually lack resources (e.g. well-trained practitioners). The demands for mental health services are in the raise so is the awareness of the need for a competent mental health system in UAE. For example, the number of clients seen at the UAE University counseling center is increasing when compared with the number of clients who sought services 4 years ago when the center started providing its services to students. The clients seen at the UAE University counseling center have shown interest in receiving therapy and working with their therapist to achieve their treatment

---

[722] Al-DarmakiF., Sayed M.,Counseling challenges within the cultural context of the United Arab Emirates. International handbook of cross-cultural counseling: Cultural assumptions and practices worldwide, 2009, pp.465-474.

[723] Bhawuk D., Toward a new paradigm of psychology. In Spirituality and Indian Psychology, Springer New York, 2011, pp. 185-202.

[724] Díaz-Guerrero R., A Mexican psychology. American Psychologist, 32(11), 1977, p. 934.

[725] http://www.apa.org/international/pi/2015/06/psychology-arab.aspx, consulted on 01.05.2016

goals. Yet, there were some clients who have expressed concerns about confidentiality and interference of their parents in their treatment (i.e. refusing the referral of their children to psychiatric care).[726] The leading centers focused on the advancement of mental health field in UAE are:

National Rehabilitation Center

National Rehabilitation Center. The center provides the program for women, which utilizes the most sophisticated, evidence-based approaches to the treatment of substance abuse by integrating dialectical behavioral therapy (DBT), mentalization-based therapy (MBT), cognitive-behavioral therapy (CBT), and psycho-education programs. A core built-in component of the program is the family therapy. Most of the mental health services are provided within the hospital setting.

The Emirates Psychological Association (EPA) was established in 2003 in Dubai by the Ministry of Social Affairs. It is the only officially recognized professional association for psychologists in the UAE. EPA's mission is to raise awareness of mental health issues in the Emirates and to advocate for the public's access to mental health services. Another mission of EPA is to serve as a liaison between governmental departments and private sectors to better serve the community.

Table 8.44 Workforce and Training

	Health professionals working in the mental health sector Rate per 100,000	Training of health professions in educational institutions Rate per 100,000
Psychiatrists	0.3	UN
Medical doctors, not specialized in psychiatry	0.11	UN
Nurses	2.12	2.12
Psychologists	0.51	UN
Social workers	0.25	UN
Occupational therapists	0.04	UN
Other health workers	0.04	NA

---

[726] http://www.omicsonline.com/open-access/mental-health-services-in-the-united-arab-emirates-challenges-and-opportunities-1522-4821-1000263.php?aid=61346, consulted on 01.05.2016

Al Jalila Foundation

Al Jalila Foundation, the UAE's first independent multi-disciplinary medical research centre focuses on five of the most pressing regional health challenges: cancer, cardiovascular diseases, diabetes, obesity and mental health.[727] The Al Jalila Foundation Research Centre is set to open in 2017 in Dubai Healthcare City.

Based on WHO`s statistics from 2006, the total expenditure on health as a percentage of gross domestic product is 2.81% and the per capita government expenditure on health is 992.0 US dollars per population. Information on expenditures for medicines for mental and behavioral disorders in UAE is unavailable.

The strengths of the mental health system in UAE include:

- Available mental health act;
- Financial support from the government;
- Extensive mental health infrastructure.

And weaknesses are:

- Insufficient human resources working in the mental health sector;
- No high educational degrees in psychology provided inside the country.

The number of clients seeking professional counseling help is increasing compared with the numbers of previous years. UAE experiences a severe shortage of qualified mental health workers. And not all of those, who work in this field, have enough education and competency. In UAE the educational choices are very limited for those, who want to pursue their degree in psychology, reduced practically to UAE University and a few public ones. And none of them does not offer PhD in psychology.

YEMEN

In November 1989, for the first time in Yemen two psychologists, Dr. Maan Saleh and Mr. Ahmed Nasser, were elected to the local council of Aden (the then capital of the democratic Republic of Yemen, South Yemen). In 1991, the first woman, a psychologist Dr. Aza Ghanim, became

---

[727] http://www.aljalilafoundation.ae/who-we-are/about-us/, consulted on 01.05.2016

the Faculty of Education Dean at Sanaa University. After the unification of North and South Yemen in 1990, Ahmed Nasser won a seat in the first elected parliament in Yemen in April of 1993. In 1997 and again in 2001, two psychologists became vice presidents of the World Federation of Mental Health for the Middle East Region (Dr. Hassen Khan and Dr. Maan Saleh). In September of 2003, Professor Ahmed Al-Sofi became the first psychologist to become the Rector of the University of Taiz. And in 2004, in Beijing China, the first Yemeni psychologist and second Arab psychologist, Dr. Hassen Khan, was elected as a board member of the International Union of Psychological Sciences (IUPsyS).[728] The field of psychology in Yemen has been fortunate to receive governmental support, albeit modest, and has also benefited from human resource development projects that have enabled Yemeni students to study psychology.[729] Mental health is not specifically mentioned in the general health policy. A mental health plan doesn't exist. Dedicated mental health legislation does not exist. Legal provisions concerning mental health are not covered in other laws (e.g. welfare, disability, general health legislation etc).National Mental Health Strategy 2014-2015 is available.[730]

There is no mental health act or legislation per se.[731] Uncodified Islamic law is the de facto guide. However, the Yemeni Ministry of Public Health and Population made some strides in the legislation in the Public Health Area. The Ministry is embracing the information age and has on its website the Arabic text of laws 1996-No.32 relating to the supplementing table salt with iodide, 1999-No.60 relating to the private health establishments.[732]

Based on WHO`s statistics from 2008, in Yemen, neuropsychiatric disorders are estimated to contribute to 9.3% of the global burden of disease.

There are 0,17 psychologists and 0.21 psychiatrists per 100,000 population (see Table 8.46.)

---

[728] http://www.apa.org/international/pi/2008/05/yemen.aspx, consulted on 31.04.2016

[729] *Ibid*

[730] http://www.who.int/mental_health/evidence/atlas/profiles/yem_mh_profile.pdf, consulted on 01.07.2016

[731] http://arabpsynet.com/Archives/OP/TopicJ20NumanGharaibeh2.pdf, consulted on 01.07.2016

[732] *Ibid*

The local academic qualification programs in clinical psychology started in 2003 by Yemeni Medical board under the Ministry of Health.[733]

Table 8.45 Availability of Mental Health Facilities

	Total number of facilities/ beds	Rate per 100,000 population	Number of facilities/ beds reserved for children and adolescents only	Rate per 100,000 population
Mental health outpatient facilities	9	0.037	UN	UN
Day treatment facilities	UN	UN	UN	UN
Psychiatric beds in general hospitals	128	0.53	25	0.10
Community residential facilities	4	0.016	0	0.0
Beds/places in community residential facilities	UN	UN	UN	UN
Mental hospitals	4	0.016	0	0.0
Beds in mental hospitals	687	2.83	0	0.0

Table 8.46 Workforce and Training[734]

	Health professionals working in the mental health sector Rate per 100,000	Training of health professions in educational institutions Rate per 100,000
Psychiatrists	0.21	0.21
Medical doctors, not specialized in psychiatry	0.23	0.27

---

[733] http://slideplayer.com/slide/679600/, consulted on 01.07.2016

[734] http://www.who.int/mental_health/evidence/atlas/profiles/yem_mh_profile.pdf, consulted on 01.07.2016

Nurses	0.13	0.15
Psychologists	0.17	0.08
Social workers	0.09	0.03
Occupational therapists	0.20	0.07
Other health workers	UN	NA

Table 8.47 Expenditures for Medicines for Mental and
Behavioral Disorders at the Country Level[735]

Type of Medicines	Expenditures at country level per year and per 100,000 population (in USD)
All the psychotherapeutic medicines	UN
Medicines used for bipolar disorders	12000
Medicines for psychotic disorders	35000
Medicines used for general anxiety	21000
Medicines used for mood disorders	33000

In 2003, the Yemeni Council for Medical Specialization under the Ministry of Health established a national academic qualification program that provides for one year of post-baccalaureate training in clinical psychology. By 2007, thirty individuals from the Sana'a governorate had graduated from this program. In Aden, the first course in this training program was inaugurated in 2006. It is also worth mentioning that there are higher education programs at the Master's level in General Psychology in the Arts Faculties of Sanaa, Aden, and Thamar universities. In Yemen, there are two types of institutions, which provide educational and training experiences in psychology (see Tables 8.48. and 8.49.) Among them, there are departments of psychology and the Yemeni Medical Council, through the Ministry of Health. There are fourteen Departments of psychology, housed in Faculties of Arts, Education or Medicine in Yemeni universities, which serve the educational, research, and accredited professional development needs for the nation. A dilemma for psychology from the Yemeni point of view is that psychology is primarily found in the Faculty of Arts. There are about 45 private mental health clinics in Yemen run by psychiatrists (see Table 8.45.) Psychologists work in a limited number of these clinics, supervised by psychiatrists. Drugs and electroshock (ECT) are the typical treatments in these setting. A few work within a collective

---

[735] *Ibid*

therapeutic team model. Unfortunately, there are no designated clinics for children. The clinical diagnosis and assessment are not standardized. The psychological tools that are available generally have been translated into Arabic and have been adapted by Egyptian psychologists. Thus, the majority of cases are diagnosed based on the individual knowledge and experience of each clinician. Successfully treating mental illness often involves the use of psychopharmacologic drugs (prescribed by psychiatrists and, in rural areas, by psychologists). While effective, the use of such medications is limited in the Yemeni situation, as they are unaffordable for most patients. The use of ECT remains widespread. Unfortunately, there are few programs and evidence-based models for treatment that are proven effective and appropriate for the culture. There are individual settings, however, where the institutional or individual initiative has led to the establishment of models that demonstrate the potential and effectiveness of psychological services in the Yemeni context. These include psychological counseling services sponsored by the Yemeni Mental Health Association in collaboration with schools and universities.

Table 8.48 Yemeni Psychologists by Degree and Employment Area[736]

Field	Degree			
	PhD	**MSc/MA**	**BSc/BA**	**Total**
Academic	45	45	49	139
Education	2	20	135	157
Health	4	35	25	64
Social Services	0	9	22	31
Other	0	50	850	900
Unemployed	0	0	2289	2289
Total	51	159	3370	3580

Telephone Hotline of the Mental Health Unit of
the Cultural Health Center Sanaa

This service is operated by the Cultural Health Center established in 1996 by the talented physician, artist, and poet, Dr. Nazar Ghanim in Sanaa in 1996. The Center ceased to function due to a financial deficit

---

[736] http://www.apa.org/international/pi/2008/05/yemen.aspx, consulted on 31.04.2016

in 1999 but reopened in May 2006. There is also a clinic for emotional guidance that is part of the Center and is currently headed by a psychologist.

Hotline Telephone for Psychological Aid (Aden)

This mental health tele-counseling service, established in 2000, is affiliated with the Yemeni Mental Health Association in partnership with the Faculty of Medicine and Health Sciences of Aden University. This service is the first officially documented service of its type in an Arab country. Five well trained and experienced psychologists work in shifts along with the President of the Association. As of 2007, the number of calls received numbered 4,072 of which 72% were from female callers. The distribution of calls according to problem type was: 6% family violence, 9% emotional problems, 4% sexual concerns, 10% disturbances of childhood and adolescence, 10% school difficulties, 35% mental disorders (e.g. schizophrenia, mental retardation), and 26% a variety of other problems.[737]

Table 8.49 Departments of Psychology in Yemeni Universities[738]

University	Faculty	Founding Date	Number of Faculty Members	Male	Female
Sana's	Art	1983	18	4	14
Sana's	Education	1975	12	8	4
Aden	Education	1970	12	6	6
Aden	Medicine	1975	5	3	2
Aden	Art	1999	8	5	3
Taiz	Education	1994	9	6	3
Taiz	Art	2003	3	2	1
Hadramut	Education	1975	10	7	3
Al-Hudaida	Education	1997	15	7	8
Thamar	Art	2000	7	6	1
Ibb	Education	1997	20	18	2
Total			119	72	47

---

[737] http://www.apa.org/international/pi/2008/05/yemen.aspx, consulted on 01.07.2016

[738] *Ibid*

School Behavioral Counseling Program

This program was established by the Yemeni Mental Health Association in 2002. It partners the Association with the Education Office of the Aden governorate and reflects a crucial goal of the Association to be responsive to the community with respect to social service issues. The program team consists of ten psychologists and social work specialists with extensive professional experience. The problems of the more than 1200 pupils served in the years between 2002 and 2006 were 66.8% emotional-behavioral, 24.1% educational, 0.9% sexual, and 8.1% school discipline.[739]

Hotline Telephone for Psychosocial and Legal Support (Sanaa)

This service, run by the Arab Human Rights Institution, was established in March of 2002. It is located in the capital city of Sanaa. The Institution operates with a team of four psychologists.

Educational and Psychological Counseling Center (Sanaa University)

This Center was established to serve students in September of 2005 with an academic and administrative team consisting of 16 individuals headed by a psychologist. Ten specialists also provide services (treatment and diagnosis) to students on a daily basis. In addition, the Center offers training courses, organizes cultural and scientific sessions, and provides consultation to mental health clinics.

Student Counseling Center (Taiz University)

The Student Counseling Center was established in May of 2006 and is located on the campus of the College of Education and provides services mainly to students but sometimes to family members. Its team consists of 17 psychologists headed by a psychologist. In its short existence, the center has provided guidance services to 155 students, male and female. The distribution of problems was: 45.1% social, 12.2% academic, 38% emotional, and 3.2% special needs.

---

[739] http://www.apa.org/international/pi/2008/05/yemen.aspx, consulted on 01.07.2016

National Mental Health Program

The National Mental Health Program was established in the late 1980s with the help of the World Health Organization (WHO) and the Ministries of Health from the North and South Yemeni governments at the time. The project concentrated on treatment in mental hospitals and on the care of mentally ill patients by qualified psychiatrists. The National Mental Health Program was established in response to recommendations put forward by the first National Workshop on Mental Health in Yemen, organized in cooperation with the International Committee of the Red Cross in October 2002. A mental health program was established by ministerial resolution was then administered as a component of the primary health care division in the Ministry of Health. The administration consists of four psychologists headed by a psychologist. In Yemen, NGOs that are chiefly focused on mental health have increased in quantity and quality since the establishment of a new Associations Law in 2001 that permitted the formation of professional organizations. According to a 2006 report there were six associations in the country headed by psychologists, comprising a membership of 1,235.[740] Most of the associations are new and struggling under a number of obstacles; nonetheless, they continue to advocate for and provide services. In the past few years, these associations have played influential roles in the campaign to combat physical, mental, and sexual violence against women and children. They have also organized celebrations for International Mental Health Day, conferences, workshops, seminars, publishing endeavors, radio and television programs, and contributions to journals and magazines through articles in psychology. Finally, they have advocated for the establishment of a formal code of ethics for psychologists, often at great personal and emotional expense that is little acknowledged and commended.[741]

Stemming from the WHO`s statistics from 2008, the total expenditure on health as a percentage of the gross domestic product is 5.63% and the per capita government expenditure on health (PPP int) is 47.0 US dollars. Expenditures for medicines for mental and behavioral disorders at the country level can be consulted at the Table 7.47.

There are two bi-annual journals published by YPA (twenty volumes), another by the Doctor and Clinical Psychologists Association (DCPA)

---

[740] Maan A., Experience of Mental Health Association in Yemen, Journal of Social Science, Aden University, 22, 2008, pp.55-62.

[741] http://www.apa.org/international/pi/2008/05/yemen.aspx, consulted on 01.07.2016

(three volumes), and two newsletters published periodically by the YMHA (thirty volumes). The Aden Central Psychiatric Hospital has also published ten newsletters. The main obstacles to publishing and printing are financial resources and the lack of technical facilities for actual printing and dissemination. Research in psychology and mental health is not well developed, mainly because of a lack of research capacity and the absence of research institutions in psychology and other mental health-related fields[742]. Most of the research in psychology is carried out at Yemeni universities by graduate (PhD and MA) students and teaching faculty. The YPA and the YMHA have taken an active role in launching research initiatives and community surveys related to a variety of mental health-related issues including violence against women and children, Qat addiction and behavior, female genital mutilation, and suicide. Lack of sustainable funding remains one of the biggest drawbacks to undertaking research.

The strengths of the Yemeni mental health system include:

- Absence of legislative mandate to encourage and coordinate mental health activities;
- No methodical up-to-date database on the mental health statistics.

Its weaknesses:

- The academic program training and accreditation of professionals are insufficient;
- Insufficient funding;

Psychology is only emerging in Yemen. Until the country develops its own research knowledge base and ensures the quality of delivering psychological services, it is not possible to speak of a properly functioning mental health system. The reconceptualization of the Yemeni mental field requires active collaboration with the regional and international organizations, as well as adaptation of foreign experience to the Yemeni clinical landscape.

---

[742] http://www.apa.org/international/pi/2008/05/yemen.aspx, consulted on 01.07.2016

PART II

THE STRUCTURE OF
MUSLIM PSYCHE

CHAPTER 9

COLLECTIVE ETHNOCONSCIOUSNESS

In The Division of Labour, Durkheim maintained that in traditional/ tribal societies totemic religion played a fundamental role in uniting members by creating the collective consciousness. Arabic ethnoconsciousness is what links a modern Arab to his/her primal ancestor. It is deeply rooted in pre-Islamic worldview and affects the self-perception and that of the world. Ghorbal distinguishes two dimensions in the Arabo-Muslim personality: one collective and the other individual. The first one is marked by an imprint of Arabicity and Islamicity (the domain of being), whilst the second is influenced by personal development (the domain of having). Any access to the individual domain should pass through the community domain.[743] The lineage of the main prophets, who are mentioned by Quran, is given in the Chart 9.1.

---

[743] https://www.cairn.info/revue-topique-2010-1-page-41.htm, consulted on 01.07.2016

Chart 9.1 Lineage of Six Imminent Prophets
(*Dotted lines indicate numerous generations*)

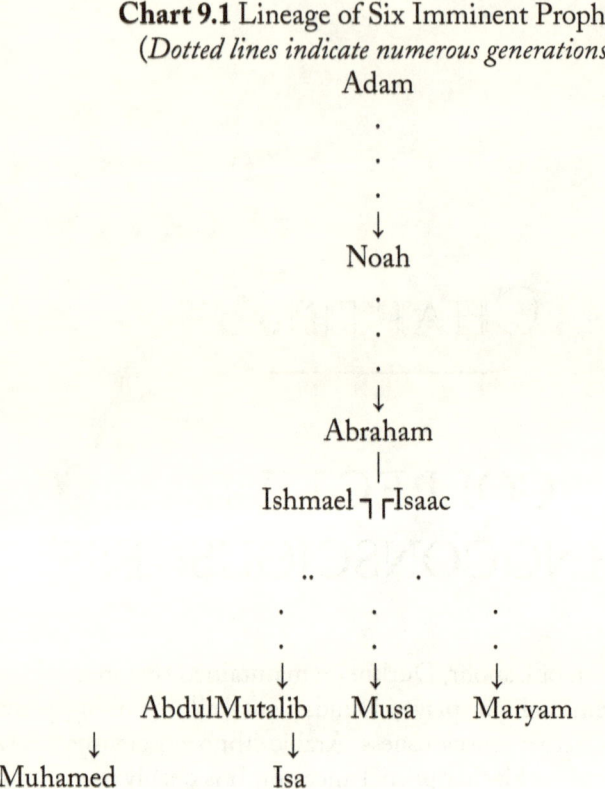

Ishmael's genealogical line descends to his son Kedar, then down to Adnan, then to the Mustariba, and Muhamed from Quraysh.

The data gathered in this chapter suggests that there exist certain fundamental elements that constitute the conception of Arabic ethnoconciousness, and, therefore, can be ranked within the following signifiers: The Other Woman-Claim of Identity-Reliance on God-Sacrifice. The return to the other woman (Hagar) and her consequent exclusion from the formal order occurs as soon as she becomes a threat to the formal order. Hagar is the foreigner who remains out of the Islamic reading. Hagar's story is a refusal of origin that led to a total denial inside the entire religion. The other woman becomes the source of double jouissance: she is clairvoyant, and her body prevents the official wife, Sara, from accessing the phallic jouissance.

The questioning of the Arabic identity continues with the story of Abdullah and Amina, who conceive their child, Mohamed, as it was ordered by Abd Al Mutalib, the father of the latter. On the way to his wife Abdullah meets Ruqiyah, a clairvoyant prostitute, who invites him to her house. However, Abdullah rejects because he was accompanied by his father. As soon as the Prophet was conceived, Abdullah returns and meets Ruqiyah again, and evokes her suggestion. However, this time, she is the one who rejects. She said that she was no longer seeing a glow between his eyebrows, which was there at the beginning (meaning: a sign of conceiving a future Prophet). This representation draws such signifiers as Father's Order-Obeyance-Other Woman-Rejection-Birth of Prophet-Revelation. If in the first case, the Other woman (Hagar) was chosen, in the second, the Other woman (Ruqiyah) was rejected.

Even though the primal ancestor of all Arabs, Abraham, did not belong to any religion, he himself was a Hernif, therefore, worshipping one God. Sarah, an official wife of Abraham, was not capable of giving birth to a child, so she offered her servant, Hagar to her husband. And this is a momentous decision of Sarah, who wants Hagar to give her a child. Sarah lends Hagar the gift of bearing her child to overcome the lack of God in her, as she was after all a prostitute.[744] There thus emerges a master-slave dialectic whereby the master agrees to form his lack into jouissance, while the slave remains in the flesh.[745] From this union, Ishmael was born, who became the first son of Abraham. However, Sarah was not ready to tolerate the other woman with a child at her home. So, Abraham was forced to expel Hagar and Ishmael from the house and leave them at the desert. Abandoned with a small child and water left for two days only, Hagar inquired Abraham, who he was entrusting herself and his son to. Abraham replied that he was entrusting them to God. So, Hagar obeyed the God's will. She went in search of water. Distressed, she was running back and forth seven times between the hills of Al-Safa and Al-Marwa. Upon her return, Hagar saw Ishmael scratching the ground with his heel, from where the water began flowing. This water spring became known as Zamzam, and the place - Mecca. At some point, a nomadic tribe Jurhum was passing by and they saw birds circling above the water, so they asked Hagar's permission to settle down, which she allowed.

Islamic tradition narrates that one night Abraham had a horrific dream as if God ordered him to sacrifice Ishmael. When Abraham confined this to Ishmael, the son accepted the God's will. As Abraham attempted to kill Ishmael, God addressed to Abraham attesting to the fact that he had fulfilled the command, and that Ishmael's sacrifice can be replaced

---

[744] http://www.academia.edu/3480874/Psychoanalysis_and_the_Veil_in_Islam_Rethinking_Truth_and_Liberation_Review_of_Fethi_Benslamas_Islam_and_the_Challenge_of_Psychoanalysis, consulted on 01.07.2016

[745] *Ibid*

by a ram. Immediately following the sacrifice ritual, Abraham received a message of the upcoming Isaac's birth. The news about the ardently-expected pregnancy of Sarah is underlined by its symbolic sense: Abraham renounces from something so that to receive something else in return. Having received the grace from God, Sarai becomes Sarah and Abram becomes Abraham: "To confirm His promise God changed the name of Abram to Abraham, and of Sarai to Sarah" (Genesis 17; 18). Both received the letter "h" in their names as the accomplishment of a promise of ancestorship of many nations. The original name Abram means a "high, or honored father," whilst Abraham means "a father of many nations". The name Sarai means "princely", whilst Sarah stands for "the princess" with its sacramental symbolic meaning of the spiritual seed.

The other day Abraham received a message from Allah stating that he and Ishmael should construct the Kaaba, "God's house", near the Well of Zamzam. The foundation stone for the Kaaba was delivered from heaven. Today this black stone is preserved in a corner of the Kabaa. When Abraham was constructing the praying house, he stood on a large rock, which Allah made soft, so that the shape of Abraham's feet would depict onit.

After his mother died, Ishmael married a woman from the Jurhum, the tribe, with who he had grown up. Once Abraham decided to render a visit to Ishmael in Mecca, however, he did not find the son at his home. Instead, Ishmael's wife came to greet Abraham. She was inhospitable and was complaining all the time. When leaving, Abraham passed a message through her to Ishmael telling to change "the threshold of his door". When Ishmael returned home, he interpreted the father's advice as that meaning to divorce his wife. Later he got married with another woman from Jurhum. Abraham once again visited Ishmael and was welcomed by Ishmael's second wife, as Ishmael himself was out. The wife was generous and offered him some treats. Abraham was pleased with "the threshold of the door", about which he notified Ishmael through his wife. When Ishmael arrived, he understood that his father meant that he should keep his wife.

The legends of Arabs' origins seem to suggest that Islam passes through a full symbolization of the real (repudiation, sacrifice etc), thus, becoming a religion of the Absolute, which was sublimated at its foundation. The God is the only solution since the origins are repudiated. Islam derivates from the foreign, being at the origins of monotheism, remains foreign in Islam[746]. The mechanism of disavowal is not about the

[746] http://www.slp-web.org/les-publications/les-articles-en-ligne/letrangere-et-son-desarroi, consulted on 01.07.2016

truth, as it is the case of denial. It does not reveal the action of negation or refusal, to recognize as it should what belongs to the register of desire. It is no longer the repudiation, which consists in repulsing of what has been accepted initially. But it gives a place to a saying that does not recognize the belonging. However, the effacing of the ancestor mother, her name and her existence from the founding text, the Quran, whilst many other protagonists of the same story are preserved there, leads to the conclusion that Islam is originally installed in the disavowal of Hagar.

Structurally, the jouissance of the primal father in all monotheisms requires that the father kills the son, which does not happen in Islam. Despite this, the essence of sacrifice is fundamentally inscribed into the logic of being a Muslim. That is to say, acceptance of one's own castration: the impossibility of having everything at the same time. Judaism was a religion of father, Christianity is a religion of son[747]. Islam is not a religion of father, nor that of the son. For instance, Benslama drew a line in Islam between the primal father and the Father-of-Genesis, the primal father is one rooted in unlimited jouissance and radical alterity. The intense and unruly jouissance of the primal father must be repudiated to allow for libidinal relations to function. Benslama argues like Freud did in Moses and Monotheism that it was Ishmael, the familial founder of Islam who was declared a part of the Arab tradition by the prophet's speech act – this act is what evokes the core dilemma of alterity that the primal father brings about for any community.Thus it was agreed: God alone is strong and good, man is weak and sinful."[748]According to Freud, therefore, the authoritarian Father-God corresponds to human childhood.[749]

Malaikat

Belief in the existence of angels is a part of the Islamic religion. In Arabic, angels are called malaika, which means "to assist". They are believed to be of large size, with wings, and from the nature of light. Quran says: "Praise be to Allah, Who created (out of nothing) the heavens and the earth, Who made the angels messengers with wings - two, or three, or four (pairs) adds to Creation as He pleases: for Allah has power over all things" (sura 35, ayat 1).

---

[747] Freud Sigmund, *Moses and monotheism*,Eastford:Martino Fine Books, 2010, p.51.

[748] Freud Sigmund,*The Future of an Illusion*, New York:W.W. Norton & Company, 1961, p. 48.

[749] *Ibid, p. 55.*

There is a strong Quranic basis to view angels as the elements of sublimation and symbols of renunciation of the personal ego. Since angels are asexual and do not reproduce, they are void of instincts, desires, and, therefore, a lack. They are complete and different from humans. The angle's sole role is to fulfill the message of Allah in the capacity of guardian of the divine order. Angels vary in their forms and nature of their responsibilities. The exact number of them is unknown.

Types of Angels

The Quran mention such angels as:

Jibril or Gabriel/Jibreel means "God is my strength", transmits revelations from Allah to the Prophets: "Say: Whoever is an enemy to Jibreel - for he brings down the (revelation) to your heart by Allah's will, a confirmation of what went before, and guidance and glad tidings to those who believe - Whoever is an enemy to Allah, and His angels and prophets, to Jibreel and Mikail - Lo! Allah is an enemy to those who reject faith" (sura 2, ayats 97-98).

Israfil or Raphael means "God heals" or "the Burning One". For the first time he blows the trumpet to announce the Qiyamat (end of the world) and for the second time to resurrect everyone for the judgement of Allah. The Quran says: "And the trumpet shall be blown, so all those that are in the heavens and all those that are in the earth shall swoon, except Allah; then it shall be blown again, then they shall stand up awaiting" (sura 39, ayat 68).

Mikail or Michael/Mikaeel/Mikhaeel means "who is like God?", is the angel, who brings prosperity, including, nourishment, rain, etc.

Izrail, or Azrael/Izraeel means "whom God helps", is the angel of death, who expels the soul from the dead body as soon as the person dies.

Kiraaman-Kaatibin or the Honourable Recorders, also called Raqib and Atid. While one of them notes down the good deeds of a human, the other writes the bad ones. Their book of deeds is revised twice a day, during Fajr and Asr; and once a year, during Nisfu Syaban.

Munkar and Nakir interrogate the dead in the grave with the three questions, which are:

Who is your Lord?

Who is your Prophet?

What is your Religion?

If the righteous Muslim answers the questions correctly (based on his/her deeds during the lifetime), then the time left awaiting the Resurrection will be pleasant. If not, the hadiths say that the bodies shall be wrapped by a large snake even before being buried. Abu narrated: "The Messenger of Allah said, "When the deceased is buried (or he said: when one of you is buried), there come to him two blue-black angels, one of whom is called Munkar and the other Nakeer. They ask him, "What did you use to say about this man?" and he says what he used to say: "He is the slave and Messenger of Allah: I bear witness that there is no god except Allah and that Muhammad is the slave and Messenger of Allah. They say, "We knew beforehand that you used to say this." Then his grave will be widened for him to a size of seventy cubits by seventy cubits and it will be illuminated for him. Then they tell him, "Sleep." He says, "Go back to my family and tell them." They tell him, "Sleep like a bridegroom whom no-one will wake up except his most beloved" until Allah raises him up. If (the deceased) was a hypocrite, he says, "I heard the people saying something, so I said something similar. I do not know." They say, "We knew beforehand that you used to say this." The earth will be told to squeeze him, so he will be crushed until his ribs are interlocked, and he will remain like that until Allah raises him up."

Ridwan is the Keeper of heaven. Quran declares, "And those who kept their duty to their Lord will be led to Paradise in groups, till, when they reach it, its gates will be opened and its keepers will say: Salamun alaikum (peace be upon you!). You have done well, so enter here, to abide therein." (sura 39, ayat 73).

Maalik is the Keeper of hell. He is assisted by nineteen guardians of hell (Zabaniyah). Allah says, "They [the people in Hell] will cry: "O Malik! Would that your Lord put an end to us!" (sura 43, ayat 77).

Dardail is the angel who flies above the earth in search of assemblies where people evoke God's name.

Muaqqibat refers to a class of guardian angels who protect people from death until the decreed time comes.

Belief in angels is an integral part of the Islamic faith. In therapy Muslims oftentimes mention "seeing" or "talking" to angels. It is wrong to consider such confessions instantly as a symptom of delusional psychosis, but they are rather to be interpreted in the context of cultural specificity.

Jinns

The Jinn are a world of their own, different from that of the humans or the angels[750]. They are called jinn because they are obscured from human

---

[750] Zarabozo Jamal, *The World of Jinn and Devils*. Boulder: Al-Basheer Publications & Translations, 1998, p. 5.

sight.[751] "Lo! He sees you, he and his tribe, from whence you see him not" (sura 7, ayat 27). There is no doubt that the jinns were created before mankind,[752] as Allah says, "Verily We created man of pottery's clay of dark mud altered. And the Jinn did We create aforetime of a flameless fire" (sura 15, ayat 26-27).The jinns live upon the same earth as humans do.[753]

The world of the jinn is a separate universe which has its distinctive features imperceptible to humans. They have a capacity for spiritual and mental influence on mankind (psychic control, possessions), however, do not necessarily apply it. Jinns share with humans the reason, understanding and the ability to opt between good or evil. They are called jinns because of their invisibility. There exist male and female jinns and they reproduce in a sexual way. Like humans, they are organized into kingdoms, states, tribes, nations, they have their own laws and religions.In the hadith transmitted by Muslim, Aisha reported that the Prophet said: "The angels were created from light, the jinns were created from fire and Adam was created, as it was described to you." The jinn is a derivate word for "majnoun", which in Arabic means "insane". The other same root words comprise:

Janin – fetus, meaning that it is always hidden;

Jénéna – garden;

Jenna - paradise;

Janan – grave.

Also in Arabic an insane person can be called as :

madroub: "struck" (by jinn);

markoub: "ridden"(by jinn);

maskoun: "inhabited"(by jinn);

mamlouk:"possessed"– not solely in a sense of possessing, but also being an owner of a place, apartment (by jinn);

masloukh: "bitten to blood" (by jinn);

malbouss: "worn" (by jinn)– as a piece of clothes, and many other examples.

Along similar lines, the name "jinn" is to be interpreted in an association with madness. In Arabic folklore jinn is attributed with powers, which are capable of causing mental illness, thus, he/she is a primary responsible for insanity. In psychoanalytical interpretation, jinn is an image of unknown, an illness itself. Jinn stands on the side of desire.

Allah has created several categories of jinns. Some of them can take on various forms, such as those of a dog or a snake. According to Abu al

---

[751] *Ibid*

[752] *Ibid, p. 6.*

[753] *Ibid, p. 24.*

Thalabah Khoushani, the Messenger of Allah said: "The jinns are of three categories: the category that has wings and can fly into the air, the category that appears in a form of a snake or a dog, and the category that can settle down or displace."Al-Shaykh al-Bani said," It was narrated by al-Shaykh Abu Tahhawi and as an authentic chain that each human is accompanied by a jinn. In this regard, Ibn Masud reported that the Messenger of Allah said, "There is none among you who does not have a companion from among the jinn."

- Even you, O Messenger of Allah?
- Even I,-the Prophet answered adding: but Allah supported me against my jinn companion and he converted to Islam and instructs me only good."

Allah has given the jinn capabilities that humans do not possess, and He told us about some aspects of their abilities such as speed of movement and displacement.[754] One jinn pledged to the Prophet Solomon that he would bring the throne of the Queen of Yemen in Jerusalem in less then a couple of seconds, just the time needed to rise from one`s place. Quran says: "O Council, which one of you will bring me her throne, before they come to me in surrender" (sura 27, ayat 39). The jinns live on the same earth as humans, in the abandoned and unclean places, such as toilets, dumps and cemeteries.The Quran teaches the Muslims the words of protection against the jinns: "And say, My Lord, I seek refuge in You from the incitements of the devils, And I seek refuge in You, my Lord, lest they be present with me." (sura 23, ayats 97-98)

In Arabic language, people do not say have "a memory like an elephant", but "a memory of jinn". The tradition reports the existence of more then seventy types of jinns, among which there are:

Asheq jinns are jinn-lovers, who transmit their sexual thoughts and desires to the possessed person.

Ghawas jinns dwell the waters.

Tayyar jinns take on a shape of birds. They are very mobile and can tour around the earth in two minutes. Shaytan, who is the jinn`s ancestor, belonged to this category of jinns.

Kadmoul Amar jinns live in dirty places.

Maqabir jinns live at the cemeteries.

---

[754] http://www.psmag.com/books-and-culture/edge-of-the-arabian-desert-the-jinn-of-oman, consulted on 21.09.2016

Amirou Beit jinns at the houses, where a man and a woman often argue.

Djallabou Attabir jinns are eager for prestige and wealth.

Attifou Nadjom jinns are jinns-children, who possess children, and sometimes, adults transforming their behaviour into infantile.

Khadimou Sirrou jinns are associates of witchcraft, and they are of two categories: Oulouwi and Soufli.

Philosophers jinns possess the scientists.

Ifrits are made of fire and dwell the earth.

Marid or blue jinns are rebellious and the most powerful jinns. In reference to this type of jinn Quran says: "They call upon instead of Him none but female [deities], and they [actually] call upon none but a rebellious Satan" (sura 4, ayat 117). It is also believed that the blue jinns were involved in a war against angels. According to the Islamic religion, when Allah ordered them to leave the human world because they had to submit it to Adam, the blue jinnsrebelled and fought for their right to stay in the human world. In the end, it is said that this war lasted a millennium, and the Angels eventually overtook the blue jinns.

Green jinns are considered to be the youngest and the weakest. Their colour is not green, that is a metaphoric reference to their place in jinn's hierarchy. They can be childish and vengeful, and, most of the time, cruel. It is believed that the green jinns enter the human world out of curiosity. One of the common Islamic assumption is that they live in holes. It is also believed that these holes lead into a subterranean jinn world.

Red jinns bring destruction under the command of Iblis. They usually manifest themselves in a form of reptiles.

Black jinns are thought of as the rulers of blue jinns. The Testament of Solomon says that at the side of King Solomon, there was a black jinn. King Solomon had total control over him, and whenever a green or a blue jinn disobeyed, it was the black jinn's responsibility to punish them.

Yellow jinns are reclusive not only from humankind but from their own kind as well, a kind of hermits in their world.

In Arabic dictionary, a word "jinn" is found as a derivative root for mental illness. It is not surprising, as the folkloric tradition has been referring to "jinns" anything unknown, including madness.

Devil

In Arabic devil means Iblis, which derives from the verbal root "balasa" (he despaired). Shaytan, which is another word for devil, derives from "shatana", meaning "the far thing"; or from "shata", which means "burned". On this subject Quran says: "And He created the jinn from a smokeless flame of fire" (sura 55, ayat 15). Some scholars believe that Iblis is the father of all of jinns, just as Adam is the father of all of humans, as mentioned in sura "Al-Kahf": "Will you then take him and his progeny as protectors rather than Me? And they are enemies to you!"

Upon his creation, Iblis lived among the angels in the heavens and obeyed Allah. He entered Paradise[755]. Iblis turned into Satan after defying the Allah`s command to prostrate in front of Adam. Iblis did not obey the symbolic order and was expelled. Thus, Iblis was cast out from Jannah. He asked to postpone his punishment until the Judgement Day, and avowed to make mankind fall. Allah`s answer followed that Iblis would not be able to mislead the righteous believers, and those, who support him would be punished in Hell. Satan was not rejected for immorality, but for questioning the divine order.

On the basis of sura 14, ayat 22 and sura 20, ayat 120 it seems fair to conclude that (on the Judgement Day) the devil has no authority over the believers, and the only thing that he did was "daaawtakum" (enticing), or "yuwaswis" (whispering in the ear). This is the only thing that the devil is able to to do to humans. And no allusion can be found in the Quran implying that hardship comes from the devil, but for the words announced by Ayoub, who was erroneously believing that the devil was purposefully burdening him. The image of Satan emerges in the following hadiths:

- It is recorded in Sahih Muslim that Abu Dharr said that the Messenger of Allah said: "The woman, the donkey and the black dog interrupt the prayer (if they pass in front of those who do not pray behind a Sutrah, i.e. a barrier). Abu Dharr said, "I said, What is the difference between the black dog and the red or yellow dog." He said, "The black dog is a devil" (Hadith Bukhari, 2:245);
- Narrated by Abdullah: A person was mentioned before the Prophet and he was told that he had kept on sleeping till morning and had not got up for the prayer. The Prophet said, "Satan urinated in his ears" (Hadith Bukhari, 4:516);
- Narrated by Abu Huraira: the Prophet said, "If anyone of you rouses from sleep and performs the ablution, he should wash his nose by putting water in it and then blowing it out thrice, because Satan has stayed in the upper part of his nose all the night" (Hadith Bukhari, 4:509);

---

[755] Zarabozo Jamal, *The World of Jinn and Devils*. Boulder: Al-Basheer Publications & Translations, 1998, p. 13.

- Narrated by Abu Huraira: Allah's Apostle said, "Satan puts three knots at the back of the head of any of you if he is asleep. On every knot he reads and exhales the following words, "The night is long, so stay asleep." When one wakes up and remembers Allah, one knot is undone; and when one performs ablution, the second knot is undone, and when one prays the third knot is undone and one gets up energetic with a good heart in the morning; otherwise one gets up lazy and with a mischievous heart." (Hadith Muslim, 1:634);
- Narrated by Jabir: I heard the Messenger of Allah saying: "Do not eat with your left hand, because Satan eats and drinks with his left hand" (Hadith Muslim).

In terms of physical appearance, Satan is extremely ugly. Allah compares the branches of the tree of Zuqqum in Hell to the heads of the devils. Allah says, "Is it better as a welcome, or the tree of Zaqqum? Lo! We have appointed it a torment for wrong-doers. Lo! It is a tree that springs in the heart of hell. Its crop is as it were the heads of the devils" (sura 37, ayats 62-65).

Shayateen can reproduce. Allah alludes to that in sura Kahf when mentioning Iblis and "his offspring"; as well as in sura Rahman, which says that there will be those in heaven whom no human nor jinn has touched, and also in numerous ayats where He talks about creating things in pairs and having spouses from among themselves. Allah evokes that devils die as well, for example, in sura Fussilat, meaning they do reproduce to keep their kind alive somehow. The devils accompany some animals, such as camels[756].Verily the camel has been created from devils. And behind every camel there is a devil[757]. Islamic mythology reveals the names of other kinds of demons, including: Azazel, Ghaddar, Al-Awar, Al-Mukhannats, Ghul, Maswath, Taaghout, Thubar, Tsabar, Ummu Syibyan, Zalnabur and others.In some early Islamic accounts, Iblis was once a powerful angel named Azazel[758]. God tells Moses that his brother Aaron should take two goats and sacrifice them: one to the Lord for sins and the second to Azazel, and send it to the wilderness. Devil appears to be on the side of seduction and realization of desire.

---

[756] Zarabozo Jamal,*The World of Jinn and Devils*. Boulder: Al-Basheer Publications & Translations, 1998, p. 26.

[757] *Ibid*

[758] Rosemary Ellen Guiley, ImbrognoPhilip, *The Vengeful Djinn*, Woodbury: Llewellyn Publications, 2011, pp. 17-18.

The Connection between Angels, Jinns and Demons

The book The Vengeful Djinn by Rosemary Ellen Guiley and Philip Imbrogno structuralized the knowledge available about the jinns, angels and demons, which can be found in the Table 9.1.

Table 9.1 The Differences between Jinns, Angels and Demons

JINNS	ANGELS	DEMONS
Have gender	Have no gender	Shape their gender
Live for thousands of years, eventually die into oblivion	Live until the end of the universe	Live longer than humans, eventually die and wither to their primordial state
Had original ties to angels	Closest beings to God	Had original ties to angels
Outcasted from God's favor	Enjoy God's favor	Outcasted from God's favor
Inhabit dirty, polluted places	Inhabit heavenly realms	Inhabit dirty, polluted places
Eat and drink	Do not eat or drink	Eat and drink
Organized in families and clans	Organized in hierarchies of powers and duties	Organized like the military
Have sex with each other	Do not have sex with each other	Have sex with each other
Shape to any form	Shape to any form	Shape to any form
Usually invisible unless they choose to be seen	Usually invisible unless they are directed to be seen	Usually invisible unless they are directed to be seen
Follow their own wills; some of the will of Iblis; converted follow the will of Allah	Follow the will of God	Follow the will of Satan
Are self-managed; some serve Iblis whilst others are submissive to Allah	Duty is to glorify God	Duty is to subvert humans
Do not speak directly to God	Speak directly to God	Do not speak directly to God
Deceitful	Messengers of God	Deceitful
Opportunistic interference in human affairs	No intervention without direction from God	Opportunistic interference in human affairs
Cause illness, bad luck, misfortune	Provide support and help	Cause illness, bad luck, misfortune

Possess humans and animals	Do not cause possession	Possess humans and animals
Can enter dreams	Can enter dreams	Can enter dreams
Knowledge of present and past but not future	Knowledge of past, present, and future	Knowledge of past, present, and future

Angels, jinns, devil are inherent signifiers of the Arabic unconscious. Even though they are unstable, they are transferable and create a specific dimension of its own.

Hyenas

None of the statements regarding dogs are found in Quran, however, the hadiths refer to them as of "impure". Per Muhammad's order, all dogs of black color were killed. Maimuna reported that one morning Allah's Messenger was silent with grief. Maimuna said, "Allah's Messenger, I find a change in your mood today."[759] Allah's Messenger said, "Gabriel had promised me that he would meet me tonight, but he did not meet me. By Allah, he never broke his promises," and Allah's Messenger spent the day in this sad mood. Then it occurred to him that there had been a puppy under their cot. He commanded and it was turned out. He then took some water in his hand and sprinkled it at that place. When it was evening Gabriel met him and he said to him:

"You promised me that you would meet me the previous night." He said, "Yes, but we do not enter a house in which there is a dog or a picture." Then on that very morning, he commanded the killing of the dogs until he announced that the dog kept for the orchards should also be killed, but he spared the dog meant for the protection of extensive fields or big gardens.

Hyenas, as well as snakes, are one of those figures, which belong simultaneously to the register of Real and Symbolic, unlike the figures of angels and jinns, which remain purely in the Imaginary register. Hyena, like any dog, is a symbolic image of impurity in Islam. Muslims avoid keeping dogs as domestic animals. Especially, a black dog is a given (by culture) object of projection of the Bad Self, obscene Self. In Islam, a dog is strongly dissociated from the positive qualities, which it personifies, for example, in the Western culture. Undoubtedly, an image of a black dog agitates the personal fears and at the same time embodies them. It could happen that a Muslim panics upon sight of a black dog or a snake, which

---

[759] Payeur Bernard, *Getting to Know Allah*, Raleigh: Lulu, 2015, p.223.

can be interpreted as a strong religious-symbolic sign transmitted to him/her.

Jannah (Paradise)

The description of Paradise follows in Quran as of the place, full of rivers of milk, rivers of wine and rivers of pure honey. The Quran precises: "For them will be every kind of fruit and forgiveness form their Lord" (sura 47, ayat 15). Then it follows: "And their recompense shall be Paradise, and silken garments because they were patient. Reclining on raised thrones, they will see there neither the excessive heat of the sun nor the excessive bitter cold, (as in Paradise there is no sun and no moon). The shade will be close upon them, and bunches of fruit will hang low within their reach. Vessels of silver and cups of crystal will be passed around amongst them, crystal-clear, made of silver. They will determine the measure of them according to their wishes. They will be given a cup (of wine) mixed with Zanjabeel, and a fountain called Salsabeel. Around them will (serve) boys of perpetual youth. If you see them, you would think they are scattered pearls. When you look there (in Paradise) you will see a delight (that can not be imagined), and a Great Dominion. Their garments will be of fine green silk and gold embroidery. They will be adorned with bracelets of silver, and their Lord will give them a pure drink" (sura 76, ayats 12-21). The Holy Book adds: "And those foremost (In Tawheed and obedience to Allah and His Messenger in this life) will be foremost (in Paradise). They will be those nearest to Allah in the Gardens of Delight. A multitude of those (the foremost) will be from the first generation (who embraced Islam) and a few of those (the foremost) will be from the later (generations). They will be reclining, face to face, on thrones woven with gold and precious stones. They will be served by immortal boys, with cups and jugs, and a glass from the flowing wine, from which they will have neither a headache, nor intoxication. They will have fruit from which they may choose, and the flesh of fowls that they desire. There will be Houris with wide, lovely eyes (as wives for the pious), like preserved pearls, a reward for deeds that they used to do. They will hear no vain or sinful speech (like backbiting, etc.) but only the saying of "Salam, Salam" (greetings of peace). And those on the Right Hand, who will be those on the Right Hand? They will be among thorn-less lote-trees among Talh (banana trees) with fruits piled one above another, in the long-extended shade, by constantly flowing water, and fruit in plenty, whose season is not limited, and their supply will not be cut off. They will be on couches or thrones raised high. Verily, We have created for them (maidens) of equal age, loving (their husbands only). For those on the Right Hand" (sura 56, ayats 10-38). The Quran reveals, "Verily, the dwellers of Paradise that Day, will be busy in joyful things. They and their wives will be in pleasant shade, reclining on thrones. They will have therein fruits (of all kinds), and all that they will ask for. (It will be said to them): "Salamun" (Peace be on you), a Word from the Lord, Most Merciful" (sura 36, ayats 55-58). It is believed that the Paradise can be entered from either of its numerous gates. The eight gates of Paradise have names. Some of these names are mentioned in Sharia texts: The "Salaah" (prayer) Gate, the "Jihaad" Gate, the "Sadaqah" (charity) Gate, the "Rayyaan"(fasting) Gate, the "Ayman" (right) Gate and the "Al-Kaathimeen Al-Ghayth" Gate, which is for the suppression of anger. The names of the rest of the Gates of Paradise are not mentioned explicitly in the Sharia texts, but have been deduced from them: The "Tawbah" (repentance) Gate, the "Dhikr" (mentioning Allah) Gate, the "Ilm" (knowledge) Gate, the "Raadheen" (those who are content) Gate and the "Hajj" (pilgrimage) Gate.As for the first four names quoted the Messenger of Allah, as saying that any Muslim who spends a couple of things of the same type, i.e. a couple of Dirhams, a couple of slaves, a couple of camels, for the sake of Allah, will enter Paradise from any gate, and would enter from the Gate of Salaa if he observed voluntary prayer as his favored act of worship: from the Gate of Jihaad if he was a Mujaahid (one who performs Jihaad) and Jihaad was his favored act of worship; from the Gate of Rayyaan if he observed voluntary fasting as his favored act of worship; and from the Gate of Sadaqah if he gave voluntary charity as his favored act of worship (Al-Bukhaari and Muslim). The evidence for the name of the fifth gate is a hadith narrated on the authority of Abu Hurayrah on the Intercession of Prophet Muhammad, on Judgment Day when the Prophet, would be asked to let those who will not be reckoned enter from the Ayman Gate (Al-Bukhari and Muslim). The sixth name was taken from a hadith narrated on the authority of Al-Hasan saying that there would be a gate in Paradise from which no one would enter except those who once forgave a wrongdoing. The name of one of the narrators in this chain of narration is not known, according to Al-Haafith Ibn Hajar. Besides humans in Paradise there live servants, houris, united families. And Allah is also present there.

The detailed description of the image of Paradise given in Islam is a sort of an attempt to address the issue of the afterlife from the side of a phantasm of returning to the mother's womb: the rivers of milk falls into instant association with the feeding breast. In the words of the Quran "... rivers of water incorruptible; rivers of milk of which the taste never changes..." (sura 47, ayat 15).

Jahannam (Hell)

One of the reason to bring attention to the religious discourse of pain and violence in the Holy Book, is not the description of the hell`s horrors, but the significance of the primal introduction of the symbolized castration. The acceptance of castration leads to relief. The castration, which is not accepted, has several models to manifest itself. Undersymbolization provokes eventual neurotization, whilst avoidance of castration leads to a paranoiac position. Those, who are in-between are the claimants of phallus. Those, who reject castration, are in phallic position.

The further studying of the Quranic descriptions of hell will allow understanding of the specificity of castration in Islam. It is depicted as a crater of concentric circles on the underside of the world that all souls must cross in order to enter paradise by way of a bridge, narrow as a razor's edge.[760] This place was designated for the kaafirs (infidels), munafiqs (hypocrites), sinful people, evil creatures, and jinns.

The Quran mentioned the punishments in Jahannam (Hell) as follows:[761]

- The burning of skin, which is to be replaced for reburning
- Garments of fire will be worn
- Boiling water will scald the skin and internal organs
- Faces on fire
- Lips burnt off
- Backs on fire
- Roasting from side to side
- Bound in yokes then dragged through boiling water and fire
- Big snakes and scorpions biting hell dwellers
- People will have their heads crushed by big hammers
- People suffering from extreme hunger and thirst.

The Islamic tradition says that the kaafirs will be desperate and will go to the guard of Hell, Hazrat Malik. They will ask him to speak to Allah of their fate. Hazrat Malik will not reply to them for a thousand years. After a thousand years, he will reply:[762] "What are you telling me for, tell

---

[760] http://www.britannica.com/topic/Jahannam, consulted on 21.09.2016

[761] Abdul-Rahman Mohamed, *The Meaning and Explanation of the Glorious Qur'an*, London: MSA Publication Limited, 2009, pp. 106-109.

[762] http://www.alzahid.co.uk/resources/Hell_$28Jahannum$29.pdf, consulted on 01.07.2016

Him Whom you have disobeyed". Then for a thousand years they will call Allah by His Merciful Names, and for a thousand years He will not reply. After a thousand years, Allah will reply, "Stay away, remain in Hell, do not talk to Me." At this time, the Kaafirs will become completely hopeless of any kind of mercy and will start screaming and crying like the sound of donkeys. First, they will cry with tears. When they will have run out of tears, they will cry with the tears of blood. There will be big gaping gaps in their cheeks due to the effects of their crying. The amount of water and pus from crying will be so much that if boats were put into them, they would start sailing. The face of Jahannamis will be so bad that if a Jahannami were brought into this world, all the people would die by looking at his face and from the foul stench. Finally, for the kaafirs, the situation will be such that for every infidel a coffin will be prepared for them to the length of their height, and then they will be put into this coffin.[763] Then, it will be set on fire and it will be locked with a padlock of fire. It will be then be put inside a larger coffin also made of fire and the gap between will be set on fire. A padlock with chains made of fire will also be put around it. It will then be put into another coffin and then also set on fire and again will be locked with a lock of fire. All this will be then put into a bonfire. Then all the infidels will think that they will never be able to withstand any other heat and that this punishment is above all punishment. There will always be punishment for them and it will never end.[764]

The Islamic tradition claims that the gates of Hell are vertical, and the levels of Hell are ranked according to the degree of torture in descending order. From bottom to top they are:

- The First Gate "Jahannam", as Allah mentions in many verses in the Quran:"They said (i.e. the hypocrites): "Don't go out for war during the heat!" Say (i.e. Muhammad) the fire of Jahannam is even hotter if you only understood" (sura 9, ayat 81). This gate is called Jahannam because the fire will scorch the faces of the men and women who enter it. Their faces will be sullen and glum. It will eat away at their flesh and Allah says: "Every time the fire eats away their flesh We will replace it with new flesh so they can taste the punishment..." (sura 4, ayat 56).

Imam As Sadi mentioned in his tafseer: "This is in response to their obstinacy and resistance in the life of this world. Just as they continued

---

[763] http://www.islam.org.uk/islam.php, consulted on 21.09.2016
[764] http://www.islam.org.uk/islam.php, consulted on 21.09.2016

to reject obedience to Allah and submission to Him, likewise the fire will continue to burn up their flesh and when it reaches the point of almost being obliterated, Allah will remove the old flesh and replace it with new flesh, a just recompense for their rebellion in this life". This is the lightest punishment that one can receive in Hell, outside of the specific punishment of Abu Talib, the uncle of the Prophet.

- The Second Gate "Ladha", as Allah says in the Quran:"There is no way out for them, except the Ladha (i.e. Fierce Blaze) will certainly scorch the inward organs and the outward flesh! It will invite everyone who turned away from following the truth, heedless of it and gathered wealth but refused to spend it in the cause of Allah..." (sura 70, ayat 15). This level of hell is called Ladha because the fire will eat away at their body parts one by one, both internally and externally. It will invite those who abandoned Tawheed (i.e. Islamic monotheism) and turned away from that which the Prophet came with.
- The Third Gate "Saqar", as Allah says:"We will throw him into the Saqar and what will make you know what Saqar is? It is a scorching fire, it spares nothing and leaves nothing behind it will shake them vehemently and over it are nineteen angels" (surat 74, ayats 26-30). It is called "Saqar" because it will eat up the flesh of the human being and not his bones. Allah mentioned:"Those in paradise will ask the criminals what has landed you all in Saqar? They will say: "We were not of those who used to pray, and we didn't feed the poor, and we used to talk vainly with those who talked vain talk; and we used to deny the Day of Recompense until death came to us and we saw the reality of all that we denied" (sura 74, ayats 40-47).
- The Fourth Gate "Al Hutamah", as Allah says:"Nay they will be thrown into Al Hutamah (i.e. Crushing Fire). And what will make you know what Al Hutamah is? The fire of Allah kindled by men and stones which scorches the hearts. Surely it is vaulted over them in pillars widely extended" (sura 104, ayats 4-9). It is called Al Hutamah because it will shatter the bones of the human being and burn the heart and other internal organs. The fire will start at his feet and burn all the way through until it reaches the heart. Allah says: "Indeed it (i.e. the hell fire) spits out sparks the size of mansions, as if they were yellow herds" (sura 77, ayats 32-33).
- The Fifth Gate "Jaheem", as Allah mentions in many verses:"Seize him and shackle him!! Then roast him in Jaheem (i.e. the hellfire) in chains that are seventy cubits long. This is because he did not

believe in Allah, the Magnificent and he did not encourage the feeding of the poor" (sura 69, ayats 30-34).

- The Sixth Gate "Saeer", as Allah says, "A group in paradise and a group in Saeer (i.e. the blazing fire)" (sura 42, ayat 7). Allah also says about the people therein: "And they will say: "If we had listened and used our intellect we would not be inhabitants of As Saeer (i.e. blazing fire). They confessed their sins but away with the companions of As Saeer" (sura 67, ayats 10-11).This gate of Hell is called As Saeer because it contains 300 castles and in each castle there are 300 houses and in each house there are 300 types of punishments.In this particular level of hell there are scorpions and snakes, ropes, chains and shackles.

- The Seventh Gate "Al Haawiyah", as Allah says, "As for the one whose scales are light, then the Hawiyah will embrace him like a mother embraces her child. And what will make you know what Al Hawiyah is? It is a kindled fire burning hot" (sura 101, ayats 8-11). This gate of hell is called Al Hawiyah because whoever enters this level of the hell fire will never come out. Allah says:"And We will call the Zabaaniyah (i.e. angels who guard the hell fire)..." (sura 96, ayat 18).

As per categories of inhabitants of the jahanam, they include:

- Disbelievers:

"But those who disbelieve and deny Our signs will be companions of the Fire; they will abide therein" (sura 2, ayat 39). "Those who have disbelieved and died while they are disbelievers will have the curse of Allah upon them and the [curse of the] angels and all of the mankind. [they will abide] eternally therein. The punishment will not be lightened for them, nor will the punishment be postponed" (sura 2, ayats 161-162).

- Hypocrites:

"Indeed the hypocrites will be in the lowest depths of the Fire; you will find no helper for them"(sura 4, ayat 145)."The hypocrites are afraid that a surah is sent down about them, showing them what is [really] in their hearts. Say, "Ridicule you! But verily, Allah will expose all that you fear". If you question them, they declare: "We were only talking idly and playing". Say: "Is it Allah and His signs and His messengers that you were mocking?" Make no excuses that you have rejected faith after having accepted it. If We pardon some of you, We will punish others because they were criminals. The hypocrites - men and women are of one another. They enjoin evil and forbid what is just and close their hands [in stinginess]. They have forgotten Allah, so He has forgotten them. Verily, the hypocrites are rebellious and perverse. Allah has promised the hypocrites men and women and the rejecters of faith the fire of Hell; they will dwell therein. It is sufficient for them. And Allah will curse them, and they will have an enduring punishment" (sura 9, ayats 64-68).

- Polytheists (Those who associate something with Allah): "Those who reject [truth] among the People of the Book and the polytheists were not going to depart [from their ways] until there comes to them clear evidence - a messenger from Allah, rehearsing pure scriptures, wherein are upright laws [or decrees]. Nor did those who had been given the scripture make schisms until after there had come to them clear evidence. And they were not commanded except to worship Allah, sincere in religion to Him, to establish regular prayer, and to pay zakah. And that is the upright religion. Those who reject [truth] among the People of the Book and the polytheists will be in the fire of Hell, dwelling therein forever. They are the worst of creatures" (sura 98, ayats 1-6).
- People of the Book (who reject Islam): "Those reject [truth] among the People of the Book are the polytheists will be in the fire of Hell, dwelling there therein forever. They are the worst of creatures" (sura 98, ayat 6).
- Arrogant Rejecters of the Truth:

"But those who reject Our signs and treat them with arrogance - they are the companions of the Fire, dwelling therein forever" (sura 7, ayat 36).

- Sinners and Criminals:

"Indeed the criminals will be in the punishment of Hell, dwelling therein forever. It will not be lightened for them, and they will be overwhelmed there in despair. And We have not wronged them, but it is they who have wronged [themselves]" (sura 43, ayats 74-76).

- The Unjust: "Then it will be said to those who were unjust: "Taste the eternal punishment. Are you recompensed except for what you used to earn?"" (sura 10, ayat 52).
- Transgressors:

"But when there comes the Greatest Event - the Day when man will remember what he strove for and the Hellfire will be brought forth for [all] to see - then for him who had transgressed and preferred the life of this world, indeed Hellfire will be his shelter" (sura 79, ayats 34-39).

• Concealers of Allah's Revelations:

"Those who conceal what We have sent down of proofs and guidance after We have made it clear to the people in the scripture - those are cursed by Allah and cursed by those who [are entitled to] curse" (sura 2, ayat 159).

• Tyrants: "But they asked victory, and disappointment is the lot of every obstinate tyrant. In front of him is Hell, and he is given pus to drink. He will gulp it but will hardly be able to swallow it, and death will come to him from every place, yet he will not die. And in front of him will be a heavy punishment" (sura 14, ayats 15-17)." [It will be said to the two angels], "Throw into Hellfire every obstinate rejecter [of Allah] - who prevented good, transgressed, and doubted, who set up another god besides Allah - throw him into the severe punishment" (sura 50, ayats 24-26).
• Murderers:

"And whoever kills a believer intentionally - his recompense is Hell to abide therein forever, and the wrath and the curse of Alllah is upon him, and He has prepared for him a great punishment" (sura 4, ayats 93).

• Persecutors of Believers:

"Those who persecute [or draw into temptations] the believers - men and women - and then do not turn in repentance will have the punishment of Hell, and they will have the punishment of the Burning Fire" (sura 85, ayat 10).

• Those who Prefer this world and Neglect the Hereafter:

"Whoever wishes for the immediate - We hasten to grant him such things as We will to whom We will. Then We have mark for them hallmark they will burn therein, disgraced and rejected"(sura 17, ayat 18).

• Those who Commit Suicide:

Abu Huraiarh narrated that the Messenger of Allah said: "He who kills himself with a steel [weapon] will be eternal inhabitant of Hell, and he will have that [weapon] in his hand and will be thrusting it into his stomach forever and ever; he who kills himself by drinking poison will sip in the fire of Hell, forever and forever. He will kills himself by throwing himself from the top of a mountain and will constantly fall into the fire of Hell forever and ever".

- Other Inhabitants:

Harithah bin Wahb narrated that he heard the Messenger of Allah say: "Shall I not inform you who the people of Paradise are? [They are comprised of] every person who is weak and taken advantage of, but if he swore that Allah would do something, He would comply. And shall I not inform you who the people of Hell are? [They are comprised of] everyone who is cruel, proud and arrogant". According to Imam Al Qurtubi, hell is so large that one must travel for five hundred years in order to get from one level to the next.

Definitely, the Muslim doctrine of the afterlife that best encourages people to lead a moral life. This idea was once enounced by an eminent Muslim scholar Averroes. Unsuccessful resolution of a symbolic castration provokes neurotization of signifiers "hell" and "paradise". Neurotization happens in such cases as 1. A person has been sinful and now is seeking a refuge (salvation) in strict religious obedience, the constant repentance for the past. 2. A person considers oneself as a believer, however, tends to disregard the Islam's pillars, thus causing an inner conflict. 3. Strictly observing Muslims, who are overcautious in pleasing Allah, a fear of committing a minor error.

CHAPTER 10

MUSLIM ARCHETYPES
AND COMPLEXES

Muslim archetypes do not differ from the universal archetypes (e.g. The Sage, The Innocent, The Warrior, etc). However, the particularity is that a Muslim archetype is always positioned in a relation to the group. The Individual is non-existent. The Prophet said that the God`s hand is with the group, which leads to the conclusion that the existence of the 'I' and the 'Subject' occupies the lesser part in the Arabo-Muslim conscious. Moreover, from the religious standpoint, the attitudes of all Arabs would be uniform, where the individual structures, therefore, remain unknown. On these grounds we can argue that:

- The dominant majority of Arab men possess a symbolic phallus, one for the whole community (in contrast to the Western world where a man has a phallus).
- When an Arab speaks from a place of current availability of resources (I am) he/she offers them to another. This is a real situation. However, frequently an Arab speaks from the Imaginary (I will) and, instead of offering, gives a promise to offer, which leads to an impossible situation, since it happens only in the Arab`s Imaginary.
- A dark side of an Arab is not an evil one, it is the unknown one. Many Muslims do not know themselves, it is ordered by collective.

- The tendencies towards twin-archetypes that co-exist side by side (e.g. angels Munkar and Nakir).
- In the Name-of-the-Father there is excluded the God`s name. In Islamic world Allah is not one of the father`s names, it is beyond, an independent substance.

The psychological complex arises on the side of the greatest lack. Under the strong manifestation of the Individual, questioning of one`s own place in the collective, turns into the complex of Mohamed, Alladin, Cain, etc., which are so frequently occurring in the modern Muslim society.

Identity "A Bedouin"

Arabic identity is determined by a tribe life, which is substantially shaped by the desert environment. In this chapter, the question under discussion is, whether, in conditions of isolation from the rest of the world, the identification passes through the incorporation of the traits of the wild desert animals, such as goats, sheeps, and camels. The Arabs have developed particular sensitivity, which allowed them to stay permanently vigilant on the background of constant danger and, luckily, preserve their lives. Even nowadays Arabs are very sensitive to gestures, movements. When greeting, Bedouin men touch their noses as a sign of particular affection and recognition.

Ibn Khaldun reveals in his Muqaddima the required length of time for the changes in the attitudes and the cultural heritage to take effect. Especially he remarks that at least four generations are needed so that to perceive the changes in the matters related to the collective "superstructure".

Bedouin`s Honour Code

Sharaf and ird
Sharaf is the Bedouin honor code for men. The honour can be gained, elevated, lost, and reconquered. Sharaf of one member implies protection of (1) the tribe`s honour; (2) ird of the women of the family; (3) protection of resources; (4) defense of the tribe (when needed).

Ird is the Bedouin honor code for women. Since the day of her birth until the wedding day a woman`s ird is to remain untouched. Ird is a signifier, which is much wider than virginity. It includes emotional, as well as conceptual chastity.

Diyafa (hospitality) is the generousity offered to the guests. If the circumstances require, Bedouin could offer a shelter and food even to the adversary. Even poor Bedouins would share the last piece they have.

Hamasa (bravery) indicates the readiness to protect one's own tribe and to fight for their safety if needed. It is closely related to the capacity to tolerate hardships, pain, including (male) circumcision.

Arabic Desert

The desert imposes as a first condition of existence — nomadism. It is not for pleasure that the Bedouin is always travelling but from stern necessity[765].The Bedouin does not exist beyond his tribe, the outside world is unknown, and, therefore, adversary to him. Faithfulness to his pledged word, honesty and frankness only concern members of the tribe, the contribules[766]. The Bedouin lives in Real and immediately reacts to its changes. The desert shaped his identity, he cannot afford to dream, because on the speed of his reaction depends his survival. He is the way he is, not because that is the way he likes, but because that is the way he is obliged to. Before Islam, Bedouin was not concerned much with the spiritual matters. He was worshipping the idols as long as they were supporting him. In the opposite case, he could even harm them, cheat by sacrificing the lesser prey than promised. Idols were needed since the desert is a dangerous place to live, and the support was expected from the Big Other. The survival depended on the unity, that is why a Bedouin is still so bound to his/her family. The Bedouin is used to be fighting for his life, and the language of force turned to be the main language for him. At the same time, the Arabs displayed a boundless loyalty to their tribes and traditions, were magnanimously hospitable, honoured the treaties, were faithful friends and dutifully met the obligations of tribal customs.[767]

As Aisha Kandisha claims, an identity of an ancestral desert man is deeply enrooted into the Arab's unconscious. And many generations of Europeanized Arabs will not be enough to chase out this image.

---

[765] Servier Andre, *Islam and the Psychology of the Musulman*, New York: Scribner, 1923, chapter 2.

[766] *Ibid*

[767] Servier Andre, *Islam and the Psychology of the Musulman*, New York: Scribner, 1923, chapter 2.

Arabic Family

The traditional Arab family is often referred to as "Arab society in miniature" for the reason that the same structure, values, and sets of relationships prevail both within the family and within the wider society.[768] Allah (Father) – mother - brothers (umma). The father as such is absent. He is present in the capacity of law.

It is a common situation with the traumatic consequences when a tradition gives parents unlimited life-long power to be in a position to control their children`s lives. For instance, to tell one`s children what to eat, who to talk to, how to behave, who to marry. Non-obedience is considered almost as a sin, so, for a dependent on his/her family child, there is no way not to obey.

Brother-Sister Love

In the closed Arabic society, the first love most frequently happens within the family, which as much frequently, grows into the official marriage. Since childhood it is common, for brothers and sisters, for example, to share one bed. This practice sometimes lasts until puberty or the marriage day. Also, such signs of emotional attachment as gentle touching, physical consolation, hugging, hair combing, hand holding and other ways of expressing tenderness, are considered as normal behaviour between brothers and sisters. Just to cite a few examples from the Middle Eastern folkloric heritage, which unfolds the affectionate brother-sister bond: the ancient Egyptian deities Osiris and his sister Isis; the Semitic religious characters Cane and Able and their twin sisters; the Arab poetess Al-Khansaa and her brother Sakhr; Prophet Mohammad's grandchildren Al-Husain and his sister Zaynab; the Abbasid Calif Haroun Al-Rasheed and his sister Al-Abbasa; the founder of modern Saudi Arabia, King Saud and his sister Nura; the main characters in Naguib Mahfouz's Trilogy, Kamal and his sister Aisha; the heroes of the Arabic folk tale "Hansel and Gretel"; Mamma and his sister Mustagheetha, and others. Despite, the abundance of incestuous examples in real life and traditional literature, the Arabic psychology is silent on the matter, as if this situation seemed to be the norm.

---

[768] Barakat Halim, *The Arab World: Society, Culture, and State,* Berkley: University of California Press, 1991, p. 118.

The child's positive relationship with the maternal uncle is a product of the love a mother has for her brother, and the strong bonds of affection between a child and his or her mother (but not with the father).[769]

Desire of a Muslim Mother

The Islamic order is not the only form of the antique world to marginalize the feminine position. From this standpoint, Islam does not differ fundamentally from other monotheisms that recognize the symbolic dignity of a woman only through the conception of a son, more precisely, in her capacity of an intermediary, who brings the son to a father. The Arabic epic tradition offers countless examples of women warriors and amazons (Princess Ain al-Hayat in Qissat Firuz Shah, the characters of Queen al-Rabab, al-Gayda, Gamra and Nitra in the Romance of Antar, Al-Samta and Aluf in Dhat al-Himma, Princess Turban in Hamza al-Bahlawan, and the female community in the Romance of Sayf).[770] According to Benslama, the "torment" of origin is an intrinsical feature of the Islamic, which came out as a result of the suppression of the feminine, which in combination with the absence of the divine paternal, accounts for Islam's extreme masculine monotheism and political radicalism. One example of the exclusion of the feminine is Hagar, who, in spite of her foundational mothering role is never mentioned in the Quran and in effect is "evicted" from the foundational discourse so that Abraham the father could be "found and reconciled" with the son to rebuild the Kaaba, Islam's holiest site[771].

A Muslim woman is no more than a phallic object of her family. Under the cover of a mother there follows a woman, not reversely. Primarily the Muslim woman appears as the Subject in her capacity of a mother. Feminine jouissance transposes onto the mother's jouissance total towards her children. So mother's desire finds satisfaction in her children. That is in relation to a mother that the children become primarily eroticized, and remain attached to her throughout the whole life, as a source of their first sensual experience. Indeed, the mother's significance is bigger than that of

---

[769] https://scholarworks.iu.edu/dspace/bitstream/handle/2022/8990/el-shamy_Arbpsy-Br-Sis-Syndrm.pdf?sequence=1, consulted on 01.07.2016

[770] Afsaneh Najmabadi, Islamicate Sexualities: Translations across Temporal Geographies of Desire. Co-edited with Kathryn Babayan. Cambridge: Harvard University Press, Middle Eastern Monographs, 2008, p.76.

[771] Benslama Fethi, *La psychanalyse à l'épreuve de l'islam*, Paris: Aubier, 2002, p.104.

the father, since the former plays a total role, whilst the latter - a symbolic one. The Prophet said that three times the most loved there shall be the mother, because the father is venerated. The strong son-mother relation can be also explained by the fact that usually after the marriage the son with his wife live at the house of his parents. So, the son basically continues living with his family, while a daughter is separated from her own family. If the traditions subdue the feminity, subjugate it to the phallic law, a woman does not easily fit into the signifier. A woman is suppressed. The price to pay is to conform with the phallic tradition, and abandon her own desire, a desire of a woman. However, it is also by means of a symptom and suffering that a woman escapes from the traditional yoke and lets herself to emerge as a woman beyond the look of Another. Yet the psychological sufferings oftentimes serve as a liberation on her way to become a woman. She is being defined in terms of the other and not as an autonomous person.[772] Like Hagar left ignored, erased from the official chronicle. Her elimination from the Quranic tradition cannot be left unnoticed. In what relation does Hagar's absence stay to the state of a woman in a Muslim society? What was eliminated (Hagar) cannot be restored. Being eliminated from the symbolic order, Hagar continues her jouissance, in which she is not restricted, in contrast to the feminine, which is ordered by the Islamic tradition. This occurrence will continue to torment the society as long as it is ignored. Islam arose from the (female) foreigner when monotheism originated, and she has remained estranged in Islam."[773]

The desire of a Muslim daughter is to belong totally to a symbolic father, that is where the sexual extremes stem from. The discourse of feminity of a Muslim woman is identic to the character of the father's interdiction.

Total Mother

Total mother, or Dominating mother, is a mother, who occupies the whole space with her presence, and whose desire is that her children do not appear as independent from her Subjects, but, rather remain as the continuation of her desire. This turns her into a phallic mother.

---

[772] Said Khalida, *Al mara al-arabiya: kain bi gheirihi am bi dhatihi?* Casablanca: Nashr al fanac, 1991, p.70.

[773] Sutton Kyra, *Islam`s Turn on the Couch: The Psychoanalytic Theorizing of Muslim Identity in France*, Connecticut: Weyslan University, 2013, p. 77.

Castrating Mother

The maternal should be reduced so that a woman could appear, without which the only possible woman, who a man faces, is always a castrating woman, who is, essentially, is a substitute for his own mother. Castrating mother is a mother who imposes the order.

Hijab

Mernissi compellingly adumbrates the theological dimensions of the veil, which she shows is a major concept in Islam that is not reducible to a strip of fabric covering the face.[774] Mernissi argues that hijab is a multidimensional concept, meaning "to hide something from sight", but also "to separate, to mark a border, to establish a threshold."[775] Among other meanings, the veil has also ethical connotations, referring to something that "belongs to the realm of forbidden."[776] "Reducing or assimilating this concept to a scarp of cloth that men have imposed on women to veil them when they go into the street is truly to impoverish this term..."[777] As Mernissi points out, the Arabic word hijab is also used with reference to the hymen, which is called hijab-al-bukuriya (hijab of virginity).[778] With reference to the hymen, hijab al-bukuriya, Derrida states, "One could say quite accurately that the hymen does not exist. Anything constituting the value of existence is foreign to the hymen." And if there were a hymen – I am not saying if the hymen existed-property value would (not be)... appropriate to it...How can one then attribute the existence of the hymen properly to a woman?[779] The hijab became an idolatrous fetish for the male elite of Islam, following the death of Prophet Mohamed.[780] The key area where the veil enters into the Islamic narrative is in the context of revelation

---

[774] Wise Christopher, *Derrida, Africa and the Middle East*, New York: Palgrave Macmillan, 2009, p. 24.

[775] *Ibid*

[776] *Ibid*

[777] *Ibid*

[778] *Ibid*

[779] Derrida Jacques, *The Ear of the Other: Otobiography, Transference, Translation*, Lincoln: University of Nebraska Press, 1988, pp.180-181.

[780] Wise Christopher, *Derrida, Africa and the Middle East*, New York: Palgrave Macmillan, 2009, p. 26.

from God to Muhammad.[781] The prohibition of veil does not come from a man, but from the women's proximity to the Prophet Muhammad's receiving of revelation. When the Prophet suspected Aisha of cheating on him with Safwan, it is the revelation (the Law) that structures the order. The sura "Light", sent immediately after this, orders that she be veiled. Another example is found in a case of Muhammad's adopted son Zaid, who had to divorce his wife because Muhammad found her attractive. This led to the prohibition of adoption in Islam – "Muhammad is not a father of any of you" is mentioned in the Quran immediately after this event. Then God says in the Quran, "Oh, Prophet, tell your wives and daughters and the women of the faithful to draw their wraps a little over them. They will thus be recognized and no harm will come to them" (sura 33, ayat 59).

When viewed from this perspective of Islamic theology, the veil is not a sign, but a thing through which the female body is partially or wholly obscured because that body has the power to charm and fascinate. In other words, for religion, it is the woman's body that is ostentatious, whereas the veil would serve as a filter that does away with and protects against the body's disturbing effects.[782]

Presence as the Absence of Father

The basic Oedipal religious theory, as developed in The Future of an Illusion, goes essentially as follows: man's initial relationship toward nature resembles the infantile prototype, in which every boy grows up to symbolically kill his father, marry his mother, and then internalize his father, whose prohibitions come to constitute the superego[783].

Islam opts for the lineage of Abraham as the real father. Despite the fact that Abraham was let out from the duty of sacrificing his son, "the paternal complex", indeed, became reactualized in Islam (e.i. the annual ritual of Hajj). Like Moses, Ishmael, (a non-Arab) is the beginning point of the Muslim lineage, making Islam's founding, not an imitation as much as it is a translation into Arabic of paternal authority.

---

[781] http://www.academia.edu/3480874/Psychoanalysis_and_the_Veil_in_Islam_Rethinking_Truth_and_Liberation_Review_of_Fethi_Benslamas_Islam_and_the_Challenge_of_Psychoanalysis, consulted on 21.09.2016

[782] Sutton Kyra, *Islam's Turn on the Couch: The Psychoanalytic Theorizing of Muslim Identity in France*,Connecticut: Weyslan University, 2013, p. 85.

[783] *Ibid, p.36.*

In Islamic discourse, the figure of a father should be contemplated upon in terms of his absence. In the world where a strong symbolic father exists, what place is attributed to a real father?

The father, who castrated, does not have a role to play afterwards (in regards to his sons). However, he is left in the historic memory. A father, who prohibits and takes pleasure in interdiction, fulfills himself in interdiction (for daughters), here he exists in present and future.

A Muslim father awaits the birth of his son, that is the very moment when he fulfills his function, celebrating oneself as a man. If a family has only daughters, a father will not experience his masculine origin. A male heir makes his father a man. A father, who is actively engaged in educating children, just alike a mother, follows an example of his mother, since his real father was absent and he transmits his mother's desire unto his own children. He did not receive a father's castration, and, therefore, will not be able to give castration to his own son(s).

A father, who does not interdict, is, actually, carries out a total interdiction, an interdiction of everything.

In the absence of a real father, an imaginary father is present (in absence there is presence). In the presence of a real father, there is presence of a symbolic and imaginatory father, which leads to the idealization of a father. Therefore, in the presence of a father there is the absence of a father, and the experiencing of one's own father like a symbol, idol, signifier, which is on the edge of symbolization for his own sons.

A son, to who it was prematurely confined that he was castrated (a "father's secret") so that to reveal his perspective of taking on a role of a castrating father in future, becomes a lost Subject. A lost Subject, to who it was confined his symbologenic castration.

An Imaginatory father is a collective fantasm. The specific of the Islamic world is taking pleasure in interdiction - jouissance of interdiction.

"Islam cut itself off from" these earlier monotheisms and from "many other vital points of the biblical-Gospel canon having to do with the loving bond between Creator and creatures"[784].There is no place for a Holy Family in Islam. This is why Islam emphasizes so much the fact that Muhamed himself was an orphan; this is why, in Islam, God intervenes precisely at the moments of suspension, withdrawal, failure, 'black-out' of the paternal function (when the mother or the child are abandoned or ignored by the biological father)[785].Without Abraham's contribution, he insists, the

---

[784] Sutton Kyra, *Islam's Turn on the Couch: The Psychoanalytic Theorizing of Muslim Identity in France*, Connecticut: Weyslan University, 2013, p.52.

[785] *Ibid, p.61.*

formulation of Islam would have been impossible. Abraham is central to Islam in three ways: the first is naming; before Islam even came into being, the Quran tells us that Abraham named Muhammad "Muslim," a word which signifies subjection to the God of Abraham. The second way, as outlined by Benslama, is "paternal filiation": Muhammad identifies Islam as the closure to monotheism, referring in the Quran to "the faith of your forbear Abraham" (sura 22, ayat 78). Finally, Abraham's third contribution to Islam derives from what Benslama calls a "ritual inscription" because Islam is the only one of the three monotheistic religions to commemorate Abraham's sacrifice. This element is crucial for the formation of the paternal complex in Islam because the renunciation of the murder of the son is continuously staged and reenacted[786]. Benslama points out that it is in "this very desire to tear himself away from the primal father" through the establishment of his own new order that Abraham, in fact, transmits the heritage of the primal father[787]. All in all, Ishmael is the son, who was abandoned by his father in the desert. Ishmael is given the gift of the promise of nationhood, but Benslama points out that this moment of gift-giving "produces a rupture through which the son is separated from the father who abandoned him[788]. In fact, there is no single schema, which would describe a figure Muslim father. Instead, there are several father figures, which are in the origins of Islam, and their relation to one another should not be considered linear or fixed but should, rather, be seen as an interplay of the transappropriation of the father.

One Man and Four Wives

The words "Man" and "Woman" appear an equal number of times in Quran, which is 24, meaning that Islam pays equal attention to both genders. Traditionally, Muslim marriages have been contracted between the closest relatives, especially cousins. Most commonly, a father's brother's son is the first contender for the hand of his female cousin, who has the right to refuse, but needs to receive his permission to marry somebody else. Traditional marriages are practiced between first, second and third cousins. Marriages outside one's tribe are not encouraged unless a tribal alliance was established. The first criteria for choosing a bride, but for her implicit chastity, is equal social status. Polygamy is permitted, which is also a sign of social status. Undoubtedly, only older and wealthy men are

---

[786] *Ibid, p.62.*

[787] *Ibid, p. 64.*

[788] *Ibid*

capable of supporting multiple households. Indeed, one reason cited for polygyny is that it allows a man to give financial protection to multiple women, who might otherwise not have any support (e.g. widows).[789] The tendency to marry many wives manifests a lack in Another. Polygamy is often characterized by competition and jealousy among co-wives as is commonly observed within plural marriage communities.[790] Usually, the co-wives have little to no contact with each other and lead separate lives in different houses, which sometimes are located in opposite parts of the city. Co-wives likely have very limited private time with the one husband they share, and thus might compete for his attention. In addition, women's self-worth is linked to the number of children they bear and, therefore, having time with their husband is also critical to their status within the family and community.[791] Usually, the first wife is selected by the fiancé's mother (that is why a wife-to-be is a mother's prototype). The second and other wives are usually selected by a man himself, and designate his own choice. The preferences for wives reflect changes that a male personality has undergone through time. If no particular changes have occurred, then, all wives, excluding the first one (since she is a mother's choice) will be resembling each other. Oftentimes all wives belong to different prototypes, and, as a consequence, are different in characters, body shapes, behaviors, which enhance and their constant rivalry. Usually, each wife is younger than a previous one. The first marriage tends to occur in 18-24 years, whilst 3 years – is an average gap between marriages. The first wife is a kind of her mother-in-law's voice and other wives are obliged to obey her. She is also the oldest one. If all wives share the same house, then they are together everywhere: they cook, clean, and even travel collectively. Thus, the polygamous family is considered as a single organism. With time their actions, even thoughts become synchronised.

The Quran says, "Ye are never able to be fair and just as between women, even if it is your ardent desire: But turn not away (from a woman) altogether, so as to leave her (as it were) hanging (in the air). If ye come to a friendly understanding, and practise self-restraint, Allah is Oft-forgiving, Most Merciful" (sura 4, ayat 129). In practice, it is almost impossible to respect equal attitude towards all wives, so there will always be a feeling

---

[789] http://fatwa.islamweb.net/fatwa/index.php?page=showfatwa&lang=A&Id=18444&Option=FatwaId, consulted on 21.09.2016

[790] Al-Krenawi Alean et al.,*The psychosocial impact of polygamous marriages on Palestinian women*, Women and Health 34.1, 2001, pp. 1-16.

[791] Committee on Polygamous Issues, *Life in bountiful: A report in the lifestyle of a polygamous community*, British Columbia Ministry of Women's Equality, 1993.

of "lack", which would be seeking to get filled in. In this regard, one Muslim woman said: "if you buy a new jumper, you will not wear an old one,"[792] and "When I think of my previous life with my husband before he got other wives after me I have a lump in my throat."[793] "If a wife wants to make slaughter (kill an animal to feed the family), she can, she should have, then, a stick between her legs."[794] "Shahpar (husband's second wife) is my rival, and how you can be nice to a rival?"[795] Oftentimes a physically healthy first wife ceases her place to another woman, as a means to revive an offense against her husband because he was initially incapable to satisfy her. So, she allows a second wife in so that to control her and in such a way to take a revenge on her husband. In an attempt to control the other woman, the excess of the radical otherness of the first wife is perceived. The rest of her life she will be demonstrating her suffering, thus, implying husband's inability to please her.

The number of wives will initially depend on a father's wish: if he had many wives, and also if he did not, but wanted to, he will transmit this desire to his son. A son might marry the first wife (mother's choice), then the second wife (father's wish), even if he did not quite want to. He will usually have as many wives as his father had, or will be constantly seeking to accomplish the father's wish. One Arab said, "I want to find the second wife because I have wanted to marry four wives even before getting married for the first time. There is nothing wrong with the first wife, we love each other. I just need another one as well. If not, I will feel bad, undervalued, unappreciated." In prevailing majority, the second wives are divorcees or financially disfavored.

---

[792] https://www.youtube.com/watch?v=IMfLzPzY2-s, documentary movie One Man and Four Wives, consulted on 01.07.2016

[793] *Ibid*

[794] *Ibid*

[795] *Ibid*

Endogamy

The practice of marrying within a specific ethnic group while rejecting all others is a common Bedouin's practice. It is the realization of an archaic phantasm of primal symbiosis and reviving Oedipus complex, where the separation is impossible.

The Other Woman

Islam is haunted by "the other woman, who has threatened to capture the son, making him an illegitimate bastard." This disavowal of the female at the origin of Islam should be understood not simply as an origin that remains static, but as a repressed core that repeats and is open. Thus, the repression of Hagar corresponds to the very basis of female subjectivity in Islam.[796] Fethi Benslama affirms that "the other woman is always the wife's double: she doubles the official wife, precedes her, supplants her from the outset in the play of maternity, and disturbs the process of difference division in the family." But it is the official wife, to who the power of the symbolic law belongs. In other words, Sarah, the official wife, is on the side of our societal norms and laws, while Hagar, the "other woman," is written out of this order.[797] Space "between-two-women" in a field of tension between the subject's desire and the mother's choice. In total then, the space-between-the-two-women narrative carries with it the establishment of "the nobility of the mother's birth, control of the other woman, and the preservation of the son's seed through the father" – these are three features that Benslama claims will have effects on Islam that remain palpable in the present day.

Eunuch

The word eunuch stems from the Greek "eune" (bed) and "ekhein" (to keep)."Eunoukhos" literally means "bed keeper". Hence, the word eunuch derives from one of his functions - to oversee the women of harem and act as chamberlain. For handling this honourable mission only castrated men were admitted. Since the Achaemenid times in the Middle East eunuchs

---

[796] http://www.academia.edu/3480874/Psychoanalysis_and_the_Veil_in_Islam_Rethinking_Truth_and_Liberation_Review_of_Fethi_Benslamas_Islam_and_the_Challenge_of_Psychoanalysis, consulted on 01.07.2016

[797] Sutton Kyra, *Islam`s Turn on the Couch: The Psychoanalytic Theorizing of Muslim Identity in France*, Connecticut: Weyslan University, 2013,p. 78.

were employed to guard the rulers` and their families` bedrooms. Eunuchs were regarded as the most loyal slaves because they were not only separated from their families and territories of origin but robbed of reproductive capability.[798] Castration itself is a removal of the testicles. In Arabic, there are different appellations of a castrated man: the term khasiya is used to describe a man with removed testicles; the term majbub designates a man whose penis has been cut, and the term mamsuh a man without both. Scholars claim that if his testicles only are cut off, then he is a eunuch; if his penis is cut off, then he is emasculated. The castration is played in three registers: privation of a virile organ (in real); the frustration of impossibility to realize one`s desire (imaginary) and castration as a ban on sexual intercourse with the harem (symbolic). Eunuch is deprived of a virile organ, however, he is not void of desire. He is the guardian of order. And he is the one, who acts on behalf of order. Hence, his sole loyalty belonged to his ruler. Eunuchs were plentiful in the Islamic empires, even though, castration is not an Islamic teaching. It is even forbidden in Islam. And still, there was hardly any area of Muslim rule in which the eunuchs did not play a chief role. They led the battles, conquered kingdoms, carried out responsible administrative duties, they were assigned posts of governors and commanders of armies. They were indispensable in the affairs of the harem. Perhaps the data most indicative of the vigour and strength of the institution of [Ottoman`s] Palace slavery are the dates on which eunuchs were admitted to the Imperial service and their names entered into the Register.[799] The more the Register's closing date is approached, the bigger the number of eunuchs was found.

The hadith 5416 by Sahih Muslim retells that Aisha narrated that a eunuch used to come to the houses of wives of Allah's Messenger and they did not find anything objectionable in his visit considering him to be without any sexual desire. Allah's Messenger one day came as he was sitting with some of his wives and he was busy in describing the bodily characteristics of a lady and saying: As she comes in front, four folds appear on her front side, and as she turns her back, eight folds appear on the back side. Thereupon Allah's Messenger said, "I see that he (the eunuch) knows these things; do not, therefore, allow him to enter." She (Aisha) said, "Then they began to observe veil from him (the eunuch)."

---

[798] http://www.encyclopedia.com/article-1G2-3403500147/eunuchs.html, consulted on 21.09.2016

[799] Toledano Ehud, *The Imperial Eunuchs of Istanbul: From Africa to the Heart of Islam*, Middle Eastern Studies, 1984, pp.379-390.

Moreover, even the Prophet Muhammad himself is said to have accepted a eunuch as a gift.[800] Abdullah ibn Masood said, "We were on a campaign with the Messenger of Allah, and we had no women with us." We said, "Why don't we get ourselves castrated?" But he forbade us to do that. Ashhab said, "Maalik was asked, Can a woman take off her head cover in front of a eunuch? Is he one of those who "lack vigour"?" He said, "Yes if he is her slave or the slave of someone else. But in the case of one who is free, then no."" Although the Quran never uses the word eunuch, the hadith and the books of the legal scholars do. Prominent scholar and Arab News' Islamic Affairs Editor Adil Salahi said, "If the eunuch is a man who has been castrated, all the rulings concerning men apply to him. If it is a question of a person being created thus, then whatever the person appears to be applied to him. If the eunuch says he is a man, or if he says he is a woman, Islam accepts this from him in things which do not give him the material advantage."

Oedipus Complex

Mernissi affirms that all Muslim men share symptoms of Oedipus complex: "In Muslim societies not only is the marital bond weakened and love for the wife discouraged, but his mother is the only woman a man is allowed to love at all, and this love is encouraged to take the form of life-long gratitude."[801] An Arab man is fixed on Oedipian phase, and emotionally stays connected to his mother all his life. He recognizes her maternal power over him, which a Muslim mother encourages as well.

Mohamed Complex

Somebody who isolates oneself from the society and restraints one`s contacts, shows the manifestations of Mohamed complex. The complex is rooted in the feelings of dissatisfaction and estrangement. One feels that he/she does not belong there, and his/her own society does not have a place for him/her. He/She judges his/her own people as inferior to him/her, believing that he/she is different. He/She manifests himself/herself in a distinctive from others manner while accusing the society of its flaws. He/She claims not to be able to grow in such conditions. He/She either

---

[800] Saad Mohamed, *Kitab al-Ṭabaqat al-Kabir*, Cairo: Maktabat al-Khangi, 2001, p.10.

[801] Zayzafoon Lamia, *The Production of the Muslim Woman: Negotiating Text, History, and Ideology*, Lenhman: Lexington Books, 2005, p.25.

---

seeks to move the country or isolates oneself from the rest of the world. He/She discovers that the society has changed after long-term seclusion. Usually, he/she turns into the activist and "fighter" for the national values, however, at distance. The complex is named after the main hero of the book by Karim Sarroub The Complex of Mohamed.

Cain Complex

In the Arabo-Muslim culture the brothers' bonds are extremely strong, and explain the fusion on the level of a group. The relation between siblings is an actual place of socialization of a child. Commonly, the older brother holds a particular status in the family. He is granted with wider authorities. Unexpectedly, there would happen a displacement of a phantasm of the killing of a father on this brother. This corresponds to the religious version of the primal murder in the history of humanity, Cain, who kills his brother Abel. One of the specificities of the Arabo-Muslim culture will be the displacement of aggressive impulses against a brother, who represents a father. The concept of Muslim brotherhood is impregnated with unconscious impulses of hatred and aggressiveness of the brothers. However, the fact that the two sections are called brothers is no proof that before its division they formed two patriarchal clans or sub-tribes tracing descent from two brothers germane.[802] It would be an entire mistake to suppose that all the Sons (let us say) of Hosein are really sprung from the loins of Hosein.[803]

Jawdar Complex

The legend narrates that Jawdar, an Egyptian fisherman, set off in search of treasure under the guidance of a Abdessamad, a Moroccan magician. The treasure was hidden deeply inside the Earth layers. Abdessamad instructed Jawdar to open the first six doors, each time reciting a relevant formula. When approaching the seventh and the last door, Jawdar was instructed to knock it. He was warned that his mother will appear saying: "Welcome, my son, home, come and greet me". "And you have to answer, -the magician adds,- do not approach me and take off your clothes." She will say, "My son, I am your mother. I have rights on you, which breastfeeding and education give. What for you want me to expose my nudity to you." You will answer, "Take off your clothes, otherwise I`ll kill you." Look then to your right side,

---

[802] Smith William, *Kinship and Marriage in Early Arabia*, Oxford: Oxford Press, 2014, p.15.

[803] *Ibid*

there you will find a spear hanging on the wall, take it off and tell her, "Take off your clothes!" She will try to implore you, don not succumb to that. Each time she takes off a piece of clothes say, "You must take off everything." When she takes off all her clothes you will decode the symbols, annul the blocks and will set yourself free. And the magician precised: "Do not be afraid, Jawdar, this is just a shade without soul." However, Jawdar, when facing mother did not dare to make her take off her last piece of clothes. He was disturbed by his mother, who kept on saying: "My son, you have gone wrong. My son, your heart is from stone. You want to dishnour me. Don`t you know that this is forbidden (haram)." Jawdar, having heard the word "haram" gave up his project, and said to mother: "Keep the cloth that hides your sex." And mother exclaims happily: "You are wrong, let`s beat him." So, Jawdar did not reach the treasure and had to restart from the beginning some time later. This time he succeeded. Once his mother was naked, she transformed into a shade without soul and Jawdar was able to reach his treasure-his own life. The story depicts well the tightly knitted relation child-mother that exists in the Muslim universe, which is nourished by interdependence throughout the whole life. The autonomy arrives with the detachment, which cannot be reached easily. The independence is acquired with the killing of unanimated shades inside oneself. The psychological maturity is an assassination of a mother. One should destroy, demystify the image of a mother inside oneself, because prioritizing mother prevents the grown child from flying with one`s own wings. Abdelwahab Bouhdiba admits that Oedipus was guilty of patricide and incest, and, therefore, punished, whilst Jawdar designates the type of behavior void of any culpability since he deals only with false apparitions. Jawdar designates a complex of imprisonment by the shade of one`s own mother, and his act personifies authentic liberation from oneself and his own mother.

Alladdin Complex

In the fairytale, Alladdin was looking for a magic solution to get rich. He was convinced that one day he would find it, however, in fact, he was not exercising many efforts for this. Thus, he was nonchalantly enjoying his life and indulging in total jouissance. Alladdin complex typifies somebody who is not interested in investing one`s labour into achieving something, so he entrusts his wellbeing to luck. This attitude is much different from tawakul (reliance on Allah), which stems from deep faith and surrender to circumstances while all personal attempts have been exhausted. Procrasting the majority of time, Alladdin is reluctant to try anything that would bring quick and easy results, not bothering about the consequences.

CHAPTER 11

CUSTOMS AND TABOOS

A custom pursues a symbolic order, which was initially imposed by the archaic father. It is offered in a payable coin of veneration to the archaic father in return for the group acknowledgment of one`s belonging to it. It resends to the notion of "father+land". Who is your father? The law of which land do you obey? The land has been identifying the man since the birth of humankind. Adam and Eva did not obey the law of the Father-of-Genesis, so they were not allowed to remain in Paradise and, thus, were chased from its gardens. It is as if via tradition a father connects his son to the land. A tradition belongs to the land. There would not have been any purpose in customs, had they not served to mark one`s territory. With this in mind, some of the customs are cited below:

1.   Pronouncing God's name before a meal or drink

First of all, by evoking God`s name before eating or drinking, a Muslim expresses gratitude to God, and, secondly, supplicates for abundance in future. The Prophet said, "Whenever anyone of you eats, he should say, "[I begin] with the name of God." If he forgets, he should then say, "Bismillah," at the beginning as well as at the end.""

2.   Doing everything with the right hand

Determining the usage of a particular hand derives from the Quranic teachings, and exemplifies *per se* a strong separator between the "people of right hand" (Allah`s adherents) and "people of left hand" (followers of Satan). The Prophet was saying, "Whenever one of you eats, he should eat with his right hand and whenever he drinks, he should drink using his right hand."

3. Greetings

The greeting "Assalaam alaikum" (Peace be upon you) expresses wishes of peace to the interlocutor, to which the addressee answers, "Wa alaikum assalaam," thus, returning back the wish.

4. Tashmeet

Tashmeet ritual dates back to pre-Islamic era, which was approved by Prophet. It is performed as follows: after a Muslim sneezes, he/she says, "Al-hamdulillah" (praise to Allah), while the people around should answer, "Yarhamukallah" (may Allah have mercy on you). In Arabo-Muslim culture sneezing means relief from some temporary disturbance, for which a Muslim thanks God, and the answer of his/her companions signifies a reminder of the fact that God's mercy and His blessings are only for thankful.

5. Trimming moustaches, removing body`s hair&circumcision

Large and unkempt moustaches have commonly been considered as a sign of arrogance. The Prophet gave the concrete instruction regarding the trimming of moustaches, the clipping of nails, removing hair from the pubic area and from under the armpits, as well as male`s circumcision, which is related to maintenance of physical tidiness.The Prophet is reported to have said, "Five things are a part of man's nature: Circumcision, removing pubic hair, clipping nails, removing hair from the armpits and trimming moustaches."

In regards to circumcision, it symbolizes the separation of a son from his mother, and, therefore, turning a boy into a man.

Islamic culture is notorious for strict prohibition of certain objects. By raising the topic of a taboo, we pass into the field of what is discarded and expelled from mentioning. Taboo is imposed by symbolic order *per se*. In Muslim culture taboos are determined along these lines:

1. Food

Muslims do not consume pork, nor pork products since they are considered impure. Other meat is prohibited unless it is slaughtered according to Islamic standards, making it halal.This method of slaughtering animals consists of using a well-sharpened knife to make a swift, deep incision that cuts the front of the throat, the carotid artery, trachea, and jugular veins[804]. The head of an animal that is being slaughtered should face the qibla upon utterance of the Islamic prayer "Bismillah" (in the name of God).

---

[804] http://halalcertification.ie/halal/islamic-method-of-slaughtering, consulted on 21.09.2016

2. Alcohol

The consumption of alcohol is viewed as a "great sin" in Islam. Supposedly, this prohibition is connected with the intoxicating and bewildering effects that alcohol has on a human, which prevents him/her from accomplishing five regular prayers in a state of sobriety. It is also believed that alcohol is banned in Islam because of its high risk of causing health malaise.

3. In relation with sex

In Islam sex between unmarried men and women is taboo, which also promptsmen and women to dress modestly.

4. Depicting human

Muslims believe in Allah as the sole Creator. Therefore, portraits are considered as attempts to accede to the place of God. Islamic scholars affirm that Mohammed forbade his companions to create portraits of him, because of fear that if those images are made, they may be worshipped, instead of worshipping Allah.

Maktoub (Fatalism)

In Islamic interpretation, fatalism is a strong belief in a fate predestined by Allah. If a man's life is predetermined, then, he cannot be free. The Asharite theory of Kasb, namely that God poses and man disposes, that God creates in man the capacity to act and that man acquires his actions through this capacity, is closer to determinism. Divine creation of capacity before action man is incapable of doing anything.[805] What is called predestination is not an intervention of divine will in human action, which would negate human responsibility and equal opportunity, but an objective field of action. Free will has its correlation not in God but in the world. God is not a limit to human free will, rather the world is.[806] The Quran stresses on both: man's free will and God's unlimited power over a human. The Islamic scholars interpret differently this issue. For example, the Determinists (Al-Jabnyyah) maintained that man's actions are determined by a higher power, God. The Asharites believed that God inscribed aforehand all man's actions. The Mutazilah differentiated between human's actions, which derive from his/her own free will, and those, which are God-given. Quran itself insists on a correlation of God's omnipotence and man's free will. Ibn Arabi disagrees with viewing the

---

[805] Hanafi Hasan, *Islam in the modern world. Tradition, Revolution and Culture*, Cairo: Dar Kebaa Bookshop, vol. II,1995, p.145.

[806] *Ibid, p.146.*

human life as a forced compulsion to certain outcomes. However, human's free will cannot be absolute, which would oppose him to God. Thereby, Ibn Arabi believed in dualism. Though Ibn Arabi occasionally tries to attribute personal responsibility to humans. In fact, the scholar denies free will even to God. For Ibn Arabi, God merely decrees what He knows must take place in accordance with the laws that have their being in Him. This understanding leads to a common misinterpretation of a concept "inshallah" (Allah willing).

According to Umar Ibn Al-Khattab: for Prophet Mohamed, iman (the faith) signified belief in God, His Angels, His Books, His Prophets, the Day of Judgement and qadar (the destiny) be it good or bad. The notions qadha and qadar are based on certain arguments, where qadha signifies divine decree, and qadar divine decision. Both concepts, according to Mohamed Ad Dahabi, constitute undeniable and indisputable principles with regard to their meaning.[807] In this light the Muslim historian exposes five main principles:

1. God precedes the existence and He knows what will happen to it even before it materializes. The following ayats read, "Indeed, Allah is Knowing of all things" (sura 9, ayat 115); "Indeed, Allah is Knowing of that within the breasts." (sura 31, ayat 23)
2. God is a Creator of everything and He has the power to create anything he wishes for, including human acts.
3. Nothing in the universe happens without God's will. The following ayats attest to that: "If Allah had willed, those [generations] succeeding them would not have fought each other after the clear proofs had come to them. But they differed, and some of them believed and some of them disbelieved. And if Allah had willed, they would not have fought each other, but Allah does what He intends." (sura 2, ayat 253)
4. A man is responsible for one's own acts and will be judged for them.
5. God is not questioned of what he wishes. Quran says, "He is not questioned about what He does, but they will be questioned." (sura 21, ayat 23)

---

[807] https://www.cairn.info/revue-topique-2010-1-page-97.htm, consulted on 21.09.2016

"Inshallah" as a Defense Mechanism, or What Does Allah Want?

According to Ernest Renan, who opposed Semites and Ariens, and who remarked that the former are very vague in terms of notion time, Laforgue affirms that Arabs do not have the notion of time[808]. He refers to the myth of the sleeping child, who could doze off for years in the mother`s womb and come out at the time when mother desired it. Instead of interpreting the whole myth, Laforgue reduces it to the dimension of real time by concealing its symbolic dimension.The tendency of delegating one`s own responsibilities to a chance, luck and higher power constitutes paralysis of personal will. Also in procrastination of fulfilling a task, an Arab demonstrates his passive-aggressive opposition.

Whatever exists has been created by the will of the Almighty. It is not for man to modify His work. If God had wished that what exists should be different, he would have made it so, irrespective of all human volition.

First of all, in analytical practice, the exactitude of rendezvous and the notion of time come into play. To a question, "Would you like a session ?" or to an affirmation, "On Monday at such time" or "Until the next week", he answered, "If God is willing."[809] In psychoanalysis an analysand attempts to escape from one`s own ambivalence and faults, he leads a psychoanalyst in a boat, leaning abusively on the divine decree like a mechanism of defense[810]. If an analysand replies me "inshallah", I ask, "what does "inshallah" means personally to you?" And many get stuck because they have never been thinking about it. Others answer. And I have come to the conclusion that there is no consensus regarding the meaning of this word. "Inshallah" for one person is totally different from"inshallah" of somebody else, varying only in graduation scale of one`s own attributed responsibility.

Types of "inshallah":

1. "Inshallah" in sense "I do not care," calculated in proportion of 100%-0%, where all responsibility is ascribed to Allah, e.g. meaning that Allah wished that I did not take medicine on time. I take no responsibility for this.

---

[808] http://jalilbennani.blog.lemonde.fr/2014/01/06/le-voyage-de-la-psychanalyse -au-maroc/, consulted on 01.07.2016

[809] https://www.cairn.info/revue-topique-2010-1-page-97.htm, consulted on 21.09.2016

[810] https://www.cairn.info/revue-topique-2010-1-page-97.htm, consulted on 21.09.2016

It is used by those Muslims, who are not used to taking responsibilities. In this case "inshallah" is usually uttered automatically even without thinking about the possibility to fulfill one`s own word.

2. "Inshallah" in sense "I will try to," calculated in proportion of 50%-50%, meaning half is my responsibility and half is Allah`s, e.g. I will try doing it, however, with the first obstacle I will give up and will not try it anymore, probably, because Allah does not want it.

3. "Inshallah" in sense "I tried to but it did not happen," calculated in a proportion of 90%-10%. E.g. I put all my strength and energy, and even more, for some time I forgot that a person is not all-powerful, and I still kept on trying, and even then it did not happen.

4. "Inshallah" in sense "I have outdone my best, and still it did not happen," calculated in proportion of (99%-1%). Such an attitude happens very rarely. After numerous failures and incredible efforts a person tries again during a significant period of time, and still, it does not happen.

Some other examples of using "inshallah" are illustrated below:
Boy: "Father, will we go to Toys 'R' Us later today?"[811]
Father: "Yes. Inshallah."
Translation: "There is no way we're going to Toys 'R' Us. I'm exhausted. Play with the neighbor's toys. Here, play with this staple remover. That's fun, isn't it?"
Inshallah is also an extremely useful tool in the modern quest for love.
Man: "So, you think we will get married?"
Woman: "Yeah, let me think about it, inshallah."
Translation: "No. Never. There is no way we are ever going to get married. Even if you were the last man on earth, I would not consider this an option and would rather the human species perish as a result of my decision"."Inshallahs" are dropped daily, for any occasions, and without. I'll get to the gym, inshallah. Yes, I'll clean up around the house, inshallah.

It can be concluded that most commonly, "inshallah" is used in Muslim community so that to escape introspection, hard work and strategic planning and instead outsource such responsibilities to an omnipotent being, who somehow, at some time, will intervene and fix the problem.

---

[811] http://www.nytimes.com/2016/04/24/opinion/sunday/inshallah-is-good-for-everyone.html?mwrsm=Facebook&_r=0, consulted on 21.09.2016

Whilst real "inshallah" stands for the situation when one has been trying multiple times excersizing one`s outmost will, and still it did not happen. This leaves space to think of what Allah wants.

Virginity

Fethi Benslama says, "[I]n the very strict tradition of keeping the hymen intact for the husband…[m]an believes that by this unique unveiling he can access woman once and for all, as if, by entering that intact depth and by removing the immaculate surface, he will succeed in "consuming" her entirely, with no remainder," no excess Other jouissance that irks him with his inability to access it for himself. He becomes the master of that loss [of a hymen, of virginity].[812] A virgin experiences fear for losing her chastity, that is when the Big Other becomes even bigger and more powerful, endowed by an ability to subdue her. He unveils the veil and eliminates any control over the object he aspires to contain absolutely. The situation in the Muslim world is presented as if from virginity a particular form of "sainthood" is born. And sainthood is of sacrificial origin. Here is present a certain idea of martyrdom, which is not alien to islam. Virginity is simply a demarcation line between sexual experience and naivety.[813] Lerner maintains that in ancient Mesopotamia, the 1780 BC Babylonian code of Hammurabi is the first legal legislation to institutionalize the sexual control of women and the patriarchal family.[814] A dominant restrictive culture and a strict moral code leave women with little to be proud of besides their virginity.[815] Virginity is an important social category and marker.[816] Virginity is also a sign of trust. In these terms, the Marvelous History of the Mirror of Virgins from the book One Thousand and One Night can serve as a reference example. The story exposes the adventures of the Sultan Zein, who, by an indication of his deceased father, set off a quest searching for a statue, which he could obtain from The Old Man of Three Islands once he succeeded in bringing him an exceptionally beautiful fifteen-year-old virgin. The Sultan found the task easy, however, The Old

---

[812] Sutton Kyra, *Islam`s Turn on the Couch: The Psychoanalytic Theorizing of Muslim Identity in France*, Connecticut: Weyslan University, 2013, p.93.

[813] Ghanim David, *The Virginity Trap in the Middle East*, New York: Springer, 2015, p.2.

[814] *Ibid, p.18.*

[815] *Ibid, p.22.*

[816] *Ibid,* p.2.

Man sowed doubt by asserting that not all virgins who claim to be such, are virgins, indeed. The Old Man granted Zein a mirror, which would help him to define the chastity of a girl simply by meditating upon her reflection in the mirror. Discerning the reflection is not a direct gaze at a woman's body, which does not transgress the personal boundaries. Zein was travelling a lot, and, finally, found one in Iraq. He fell in love with her, however, had to bring her to The Old Man, as promised. Having seen the young woman, The Old Man turned into a guardian angel and replied, "Since the day of your birth I have been protecting you and assuring your happiness, however, total happiness is not possible without a beautiful virgin with an excellent soul. This triad is the utmost treasure." In the story Shahrezade by acceding to the desire of King Shahryar to hear "a marvelous story," reveals sincerely that virginity exists only in fiction. It remains simultaneously a phantasm and reality, however, it has only the sense, which is projected upon it by the Other.

The question of a lack, a central notion in psychoanalysis, is a key to unlocking the concept of virginity in the Islamic society. Especially, in the light of three registers Real-Symbolic-Imaginatory, which were elaborated by Lacan in three possible forms:

- Castration as a symbolic lack of an imaginatory object;
- Frustration as an imaginatory lack of the real object;
- Privation as a real lack of the symbolic object.

Virginity can interplay in three of these axes. There is virginity as a constant, being referred to the Real; the virginity as a reference on the side of identifications in the Imaginatory; and signifying virginity of the inscription in the Symbolic chain.

Actually, Quran mentions virginity only in two cases: firstly, when talking about Paradise, where women become virgins again after each night of love. Secondly, in the ayats mentioning Maryam, the mother of Isa. Moreover, among thirteen wives of Prophet, only Aisha was virgin, who was married off before her puberty. Therefore, virginity is not an Islamic religious conception, but rather a consequence of patriarchal society dominance.

Female's Circumcision

It is believed that female genital mutilation was already known in the Pharaonic Egypt. As recent as the 1950s, clitoridectomy was practiced in Western Europe and the United States to treat perceived ailments including hysteria, epilepsy, mental disorders, masturbation, nymphomania, and melancholia.[817] Female genital mutilation is a common practice in a number of Muslim countries. The 2008 WHO estimates a prevalence of 23% among women in Yemen, 71% in Mauritania, 90% in Sudan, 93% in Djibouti, 96% in Egypt, and 98% in Somalia.[818] Besides, it is still being widely practiced in Iraq, Malaysia, Oman, Pakistan, Palestine, Senegal and UAE, even though, some of these countries have banned FGM by law. While the health consequences of FGM vary widely from setting to setting according to type and prevalence, its persistence illustrates continuing control over the female body and restraint of feminine jouissance. It is an act of privation of the "feminine" because it is considered dangerous. Also, it is thought to ensure virginity before marriage and fidelity afterward, and to increase male sexual pleasure.[819] The psychological stress of the procedure may trigger behavioural disturbances in children, closely linked to loss of trust and confidence in caregivers.[820] Eventually, women are submitted to a permanent feeling of anxiety, depression and sexual dysfunction.

Feminism

The Islamic feminism differs from the secular one since it is inscribed in the religious tradition. Justice in Islam means everything being in its proper place, not, forcibly, equal. Therefore, the Islamic feminism is not that much about equalizing the genders` roles, as allowing woman an active role in the patriarchal society. Practically speaking, feminism aims at the subversion of patriarchal social arrangements and enabling women into the domains, which were previously massively presided by males. Thus, creating opposition to the patriarchal tradition.

Specificities of Islamic feminism:

-   Strong support in favor of the veil. Both men and women now consider veil as a symbol of Islamic freedom;
-   Islamic feminists advocate for women to be allowed to pray beside men without a partition as they do in Mecca;

---

[817] http://www.unfpa.org/resources/female-genital-mutilation-fgm-frequently-asked-questions#consequences_childbirth, consulted on 01.07.2016

[818] http://hdr.undp.org/en/reports/regional/arabstates/name,3442,en.html, consulted on 01.07.2016

[819] http://www.unfpa.org/resources/female-genital-mutilation-fgm-frequently-asked-questions#consequences_childbirth, consulted on 01.07.2016

[820] *Ibid*

- Equality in leading prayer. For instance, on March 18, 2005, Amina Wadud led a mixed-gender congregational Friday prayer in New York City.

Ergo, Islamic feminism is a passover from feminine passivity into activity, while remaining in Islamic order.

Democracy

Till very recent a symptom has been tabooed in Arab community due to its social unacceptability, just very much like democracy itself. Indeed, Islamic religion and Bedouin culture control all aspects of a human life. However, it is not a question of co-existence of democracy and religion in as much as it is that of the archetypal figure of the father, who either willingly enables this co-existence or largely obstructs it. It can be truly said that the democracy in Arab countries has got the face of the national leader. And it is accorded in proportion just enough to be considered democracy. However, in certain countries (e.g. Algeria, Syria, Somalia), it is not sufficient as for the practice of psychoanalysis. Shall it be reminded that Quran is not, like Bible or Gospels, a narrative of a human, but it is a word of Allah? Therefore, Quran cannot be criticized, nor amended. The maintenance of the rigid order requires the presence of a strong leader. So, a signifier "democracy", from one side, is in the domain of the father's desire (which encourages democracy), and from the other side, in the domain of his capacities (which preserve it from exceeding the allowed). As the consensus of these conditions, psychoanalysis can function in an Arab country.

Sexuality

The Islamic world draws an explicit line between private and public, the transgression of which is severely punished by law. Even though Islam recognizes and accepts human sensuality, it is cautiously protected from the Other. As a source of pleasure, sexuality is permitted, and, therefore, fully "covered" (protected) from public access, which creates a particular order for enabling jouissance. There is for, example, no celibacy or monasteries in Islam where believers can withdraw from the world.[821] Celibacy is

---

[821] https://en.qantara.de/content/islam-and-psychoanalysis-a-tale-of-mutual-ignorance, consulted on 01.07.2016

not considered as an accepted practice.[822] Despite this, Alriyadyh Arabic language daily, citing an unnamed medical study in the Gulf Kingdom, said nearly 12% of Saudi Arabia's 20 million national men are suffering from impotence and that 80% of the cases are associated with psychological problems.[823] According to the study, Arab countries spend more than 10 billion dollars on Viagra and other anti-impotence medicines every year and that Saudi Arabia alone spends over 1.5 billion dollars. It is followed by Egypt and the UAE, which spend about 500 million dollars respectively.[824] Europeans condemned Islam for its acceptance of human sexuality when Victorian morals dominated Europe. When Freudian ideas were popularized, Islamic limitations for sexual rapports were severely criticized. A strict ban on free expression of one's sexuality could also be viewed as a cause of ongoing wars and violence in the Muslim world.

---

[822] http://applications.emro.who.int/emhj/0703/emhj_2001_7_3_336_347. pdf?ua=1

[823] https://wikiislam.net/wiki/Muslim_Statistics_-_Health_and_Disability, consulted on 01.07.2016

[824] http://www.emirates247.com/news/region/saudis-6th-largest-consumers-of-sex-drugs-2012-03-04-1.446439, consulted on 01.07.2016

CHAPTER 12

THE MUSLIM EXEGESIS

Quran has an inner meaning, and this inner meaning conceals an even deeper meaning inside, which contains yet a deeper meaning and so on (up to seven levels of meaning). The interpretation of sense of Quran is named tafseer, or Muslim exegesis. In Islamic context it is understood as uncovering of the hidden. Tafseer enables proper understanding of the word of Allah, and the Muslim unconscious as well. Before any other sources, which can bring light to the Muslim unconscious, such as, the tales, the proverbs, the customs etc., the first and foremost there comes Quran, then sunna, and reports of sahaba (companions of Prophet).

- The Quran explained by the Quran means that all possible questions, which might arise, are already explicated in the Holy Book. For instance:

"Then learnt Adam from his Lord words of inspiration, and his Lord turned towards him, for He is Oft-Returning, Most Merciful." (sura 2, ayat 37)
These "words of inspiration" are clarified by the Quran as follows:
"Our Lord! We have wronged our own souls. If Thou forgive us not, and bestow not upon us Thy mercy, we shall certainly be lost." (sura 7, ayat 23)

- The Quran explained by the Prophet. Muhamed himself was meditating upon the meaning of the sent verses, and if their

336

meaning was vague to him, he was asking Angel Gibrael for explanations. Also, the followers of the Islamic faith were addressing to Muhamed for clarifications. For example:

"And eat and drink until the white thread of dawn appears to you distinct from its black thread. . ." (sura 2, ayat 187)

Narrated Adi b. Hatim: I said, "O Allah's Apostle! What is the meaning of the white thread distinct from the black thread? Are these two threads?" He said, "You are not intelligent if you seek for the two threads". He then added, "No, it is the darkness of the night and the whiteness of the day."

- Reports of sahaba close the three most viable sources of Muslim exegesis. Among the most trusted followers, known for their knowledge, were: Abu Bakr, Umar, Uthman, Ali, Ibn Masud, Ibn Abbs, Ubay b. Kab, Zaid b. Thabit, Aba Musa al-Ashari, Abdullah b. Zubair.

This chapter will also look into the traditional sources of the Arabic mentality, which stay rather on its cultural side (Arabic), rather then religious (Muslim).

Concept of Id, Ego and Superego of Arab People

"Superego is an heir of the Oedipus complex," thus, in one single phrase Freud resumed the very essence of the superego. The superego is unconscious. And this is the parental authority, interiorized during the Oedipus, and differentiated inside I as one of its parts is called superego. The superego of a modern Arab is often projected onto the state. In less authoritative authority the super-ego is projected onto the collective authority. Indeed, the Arab state is expected to exercise as much of the authority on their citizens as the parents on their child. Since the majority of Arabs are modified in their superego, this means that the more authoritative is the state, the higher degree of authoritarianism will appear in the Arab mentality.

Freud's structural and topographical model of personality is very much in-line with the Islamic concept of Nafs. Three states of the self are mentioned in the Quran, including Nafs–e-Ammara, Nafs-e-Mutmainnah and Nafs Lawwama.

Nafs–e-Ammara is prone to the lower aspects of the self, and corresponds to the hedonistic Id, impulsive part of the psychic apparatus that operates on the "pleasure principle". It is the source of basic impulses, which seek immediate pleasure and avoid pain. According to Freud the Id is unconscious by definition: "It is the dark, inaccessible part of our personality, what little we know of it from what we have learned from our study of the dreamwork and of course the construction of neurotic symptoms, and most of that is of a negative character and can be described only as a contrast to the ego. We approach the id with analogies: we call it a chaos, a cauldron full of seething excitations. ... It is filled with energy reaching it from the instincts, but it has no organization, produces no collective will, but only a striving to bring about the satisfaction of the instinctual needs subject to the observance of the pleasure principle."[825] Islam seeks to control Nafs–e–Ammara. In fact, the highest struggle (jihad) in Islam is the struggle against one's Nafs (Jihad bin Nafs). Nafs-e-Ammara is mentioned in sura 12, ayat 53.

Nafs-e-Mutmainnah is analogous to the ego, which is the part of the psyche most directly reflected in the person's actions. The ego represents what may be called reason and common sense, in contrast to the id, which contains the passions ... in its relation to the id it is like a man on horseback, who has to hold in check the superior strength of the horse; with this difference, that the rider tries to do so with his own strength, while the ego uses borrowed forces.[826] Islamic tradition believes that in order to achieve the state of tranquility and peace one has to awaken the remorseful self (e.g. through sincere repentance) and control the lower commanding "self" (through self-discipline). Nafs-e-Mutmainnah is described in sura 89, ayats 27-28 as the state of inner peace, happiness and satisfaction.

Nafs Lawwama is viewed as the superego, which contains internalized societal and parental standards of "good" and "bad", "right" and "wrong" behaviour. It includes conscious appreciations of rules and regulations as well as those incorporated unconsciously. According to Freud, "The superego retains the character of the father, while the more powerful the Oedipus complex was and the more rapidly it succumbed to repression (under the influence of authority, religious teaching, schooling and reading), the stricter will be the domination of the super-ego over the ego later on—in the form of conscience or perhaps of an unconscious sense of guilt."[827] In Islam this state corresponds to the self when it becomes aware

---

[825] Freud Sigmund, *New Introductory Lectures on Psychoanalysis*, London: Penguin Freud Library,1933, pp. 105–106.

[826] Freud Sigmund, *The Ego and the Id, On Metapsychology*, London: Penguin,1991, pp. 363–364.

[827] *Ibid*

of wrong-doing and feels remorse. Nafs-e- Lawwama is evoked in sura 75, ayat 2, as a self-reproaching self.

According to Islamic thought, the process of human mental and spiritual development is a constant evolution from a purely self-gratifying stage (nafs-e-amareh) to a stage of inner peace and self-assuredness (nafs-e-mutmaennah).[828] This passage is filled with self-doubt, self-accusation, and self-acceptance.

If we follow the Freudian text further, in fact, it is not easy to distinguish who from I and super-ego is at the origin of another. For example, in the book I and Id, the superego appears as the consequence and the reason of an agreement between the identifications of I. Freud insists on the structural ambiguity of superego. He speaks of "double faces", which could be the face, who is, and the face who is not. Likewise, the superego participates in the game of illusion and disillusion. What are the faces of superego? The superego is double-faced; from one side-encouraging and motivating, and from the other destructing and tyranic. The face of an Ideal Father is an Archaic Father, who says, "Keep on, do your best." Whilst the Archaic Mother, who is the Desiring Mother, wants to devour her child and she says, "You are nothing, who are you taking yourself for?" The figure of Seducing Father, integrated by love, says, "Let it happen." The superego fulfills three functions: auto-observation, conscious moral and the ideal. The other category of the superego, the tyranic superego, does not solely represent the exterior reality in the eyes of I, but also the infernal world of jouissance, that is to say, the world of Id. The superego consists of two blocs: The conscience and the ideal self. The conscience causes the feeling of guilt if ego diverts from the superego`s prescriptions. And the Ideal I is the image of how one should behave so that to be loved by the other. There is also another instance, which is called I Ideal, which represents the ideal image of how I see myself for myself. The superego is at once injunction and interdiction, which imposes the articulation of these two opposing faces and their concordance so that to allow I to reconstruct its future. Between I and superego exists a sadomasochist relation, a concept, which operates anthropomorphisation, the personnification[829] of the instances (superego=father; censorship=mother) and acts on the level of intersubjective relations. In fact, the function of superego is exceptional, since it is the one, which establishes the link between the culture and ethics

---

[828]   http://applications.emro.who.int/emhj/0703/emhj_2001_7_3_336_347. pdf?ua=1,consulted on 21.09.2016

[829]   Freud Sigmund, Personnages psychopathiques à la scène, Résultats, idées et problèmes, Paris: PUF, 2006.

of the society. The primary question is to know the way, which would allow I and superego to fix the sufficiently functioning distance.

Concept of Fitra

The Arabic term nafs (self) signifies individual personality and the term fitra (nature) indicates the human nature. Indeed, a cornerstone concept for understanding a human nature from an Islamic perspective is "Fitra". It embodies the man in his primeval state and natural predisposition. Here the primeval state is related to the initial spiritual experience, which stems from a belief that all souls made a pledge with Allah long before they were born on the Earth, acknowledging Him as their Lord (sura 7, ayat 172). Charles Morris attributes fundamental significance to the soul's pre-natal experience, just as big as Freud to the impact of childhood on the development of psychic symptoms in adulthood. Therefore, the natural predisposition of a man is a state of submission to Allah. The religious experience symbolizes a form of recognition rather than discovery. Quran says, "He the Prophet enjoins on them that which they themselves sense as right, and forbids them that which they themselves sense as wrong" (sura 7, ayat 157). Due to the initial experience of union with Allah, a part of the individual seeks that union again. Often this quest starts with a search for the meaning of life. According to the Quran, the eternal aspect of each individual, the soul, is on a journey and passes through various stages in life. The final destination of this journey, as well as its beginning, is Allah. Quran says, "And now you have returned to Us alone, as We created you at first, leaving behind all that we bestowed on you" (sura 6, ayat 94).

The Arabic Mythology

The Arabic mythology includes myths, legends, fairy tales, proverbs, sayings, beliefs and other folklore material of Arab people. Arabian mythology is a primal source of the Bedouin unconscious. Besides, it is possible to claim that the world vision for a majority of Arab people remains based on mythological beliefs. It can be explained by the fact that scientific concepts have not yet overthrown the most primitive perceptions. The Table 12.1. shows the existent elements of the Arabic culture, which were brought in by different world cultures.

The distinctive feature of the Arabic mythology is the figure of Allah. Allah, as a supreme power, is omnipotent over the hero's destiny. God can respond to the main hero's prayers and grant him wealth, or, on the contrary, punish him for committing the evil acts.

Whilst a woman is viewed exclusively in a relation to a man (father, brother, or husband). She is either described as a good wife, who is a loyal companion to her husband, or, as a bad one, who is constantly interfering with her husband's plans. The woman's honor, virginity, is her most precious value before getting married, and her loyalty to her husband afterwards.

Another popular character is the King, who epitomizes the most powerful earthly figure. He is not subdued to justice, nor to any laws, only to his proper will and desire.

Moreover, the Arabic fairy tales are abundant in the presence of supernatural forces. Jinn, Jinniyeh, Ifreet, Ghouls, Ghouleh, Giants, Satan, Angels and other mythological creatures get in contact with the main heroes in order to test, guide, seduce, confuse, or even attempt to kill them. However, in the end, good forces turn to be more powerful than evil forces. Apart from creatures with super powers, there are magical objects, like a ring, a lamp, a crystal ball, or a flying carpet.

Arabic heroes pay high attention to certain numbers revealed to them throughout the story, which have particular spiritual meaning. For example, the numbers three, seven and forty appear in such connotations as: "seven days and nights," "three days of hospitality," and "forty doors to open", etc.

Arabic folktales are marked by violence. Many scenes of detailed struggle augment as the hero moves closer to one's goal.

In general, the Arabic folklore praises such values as kindness, hospitality, bravery, honor, generosity, and others.

This said Arabic fairytales can be divided into several categories, notably, about:

Heroism, which allows a human to feel oneself superpowerful. The Bedouin legends amassed a great collection of myths about a winner, who was considered to be a superhuman (owing to his loyalty, strength, smartness, and not supernatural powers).

Kings or other notable persons, where they appear as extremely powerful figures, who can influence the destiny of the main hero. Oftentimes the Earthly power of a King is counterposed to the supernatural powers or distinctive qualities of a hero, which, in the end, win the bid.

Warfare, where the adroitness and remarkable bravery of the main hero are extolled.

Religion, which helps a main hero in overcoming life troubles.

Supernatural forces, which oftentimes help the main hero to achieve his principal goal in return for a certain service rendered to them.

Juha, satiric stories, which are based on real or semi-real anecdotic plot. This genre appeared after the Bedouins moved to the urban life, since desert life did not offer a context for jokes. So, this genre of stories stands for a big shift, which happened in Arab perception.

Love stories, which usually depict sufferings and torments of the main hero, who is afflicted by unhappy love, which is not meant to materialize. This high and idealized love lives purely in imagination. The love leads to delirium, then madness, or even death. Arabic love stories are full of sensual elements, which seduce a hero in his ultimate search for pleasure. The longing for volition in love, for attainment of love's greatest ecstasy, was to linger for centuries in the Arab soul, transcending the rich urban centuries of the empire, with their abated, colourful male sexuality, their open negotiations with the erotic, to surface again in various periods and areas of the Arab world, then assert its hard command among modern Arab poets and writers of fiction in the first half of the twentieth century.[830]

Arabic Tale "Nur al-Din Ali and His Son Badr al-Din Hasan"

A long time ago there was a King of the Kings of the Banu Sasan in the islands of India and China, a Lord of armies and guards and servants and dependents[831]. He had only two sons, an older and a younger one, who were both courageous men. The older son King Shahryar succeeded to the throne, and he made his younger brother, Shah Zaman hight, King of Samarkand in Barbarian land. And each ruled his own kingdom with equity and fairness.

Table 12.1 Examples of Certain Mythological
Influence of Other Civilizations on Arabs

Sumerian/ Mesopotamian/ Babylonian/ Assyrian	Persian	Indian	Egyptian	Greco-Roman
Metal amulets	Shell amulets to avert the evil eye	Stone amulets	Reincarnation	Crystal amulets

---

[830] Jayyusi Salma,*Classical Arabic Stories: An Anthology,* NewYork: Columbia University Press, 2012, p.14.

[831] https://www.library.cornell.edu/colldev/mideast/arabnit.htm, consulted on 21.09.2016

Curative knots	Astrology	Sacred danse	Sacred animals	Belief in an underworld
Incense for purification	Zodiac		Kings were gods	Numerology
Lucky / unlucky days Lucky / unlucky numbers			Magic	

But at the end of the twentieth twelve months the elder King yearned for a sight of his younger brother and felt that he must look upon him once more.[832] Following the advice of his Minister, the King started preparing the gifts for his brother, instead of going to see him. Also, he wrote a letter to Shah Zaman, which ended with these words: "We, therefore, hope of the favor and affection of the beloved brother that he will condescend to bestir himself and turn his face upward. Furthermore, we have sent our Wazir to make all ordinance for the march, and our one and only desire it is to see thee ere we die. But if thou delay or disappoint us, we shall not survive the blow. Wherewith peace be upon thee!"[833]

As soon as the Wazir delivered the letter, Shah Zaman read it and said, "I hear and I obey the commands of the beloved brother!" adding to the Wazir, "But we will not march till after the third day's hospitality." But when the night was half-spent he bethought him that he had forgotten in his palace somewhat which he should have brought with him, so he returned privily and entered his apartments, where he found the Queen, his wife, asleep on his own carpet bed embracing with both arms a black cook of loathsome aspect and foul with kitchen grease and grime.[834] He said, "If such case happens while I am yet within sight of the city, what will be the doings of this damned whore during my long absence at my brother's court?"[835] So, he cut the two with his sword and gave orders for immediate departure. When Shah Zaman approached the capital of his brother, Shahryar came to meet him. However, the elder could not but see the change of complexion in the younger and questioned him of his case, whereto he replied, "This caused by the travails of warfare and my

---

832 *Ibid*

833 https://www.library.cornell.edu/colldev/mideast/arabnit.htm, consulted on 21.09.2016

834 *Ibid*

835 *Ibid*

case needs care, for I have suffered from the change of water and air! But Allah be praised for reuniting me with a brother so dear and so rare!"[836] In a few days, Shahryar left for hunting and his brother stayed at palace thinking sadly about his wife's betrayal. During that time he witnessed the Shahryar's wife betraying her husband. Now when Shah Zaman saw this conduct of his sister-in-law, he said to himself: "By Allah, my calamity is lighter than this! My brother is a greater King among the Kings than I am, yet this infamy goeth on in his very palace, and his wife is in love with that filthiest of filthy slaves. But this only showeth that they all do it and that there is no woman but who cuckolded her husband. Then the curse of Allah upon one and all, and upon the fools who lean against them for support or who place the reins of conduct in their hands!"[837]In the following days, he began recovering his healthy condition. When his brother came back from the chase ten days after Shah Zaman told him, "Know, then, O my brother, when thou sentest thy Wazir with the invitation to place myself between thy hands, I made ready and marched out of my city. But presently I minded me having left behind me in the palace a string of jewels intended as a gift to thee. I returned for it alone and found my wife on my carpet bed and in the arms of a hideous black cook. So I slew the twain and came to thee, yet my thoughts brooded over this business and I lost my bloom and became weak. But excuse me if I still refuse to tell thee what was the reason of my complexion returning." Thereupon Shah Zaman told Shahryar all he had seen about the wife of the latter, ending with these words: "When I beheld thy calamity and the treason of thy wife, O my brother, and I reflected that thou art in years my senior and in sovereignty my superior, mine own sorrow was belittled by the comparison, and my mind recovered tone and temper. So, throwing off melancholy and despondency, I was able to eat and drink and sleep, and thus I speedily regained health and strength. Such is the truth and the whole truth."[838] King Shahryar answered, "O my brother, I would not give thee the lie in this matter, but I cannot credit it till I see it with mine own eyes." Shah Zaman suggested that next time he would pretend getting ready for hunting, and instead, would hide in Shah's Zaman room. In next days the brothers disguised themselves and returned secretly by night to the palace. They were observing the Queen and her lover satisfying their lust. When King Shahryar saw this infamy he cried out: "Only in utter solitude can man be safe from the doings of this vile world! By Allah,

---

[836] *Ibid*

[837] *Ibid*

[838] *Ibid*

344

life is naught but one great wrong."[839] He added, "Let us up as we are and depart forthright hence, for we have no concern with kingship, and let us overwander Allah's earth, worshiping the Almighty till we find someone to whom the like calamity hath happened. And if we find none then will death be more welcome to us than life."[840] During their journey, they encountered a Jinni. He then set down the coffer on its bottom and out of it drew a casket with seven padlocks of steel, which he unlocked with seven keys of steel he took from beside his thigh, and out of it a young lady to come was seen, whiteskinned and of winsomest mien, of stature fine and thin, and bright as though a moon of the fourteenth night she had been, or the sun raining lively sheen.[841] When she perceived the Kings, she said, "Come ye down, ye two, and fear naught from this Ifrit."[842] She ordered them to futter her. When they had dismounted from her, she said: "Well done!". She then took from her pocket a purse and drew out a knotted string whereon were strung five hundred and seventy seal rings, and asked, "Know ye what be these?"[843] They replied that they did not know. Then quoth she, "These be the signets of five hundred and seventy men who have all futtered me upon the horns of this foul, this foolish, this filthy Ifrit. So give me also your two seal rings, ye pair of brothers."[844] When they passed their rings to her, she said, "Of a truth this Ifrit bore me off on my bride night, and put me into a casket and set the casket in a coffer, and to the coffer he affixed seven strong padlocks of steel and deposited me on the deep bottom of the sea that raves, dashing and clashing with waves, and guarded me so that I might remain chaste and honest, quotha! that none save himself might have connection with me. But I have lain under as many of my kind as I please, and this wretched Jinni wotteth not that Destiny may not be averted nor hindered by aught, and that whatso woman willeth, the same she fulfilleth however man nilleth." Even so saith one of them,

"Rely not on women,
Trust not to their hearts,
Whose joys and whose sorrows
Are hung to their parts!

---

839   https://www.library.cornell.edu/colldev/mideast/arabnit.htm, consulted on
        21.09.2016
840   *Ibid*
841   *Ibid*
842   *Ibid*
843   *Ibid*
844   *Ibid*

Lying love they will swear thee
Whence guile ne'er departs.
Take Yusuf for sample,
'Ware sleights and 'ware smarts!
Iblis ousted Adam
(See ye not?) thro' their arts."[845]

Afterwards they returned to the Palace of King Shahryar, which they on the third day. Shahryar instructed to send for the Chief Minister, the father of the two damsels, saying: "I command thee to take my wife and smite her to death, for she hath broken her plight and her faith."[846] So, she was executed. He also swore that whatever wife he married he would abate her maiden head at night and slay her next morning, to make sure of his honor. "For," said he, "there never was nor is there one chaste woman upon the face of earth."[847] During three years he continued marrying a maiden every night and killing her the next morning, till folk raised against him and cursed him. One day the King ordered his Chief Wazir, the same who was charged with the executions, to bring him another virgin. He was anxious because he had two daughters, Sheherazade and Dunyazade. On that day Sheherazade told her father: "Why do I see thee thus changed and laden with cark and care?"[848]

When the Wazir related the story to her, she answered, "By Allah, O my father, how long shall this slaughter of women endure? Shall I tell thee what is in my mind in order to save both sides from destruction? I wish thou wouldst give me in marriage to this King Shahryar. Either I shall live or I shall be a ransom for the virgin daughters of Moslems and the cause of their deliverance from his hands and thine."[849] The Wazir was furious and ended with: "In very deed I fear lest the same befall thee which befell the bull and the ass with the husbandman."[850] "And what," asked she, "befell them, O my father?"[851] Whereupon the Wazir began the tale.

---

[845] *Ibid*

[846] *Ibid*

[847] *Ibid*

[848] https://www.library.cornell.edu/colldev/mideast/arabnit.htm, consulted on 21.09.2016

[849] *Ibid*

[850] *Ibid*

[851] *Ibid*

Some Types of Folkloric Creatures

The Arabic mythology is abounding in mystical figures. Just a few of them are mentioned below:

Abgal -a god of the desert.

Alladdin is a proprietor of a magic lamp in The Arabian Nights. The jinn, who lived in the lamp could fulfill any Alladdin's wish, including assisting him to get married with a beautiful princess, Badr al-Budur. After her father died, Alladdin became the emperor of China.

Alasnam is an owner of eight precious statues in The Arabian Nights. He also had a magic mirror that could detect if a maiden was virgin.

Ali Baba is a hero of a story in The Arabian Nights, who found out the password (Sesame or Simsim) to the robbers' cave and stole their treasure.

Amina is an evil ghoul in The Arabian Nights, who was humiliating her three sisters: she was leading them on leads like dogs.

Apples of Samarkand- Apples that could heal any ill person.

Bahamut - a vast fish that supports the earth with a head of a hippopotamus.

Barmecide's Feasts is a meal at which the beggar Schacabac is offered empty plates instead of promised treats.

Buraq - a winged creature with a very wide stride: it could place its hooves at the farthest boundary of its gaze. He carried Muhammed and Abraham on his wings when travelling between cities.

Dandan - is a mythical largest marine creature.

Iram is a golden city in the mountains of Yemen, which was invisible to humans. However, once it was seen by a man called Abdullah who appropriated some of its treasure before the city disappeared again at dawn.

Khaleel - a man who owned a cat which spoke in Arabic.

Kujata. In order to ensure the stability of the world, God ordered a huge angel to fly beneath the lowest layer of the earth and place it on his shoulders, however, his feet did not have support. So God created a rock of ruby, and placed this rock under the feet of the angel. But there was no support for the ruby. So God created a big bull called Kujata to keep the ruby. But there was no support for the bull. So God created a giant fish called Bahamut to support the bull.

Nasnas - is a half-human, half-demon.

Rukh -a gigantic bird.

Sandwalker - a creature in the form of a giant crab, which devours camels.

Therefore, Arabic legends and folktales reflect the culture's history, social customs, and religious beliefs. Faith in God is the common characteristic of Arabic tales, which is usually expressed through the main hero, who achieves the goals owing to his strong and unshakable trust in God. The tales teach that "patience is the key for success," "loyalty brings reward", etc. The Arabic mythology constitutes a foundation of the archetypal self-expression.

Islamic Symbols

Indeed, no official Islamic symbols exist. Quran excludes from the divine mentioning any allusion to symbolization. However, with time, as a result of interacting with other peoples and religions, several different representations came to stand specifically for Islam. Some of them are referred to below:

Allah`s calligraphic name inscribes into the ornamental tradition of Arabic writing, which, all together venerates the Creator and does not transgress the ban on depicting humans.

Crescent and star symbol was borrowed from the Sumerian civilization, where it was associated with the sun God and moon Goddess. Later the symbol was adopted by the Ottoman Empire as their identification sign at the battlefield. As the Ottoman Dynasty grew into the main political power of the epoch, inevitably, the symbol would be associated with the Muslim population as well.

Khamsa (Fatima`s hand, Hamesh hand) is a protective talisman, which is believed to symbolize five pillars of Islam. In Arabic, the name khamsa means "five". Its other name, the Hand of Fatima, is named for the beloved daughter of Mohamed. The eye in the middle of the hand is considered to protect against the "evil eye".

Letter Nun is the fourteenth letter of the Arabic alphabet, which is derived from a pictogram of a snake.

Rub al Hizb is the particular eight-pointed star used to mark the end of passages in the Quran.

But for the representations, certain colors also have their meaning in Islam. For instance, the colours green and white are strongly associated with Islam since many centuries. The color green is mentioned in several Quranic verses as the color of clothing in paradise. During the times of the Islamic Caliphate, the Umayyad Caliphate took on white flags while the Abbassid Caliphate had black flags. The colors of Pan-Arabism, which can be found in the majority of Arab national flags, are: red, white, green, and black.

Arabic Proverbs

From various sources of Arabic world perception, its folk wisdom goes in front. The proverb contains the concise and essential moral, inherited from previous generations. Some of the Arab proverbs say:

- "Give your friends your money and your blood, but do not justify yourself. Your enemies will not believe it and your friends will not need it."
- "Unity is power."
- "Go with the lesser of two evils."
- "The smarter you are, the less you speak."
- "Be patient and you will get what you want."
- "There is always tomorrow."

Why would ancient Arabs transmit and interpret the happenings in their life, would it not be the very true of the Subject? Jung remarked the abundance of the symbolic epitomized by tales, legends, sayings, which for thousands of years helped people to make sense out of their perception and feelings, is, in fact, the key to collective mind, and the self in the broadest sense. His larger concept of the self is also based on the idea that humans are an image of universal layers of consciousness. And to comprehend the essence of each person, one should refer to collective wisdom.

CHAPTER 13

THE STRUCTURE OF ARABIC LANGUAGE

When we talk about Arabic as the mother language, we speak about the culture, the symbolic, in which a human is inscribed even before his/ her birth. Arabic calligraphy is characterized by sophisticated motifs and sumptuous ornaments. The Alexandrian philosopher, Euclid, called it a "spiritual technique". Arabic alphabet is a derivative of the Nabataean variation of the Aramaic alphabet, which descended from the Phoenician alphabet. The structure of Arabic language is a key to Muslim unconscious.

Specificity of Arabic language:

- Letters are written from right to left.
- Numbers are spelled from left to right.
- For the 28 letters, there are 18 shapes, 8 letters share the identical shape.
- Dots, short strokes, and other diacritic signs are used to mark the difference between identically shaped letters.
- Consonantal root system. Vowel signs are optionally indicated.
- No capital letters.
- Parsing. Words are formed from a root set of three consonants.
- There is no analogy to the letters P and V.

Grammar

Knowing the psychological state of the receiver of the message, a reporter can accordingly adjust his or her text. So, in Arabic there are three categories of audience:

1. Open-minded (khali al-dhihn), who do not need to be persuaded in the veracity of the message. No affirmation tools are used here.
2. Doubtful (mutaraddid), who distrusts the message. In this case affirmation tool is used by adding an affirmation particle ("in"). For instance: Verily, Sameer is ill: In Sameer mareedan. Moreover, the affirmation particles are often used to punish, threat.
3. Denier (munkir), who disbelieves the message. In this case no affirmation tool shall be used, instead, a basic sentence form can be used.

Another particular feature of Arabic language is a double negation. Repetition of negation reinforces negation. For example: No no I do not want this: Lya, lya ana oreedo zelika

A Verb "To Be"

The structure of the Arabic language is marked by the absence of the verb "to be", therefore, the absence of classical Cartesian cogito. From this aspect, the Arabic language is not positioned as temporal, alike the Western languages, but aspectable (accomplished or unaccomplished) and temporal. The verb "to be" (kana) is addressed to the past, however, to the present and the future. The ayat "Allah was omnipresent and wise" signifies that Allah, in fact, is and will be omnipresent and wise.

Parsing

Most Arabic words consist of a three-letter root, which constitutes the basis for nouns, verbs and adjectives. A root word is called "mada" meaning subject matter. When a new word is created on the basis of "mada", other letters are added to form a new meaning, with the preserved characteristics of the primary word root. Also, the insertion of vowel sounds into the root word gives a more precise and specific meaning.

Metaphors

It looks as if in the Arabic language the metaphors are placed in the domain of death. It is not solely an issue of linguistic difference, but it is an epistemological detection because it reveals the most disguised rapport, which exists inside the language between the death and the sex[852]. Muslims live more in symbolic, this is what immediately triggered off when any new event occurs: new experience is compared to what was already symbolized. The Muslim discourse occurs in the life-after (Imaginary register), not here and now. It is placed between "what will happen after the death" and "negation of present life". That is why it is impossible for a Muslim to console the religion with the real. Usually, it is a total negation of real. If partial consolidation happens it can lead to neuroses and psychosis. Possible ways of total consolidation between religion and real is the integration of real into religion, and not religion into real.

Greeting "Assalam aleikoum" is evoking final rest, therefore, death. Wishing each other final peace. "They will not hear therein ill speech or commission of sin. But only the saying of: "Peace! Peace!"" (sura 56, ayats 25-26). We are living the psychoanalysis as a metaphor of the translation and translation as a metaphor of the psychoanalysis[853].

Words (Related to Love), Which Do Not Exist in Other Languages

There exists a great abundance of words to describe love in Arabic, which varies in degree of its intensity. Just a few of them are exposed here:

Hawa describes the initial attraction. The term comes from the root word "h-w-a" - a transient wind that can rise and fall.

Alaaqa describes the following stage. It comes from the root word "a-l-q" meaning "to cling on to", that is to say when the hearts begin attaching to each other.

Wajd– a strong emotion, which can also be platonic

Ghazal– romantic affection on the level of flirting

Kalaf-infatuation, which means, amongst other things, to become red (in the face).

Ishq - a blind desire

Hubb- love, which comes from the same root as the word "seed", meaning a potential for growth

---

[852] Nached Rafah, *Histoire de la psychanalyse en Syrie*, Topique 1/2010, №110, pp. 117-127.

[853] *Ibid*

Sabwa-sensual love

Shaghaf- all-consuming love

Sababa-ardent love

Gharam- passion

Huyum- the complete loss of reason

Lawaa- agony from love

Taym- loving to the point when a lover becomes emotionally and psychologically enslaved by the beloved one, an obsession.

Jawaa-a chronic illness caused by love.

Tadleeh – when a heart is destroyed by chaos, which results from love.

Tuqburni – The literal translation is "You bury me," referring to a love so deep one cannot imagine living without one's partner.

Exported Words

English has many words acquired either directly from Arabic or indirectly from Arabic words that have entered into Roman languages before passing into English. Examples include: racquet, alchemy, alcohol, algebra, algorithm, alkaline, (the article "al" in Arabic denotes "the"), amber, arsenal, candy, coffee, cotton, ghoul, hazard, lemon, loofah, magazine, sherbet, sofa, tariff – and many more[854].The algebraic letter "x" that represents an unknown number, originates from the Arabic word "shay" (thing), which eventually became translated to "xay" in Spain, leading to its final abbreviation and use in algebra as "x".[855]

Dialects

The Arabic dialect (lahja), which differs from country to country, from tribe to tribe, neither resembles the Classical Arabic (fos-ha), the language of Quran. For a psychoanalyst, the dialect is the mother language, the language, in which a patient pronounces spontaneously the most intime, or behind which he/she hides because of shame.

Specificities of Pronunciation

There exist certain sounds that cannot be found in other languages, such as "ح", which is a "h" sound as in "hub" (love). For example, letters

---

[854] https://www.britishcouncil.org/voices-magazine/surprising-facts-about-arabic-language, consulted on 01.07.2016

[855] *Ibid*

"ayn" (ع), "kh" (خ) and some others are similar to the sounds of nomadic animals (i.e. camels with deep throat vocalization).

Zagroota

Zagroota, (plural = zaghareet) is the traditional wailing scream of the Arabic women. It is a traditional feminine way of expressing appreciation, happiness, joy.

CHAPTER 14

ISLAMIC ARTS

Freud considers that an artist works out a fantasm, which inhabits him/her, and assigns it a form transmissible to all. An artist purifies a phantasm from shame so that a spectator/reader would not have to defend oneself.

Lacan says that creation is something that targets the vacuity: a Thing. It is an attempt to give a shape to something, which escapes the representation.

For Anzieu, the process of creation is based on employment of something, which was not applied before, for instance, childhood memories. The artwork would be an attempt to weave the tissue with an aim of filling in the vacuity and, thus, creating a form.

Freud is located more on the side of the Imaginatory-Symbolic. Lacan is based on the level of Real. Whilst Anzieu is purely in the Imaginatory dimension. That said, could a phenomena of Islamic art be inscribed into any of these theories on artistic sublimation? To answer this question, one should keep in mind that Islamic art arose out of a need for new aesthetics, which would embody the essence of Islamic faith. The Islamic art was meant to raise the awareness of God, the raison d'être, of any Muslim. The term Islamic art is not used merely to describe religious art or architecture but applies to all art forms produced in the Islamic world. Muslims do not accept the proposition that Jesus is God, so it follows that the ban on graven images remains relevant[856]. That is also why images cannot be

---

Wise Christopher, *Derrida, Africa and the Middle East*, New York: Palgrave Macmillan, 2009, p. 19.

355

fashioned of prophets, and why mosques are adorned with calligraphy from the Quran, but not images of Muhamed, Jesus, Moses and other important figures[857]. Since depicting humans is strictly prohibited in Islamic art, the arts took on another mode in a form of calligraphy, arabesques, which are not simply meaningless shapes and writings. They have their own symbolic meaning. The centre of the Islamic artistic tradition lies in calligraphy, a distinguishing feature of this culture. Calligraphy, along with geometric and vegetative motifs, has become a sort of signature of the Islamic art. The weaved tissue of ornament resembles a veil under which the representation of a human hides. Islamic art forms give impression as if they were deliberately designed to bewilder, and not to expose. Crafts and decorative arts are regarded as having full art status, whereas painting and sculpture are not thought of as the noble forms of art.In Oriental tradition, the masterpieces were rather left anonymous. Nobody will ever know the names of those who embellished the exquisite pieces of art of the Ottoman empire. This philosophy strives to bring freedom from oneself. Besides that, a piece of art is considered to be an act of worship, which is based on the following hadith: "God is beautiful and He loves beauty". Some mosques astonish with grandiosity and fantasming about the Islamic dominance. Islamic art interplays in all three dimensions: realization of fantasm, the filling in of the vacuity and shaping into a form.

Architecture

A building is the construct, which fills in the vacuity. The architectural algorithm may turn the vacuity either into profane or sacred space. The signifier becomes the signified. The first built mosque in the world is called The Qubaa Mosque, which derives from the word "qabaa"- to build. Also "quba" means a dome. Indeed, the Islamic architectural propensity towards the round and oval shapes is very famous in contrast to the Gothical punctuated building. The Islamic architectural styles have evolved through centuries, with a few features remained unchanged till nowadays, especially:

Arch of the mosques resembles a curved back of a Muslim praying. Another reason can be related to the Arab`s love of the palm tree,[858]whose flowing curves of the branches were imitated in the arches.The Islamic architecture favours semi-circular, horseshoe, pointed, ogee, cusped and multi-foil arches.

---

[857] *Ibid*

[858] Scott Samuel, *History of the Moorish Empire in Europe*, Philadelphia: J. B. Lippincott Company, 1904, p.54.

Dome has a form of circle, with repeating decorative arabesques. Ernst Grube, in explicating what he thought Islamic architecture was, wrote the following about the dome: "The dome appears to be a general symbol, signifying power, the royal city, the focal point of assembly."[859] For example, the Dome of the Rock (Qubbat al-Sakhrah) in Jerusalem is one of the representative buildings of Islamic architecture.

Vaulting aligns with the concept of unity (tawhid), which points out to the final destination of all pathways, which cross at the sole centre.

Iwan is the vaulted hall space, a sort of gateway leading to the entrance of the mosque.

Courtyard (sehan) is based in the centre of the building, usually with a fountain encircled by the garden.

Ornaments. Arabesques (islimi)

Islamic art frequently adopts the use of geometrical flora or vegetal designs in a repetition known as arabesque. Nonrepresentational motifs of Islamic architecture have always been ordered repetition, radiating structures, and rhythmic, metric patterns. Could the ornamental paintings be considered as a way to fill in the Other, to tie the untied into one? Because circles have no end they are infinite - and so they remind that Allah is infinite. Complex geometric designs create the impression of unending repetition. The repeating patterns also demonstrate that in the small you can find the infinite ... a single element of the pattern implies the infinite total.

The spiritual and temporal life of Muslims is regulated in circles. A basic arabesque ornament, the three intertwined circles, which resemble the Baromean knot, also represent the constant revolving movement of the believer's life towards God.

Indeed, the typical expression of Muslim art is the arabesque, both in its geometric and in its organic form—one leaf, one flower growing out of the other, without beginning and end and capable of almost innumerable variations, only gradually detected by the eye, which never lose their charm.

---

[859] http://www.hurriyetdailynews.com/the-dome---symbol-of-power-.aspx?PageID=238&NID=60863&NewsCatID=438, consulted on 01.07.2016

Dance

In the Middle East, dances make up a part of everyday life, weddings, feast days, and family gatherings. Dance thrived during the Golden Age of Islamic civilization. Since that epoch in different social classes distinct styles evolved. The lower-class dancers performed natural and rough movements, while the upper-class dancers developed more a refined and graceful style. Traditional Arabic dance is a collective symbiosis, where the personal ego disappears. There can be defined such types of Arabic traditional dances as:

Line Dance

This type of dance is performed by both men and women, however, separately, from the opposite gender. The main movements consist of heavy steps, stomping and kicking. The dancers are usually motionless from the waist up to the head. Previously, line dances could have been enacted by entire villages, and the neighbours would join in at any time, thus, letting the "line" expand. That is one of the reasons, which stands behind the shape of the dance. The most popular line dance is dabka.

Circle Dance

Circle dances are acted out by both men and women in separate circles. Sometimes a circle of women is formed inside a circle of men or vice versa. Circle dances symbolize unity (tawhid) and infinity without a beginning or an end.

Women's Dance

The exclusively women dances involve one woman dancing alone or several women dancing simultaneously. Styles, costumes and message of the dance vary across regions.

Men's Dance

The men's dance is dedicated to the religious theme, war or battle, which is performed both in groups or in solo format.

Folk Dance

This style originated among the tribes and is traditional to their culture and community. Also, the folk dance includes Khaleeji (Gulf countries), Ouled Nail and Guerda (Maghreb) and other styles.

Khaleeji

The dance is performed by groups of women, dressed in a shuffling gait, who swing and toss their hair. This dance does not have the hip movements and the performance varies from region to region.

Ouled Nail

The dance took on a name of a tribe in Algeria, which is famous for their distinguished dance style, which involves small, rapid foot movements paired with brisk torso and hip movements.

Guerda

It is rather a ritual dancing, which is acted out on the knees. It starts with a head, which remains covered, passes into flicky movements of the hand, paralleled with swaying of the head.

Sheikat

The name of the dance derives from a word "sheikha" (plural "sheikat"), a definition in Arabic for an old woman. Traditionally, the dance is performed on the eve of a wedding by a group of older women, which includes all those movements, which a future wife is supposed to work out to satisfy her husband at night.

Performance Dance

It is a form of a theatrical play, the examples of which include raks sharki, belly dance etc. Indeed, the traditional Arabic dance is performed in groups, while solo is usually acted as a theatrical performance. The dancer literally reflects the music, while the different body parts react to different rhythms. The dancer communicates one's emotions through facial expressions, in particular, with the eyes, which are a vital component of any Arabic dance. Another distinctive body part in the Arabic dancing is the torso, the area, where the rhythms are born and are most frequently displayed. Also, there is a profound connection between the hips and the sounds of the drums, since the hips move in the rhythm to the main drumbeat.In all traditional Arabic dance the legs are supposed to be covered, otherwise, it is considered to be inappropriate. Most definitely, Arabic dance is an abstract performance, behind which there stands emotional self-expression, rather than the narration of a story.

Thereupon, Islamic arts focus on the spiritual representation of beings and objects, and not their physical form.

Chapter 15

IN THE NAME OF ALLAH. ATHWART ALLAH

In Islam, the Kingdom of God is in Heaven and on Earth, not only a Kingdom in the Heavens (Christianism), or a Kingdom on Earth (Judaism). Islam starts with the evocation "lya illaha ilya Allah," which can be split into two parts. The first one is a negative statement: "La illaha", which means "No gods". The second is an affirmative one: "ilya Allah," which means "except God". The first one is denial of polytheism, including any substitutions for God. The second one is the acknowledgement of existence of the One and Only God. Therefore, in order to be a Muslim, a double act of consciousness is required.

The conflict between traditional values and modernity has generated a phenomenon of Suppressed God. And God, as an omnipresent figure in Muslim society, is being submitted to the mechanism of suppression. Deliberate neglect of religious prescriptions in a state of full awareness of punishment incites the neurotization of modern Muslims, who are stuck between desire and fear. They suffer under the burden of their guilt feelings, which only grow stronger.[860]

---

[860] https://en.qantara.de/content/islam-and-psychoanalysis-a-tale-of-mutual-ignorance, consulted on 01.07.2016

The Economy of Death

The economy of death is constructed around the perception, attitudes and a specificity of death in Islam. Since the first days of life, a Muslim already prepares oneself to die. Reaching Paradise after the death turns into the overriding obsession. There even exist imaginary coins called "hasanat", which, a Muslim gains after accomplishing a good deed. The calculation is simple: the more "coins" were gained during the life, the higher reward is believed to be expected in the afterlife. Unsurprisingly, obsessive-compulsive rhetoric is strongly supported by the religious leaders, society and family.

The definition of death in Islam is the departure of the soul from the body in order to enter the afterlife. In 1986, at the third International Conference of Islamic Jurists in Amman, Jordan, a fatwa number five was issued, which states that "A person is considered legally dead and all the Shariah's principles can be applied when one of the following signs is established:

(i)   Complete stoppage of the heart and breathing which are decided to be irreversible by doctors.
(ii) Complete stoppage of all vital functions of the brain which are decided to be irreversible by doctors and the brain has started to degenerate.

Muslims believe that the soul returns to his or her creator (sura 2, ayat 156). If death occurs in a hospital, the face of the deceased person or his/her bed should be turned toward Mecca. The clothes are removed by same gender family members and the body will be covered by sheets. The family quickly prepares the arrangements for washing (ghusl) and Islamic burial, wich usually happens within 24 hours. In Islam, the body is sacred and belongs to God, therefore, embalming and cremation are forbidden in Islam.

Fear of Life

Fear has come to occupy a big part in the life of modern Muslims, which pushes them towards a new paradigm of life perception and their place in it. To Freud, fear constitutes personal choices in matching assumptions and feeling from the past with the present and the future and in differentiating the common features of the stories, which have passed and have yet to be initiated. Accordingly, a human can demonstrate a completely new set of values, where certain goods are given priority over the ancient ones. Muslims consider death as the continuation of life, and not its end. They believe that leading a pious life and observing the Islamic canons will eventually assure them the eternal delightful after-life. In anticipation of perpetual rewards, there are Muslims who do not dare, even fear to live on the Earth. Their minor steps are filled with remorse, a feeling of guilt or, even collective panic. A Muslim remains under constant pressure with a sole wish to die since this is what merely left for him/her. Consequently, a Muslim leads a life (as if) in preparation to death. Therefore, two opposite tendencies prevail (1) suppressing one`s own desires in aspiration of getting a place in paradise; or (2) suppressing the idea of death and the afterlife punishments, so that to surrender oneself to life pleasures. Both positions result in neurosis. Moreover, fear has been an inalienable component of an Arab culture: a fear of God, a fear of King, a fear of husband/wife, that is to say, there has always been a pretext to nourish the fears of an individual. In the modern Arab history nothing has been more powerful than the state in preserving and supporting the system of massive fear.

In Orientalism, Edward Said attributes to the fear of being inferior, the exodus or escape of an Arab man from one`s own identity, which also causes massive depressions all around the region.

The Culture of Martyrdom

In Islam, the concept "shahada" (martyrdom) relates to the notion "jihad" (holy struggle), "al-amr bil-maruf" (telling apart right from wrong) and the "path of Allah". Shahada can also be interpreted as a consecutive act of witnessing-testifying-struggle-martyrdom. Witnessing that there is no God but Allah (lya ilaha ilya Allah), testifying that He is the Only God (tawheed), struggling for the righteousness (birr)-dying as a witness (shahid). Shahid sacrifices one`s own life in a name of Allah testifying that He is the God; He is All-Powerful; and to Him we return. Anas bin Malik narrated that the Messenger of Allah said, "Who seeks martyrdom with sincerity shall get its reward, though he may not achieve it" (Sahih Muslim). Therefore, shahada is singled out by the intention. Raashid ibn Hubaysh narrated that the Messenger of Allah entered upon Ubaadah ibn al-Saamit when he was sick and said, "Do you know who is a shaheed (martyr) in my ummah?" The people remained silent, then Ubaadah said, "Help me to sit up." They helped him to sit up, then he said, "O Messenger of Allah, (is it) the patient one who seeks reward from Allah for his patience?" The Messenger of Allah said, "Then the martyrs among my ummah would be very few. Being killed for the sake of Allah is martyrdom, the plague is martyrdom, drowning is martyrdom, stomach disease is martyrdom, and if a woman dies during the post-partum period, her child will drag her to Paradise by his umbilical cord." Since Quran promises eternal life to a shaheed (sura 3, ayats 157-58, 169-71), the presence of Allah (sura 3, ayats 157-58), and after-life rewards (sura 4, ayats 74, 95-96; sura 47, ayat 4), martyrdom is considered as an act of honour. The elevation of a place of a martyr in Muslim society has engendered the notion of deliberate martyrdom. The premeditated suicide-attacks make part of the strongest impulses of I, which do not even change their "destiny", as Freud formulated it in 1915. The specificity of the choice of bomb suiciders is not to live but to die for the imagined future. Indeed, deliberate martyrdom is is a voluntary death for non-pathological reasons. The suicidal assaulter does not reveal clinical psychopathology by consciously choosing to die and to inflict a death toll for the enemy side, but stands on the side of a loss of one's own identity and social detachment. It can also be a question of a false identity, and, in particularly, from this place, one attacks the other for his "otherness". There can be structured two types of suicidal attackers: 1. The type which dies "for" a certain cause. 2. Type, which dies "against" particular circumstances. To the first type belong the attacks aiming to defend the motherland, or obtain the independence (e.g. Palestinian suicidal attacks). Whilst into the second type fit all narcissistically wounded suiciders, who refuse to accept the values of modern society, which makes them renounce their place in it. The terrorist organization resembles the household structure and takes on a role of a family for every single member. By committing an act of a suicidal attack they express their revolt against the society, and also serve as a spokesperson on behalf of their group.

Act of martyrdom is a sublimated desire to kill God, which is strongly connotated with a rigidly normalized system of tribal life values, from which a neuroticized Subject cannot escape, but through death. In these terms, modern martyrdom is viewed as a magical resolution. Since, suicide as a voluntary act, is forbidden in Islam, it has taken on another form, which is martyrdom. Even though each case is different, still, there exists a symptomatic complex, which can be described with regard to the following conditions:

Paranoia, more precisely, the paranoid-schizoid position, which is responsible for the persistence of the infantile stage (according to Melanie Klein), incites the Subject to suspicion, projected on the Other and justified by self-defense. Projection of insupportable interior elements on the exterior object, a typical infantile mechanism of defense, is activated when I of an adult is ruined. Therefore, the "good self" is idealized and the "bad self" is split up and projected outside.

Shame and humiliation, which precede the passage to act, play decisive roles in modern culture. Both feelings stand for the impossibility to conclude one's own narcissistic contract. Also, the attacker, who pertains to the first type, with his/her body and life tries to cover the democratic deficit of his motherland.

Communication signifies the message, transmitted by the martyr's death to the adversary.

Identification: some analysts view the lack of confidence as one of the reasons, why adolescents adhere to terrorist groups. According to Peter Olsson, the fact of belonging to the group consolidates identity and gives sense to one's own existence. The scientist also argues that young people might be charmed by the charisma of a group's leader, who also represents a strong father's figure, and might assume for them the parental role.

Khosrokhavar concluded, "Hegel believed that the struggle for recognition indicated the confrontation between the master and a slave. In fact, the slave is dead, and no person is left, over who his hegemony could be exercised. The modern martyr opens new space of intelligibility, the struggle for recognition passes through the death, making an appeal to the sacred."

Narcissistic wounds are left by the deficiency of the favourable environment necessary for the sane development of an individual, according to Winnicott. From the standpoint of Kohut, the lack of maternal empathy may also create a narcissistic wound, which perturbates the development of a child. One of the consequences might be the persistence of infantile grandiose fantasms. The other consequence is a failure of interiorization of the idealized paternal image. Anyways, the desire to destroy originates from the wound and narcissistic ferocity. This ferocity is principally directed against the ruined I, and could mark the regression to the infantile narcissism. By expressing the fury of their community they evoke the impulse of death, which can be set off in the most favourable moments, especially when they are associated with Eros, that is to say under the pretext of idealism and patriotism, as Freud mentions it in the Civilization and its Discontents.

Sacrifice, duty, and donation: some believe that the modernity has created its own enemy. By committing a suiciding attack, a martyr renounces his/her object. As Lacan put it, "…the sacrifice signifies that in the object of our desires we try to find the testimonial of the presence of the desire of that Other, the obscure God."

In accordance to the basis of Islam, a believer, who gives his life in the combat for a cause of God is a martyr. [861] However, it is not mentioned that the one who goes for one's own death deliberately through suicide (a prohibited practice by Islam) and kills the civilians, may accede to the same glory.[862] Like all fanatics, they [followers of Al-Qaeda] believe that they enjoy a monopoly on truth and that those who disagree with them are not merely mistaken, but wicked or mad.[863] As Freud (1921) has already shown, the one, who projects his ideals on the other feels as if he shares the greatness, which he attributes to the leader: he feels that he grows narcissistically owing to this link of idealization through identification with the leader.[864] The idealization in this sense is accompanied by identificational movement, which allows for important narcissistic gratification.[865] And the image of Shaheed contributes to the production of an ideal, which the Subject appropriates.

Extremism: a Flee from Allah?

Extremism is the ideology of a damaged ideal. For this reason, it appears to be so appealing to the teenagers and young adolescents. An extremist is the one who takes the Quranic ayats in their isolation while disregarding the entirety of the Holy Book, which causes fitna. Extremism is a compensated failure of self-assertion. In this context, it seems relevant to cite the unpublished letter of Edward Edinger On the Psychology of Terrorism, written in 1995. It says:

Terrorism is a manifestation of the psyche. It is time we recognized the psyche as an autonomous factor in world affairs. The psychological root of terrorism is a fanatical resentment – a quasi-psychotic hatred originating in the depths of the archetypal psyche and therefore carried by religious (archetypal) energies. A classic literary example is Melville's Moby Dick.

---

[861] Casoni Dianne et al.,*Comprendre l'acte terroriste*, Québec:Presses de l'Université du Québec, 2003, p.29.

[862] *Ibid*

[863] *Ibid, p.31.*

[864] *Ibid, p.87.*

[865] *Ibid*

Captain Ahab, with his fanatical hatred of the White Whale, is a paradigm of the modern terrorist.

Articulate terrorists generally express themselves in religious (archetypal) terminology. The enemy is seen as the Principle of Objective Evil (Devil) and the terrorist perceives himself as the "heroic" agent of divine or Objective Justice (God). This is an archetypal inflation of demonic proportions which temporarily grants the individual almost superhuman energy and effectiveness. To deal with terrorism effectively we must understand it.

We need a new category to understand this new phenomenon. These individuals are not criminals and are not madmen although they have some qualities of both. Let's call them zealots. Zealots are possessed by transpersonal, archetypal dynamisms deriving from the collective unconscious. Their goal is a collective, not a personal one. The criminal seeks his own personal gain; not so the zealot. In the name of a transpersonal, collective value – a religion, an ethnic or national identity, a "patriotic" vision, etc. – they sacrifice their personal life in the service of their "god." Although idiosyncratic and perverse, this is fundamentally a religious phenomenon that derives from the archetypal, collective unconscious. Sadly, the much-needed knowledge of this level of the psyche is not generally available. For those interested in seeking it, I recommend a serious study of the psychology of C.G. Jung.

An image of Islam can be easily distorted by misinterpretation given by the tormented Subject. Underexcessive fear of Allah there is hidden nothing more than a desire to abandon God, and, thus, renounce the weight, which responsibility towards religion, poses. The stronger the desire is, the more radicalized the Self becomes.With the rise of the Islamic fundamentalism and terrorism in the past decades, many people associate Islam with violence, and images of violent Jihadists and Islamic terrorists, who have been fueling negative projections and demonizations of Islam and feelings of hatred and cultural complexes around the world.[866] Terrorism can be viewed as an acting-out of the intrapsychic conflicts in the external paradigm. In these terms, Slavoj Žižek said:

Any critique of Islam is denounced as an expression of Western Islamophobia, Salman Rushdie is denounced for unnecessarily provoking Muslims and being (partially, at least) responsible for the fatwa condemning him to death, and so on. The result of such stances is what one should

---

[866] Kiehl Emilija, *Copenhagen 2013 - 100 Years On: Origins, Innovations and Controversies: Proceedings of the 19ᵗʰ Congress of the International Association for Analytical Psychology,* 2015.

expect in such cases: the more the Western liberal Leftists probe into their guilt, the more they are accused by Muslim fundamentalists of being hypocrites who try to conceal their hatred of Islam. [T]his constellation perfectly reproduces the paradox of the superego: the more you obey what the Other demands of you, the guiltier you are. It is as if the more you tolerate Islam, the stronger its pressure on you will be. What this implies is that terrorist fundamentalists, be they Christian or Muslim, are not really fundamentalists in the authentic sense of the term-what they lack is a feature that is easy to discern in all authentic fundamentalists, from Tibetan Buddhists to the Amish in the US: the absence of resentment and envy, the deep indifference towards the non-believers' way of life. If today's so-called fundamentalists really believe they have found their way to Truth, why should they feel threatened by non-believers, why should they envy them? When a Buddhist encounters a Western hedonist, he hardly condemns. He just benevolently notes that the hedonist's search for happiness is self-defeating. In contrast to true fundamentalists, the terrorist pseudo-fundamentalists are deeply bothered, intrigued and fascinated by the sinful life of the non-believers. One can feel that, in fighting the sinful other, they are fighting their own temptation. The passionate intensity of a fundamentalist mob bears witness to the lack of true conviction; deep in themselves, terrorist fundamentalists also lack true conviction-their violent outbursts are proof of it. How fragile the belief of a Muslim would be if he felt threatened by, say, a stupid caricature in a low-circulation Danish newspaper? Fundamentalist Islamic terror is not grounded in the terrorists' conviction of their superiority and in their desire to safeguard their cultural-religious identity from the onslaught of global consumerist civilization. The problem with fundamentalists is not that we consider them inferior to us, but, rather, that they themselves secretly consider themselves inferior. This is why our condescending politically correct assurances that we feel no superiority towards them only makes them more furious and feed their resentment. The problem is not the cultural difference (their effort to preserve their identity), but the opposite: the fact that the fundamentalists are already like us, that, secretly, they have already internalized our standards and measure themselves by them.

In other words, it is the need of the individuals to have enemies in order to deal with their projected aggression, which stems from their death instinct. In the opinions of Arabs, the modern Muslim world is full of provocative violent aggressors, for example:

- The occupants of the Arab lands. Under this category fall Palestine, Afghanistan, Kashmir, as well as KSA and Turkey, which are invaded by the presence of Other and stay permanently controlled.
- Internal oppressors and dictators. Privation from a symbolic object by the Big Other, which is the Archaic figure of the father.
- Rich inside Muslim societies. The imaginary phallus, about which one thinks that if he does not have it, then, definitely, the Other must have it; while the Other thinks that he, indeed, might have it.
- Dismantlement of the Muslim world. The separation from the Archaic Father, after which each single Muslim umma is faced with a need to undergo its own process of self-assertion.
- Westernization of Muslim societies is perceived as a threat to the Arab cultural identity. The polarity between the Self and the Other has reached its point of no return. As long as the relation between the Center and the Periphery proceeds in the logic of master and disciple, the complex of superiority will be aggravating the complex of inferiority in the Other. It is sad that often the Arabs exaggerate the danger of "the Other", thus attributing him with one`s own person unresolved conflicts, fears, and auto-generated aggression

The extreme form of power is All against One, the extreme form of violence is One against All[867]. Subsequently, in the Arab world, the question arises as to the transformative capacities of the damaged ideal, and if it can hamper the ideology of hatred.

Jihad and Jihadism

Jihad is the most misunderstood and deformed concepts of Islam. And it is often translated to denote holy war. In fact, jihad represents resistance to one`s own impulses and dominance over the Id. The derivative root word is "j-h-d", which signifies an effort. Jihad engages the mechanism of Super-Ego, which is responsibilized to take control over the Id. Islam differentiates four ways in which the duty of jihad can be fulfilled: by heart, tongue, hand, and sword. The first consists in a spiritual purification and overcoming the inducements to evil. The dissemination of knowledge about Islam through the tongue and hand. The fourth way consists in fulfillment of one's duty by waging war against unbelievers and oppressors

---

[867] Arendt Hannah,*On Violence*, Boston: Houghton Mifflin Harcourt, 1970, p.42.

of the Islamic faith. Also, jihad is divided into: "great jihad," "medium jihad" and "lesser jihad". The greater jihad stands for a struggle against oneself (sura 2, ayat 256; sura 5, ayat 105). For example, when a person experiences depression the challenge of changing their negative cognitions may be considered jihad.[868]The medium jihad implies social struggle to allow the better financial maintenance for one`s own family (sura 8, ayats 59-60). And the lesser jihadis fighting against an outer enemy (sura 9, ayat 5). It becomes obvious that military jihad is not at the core of the Islamic doctrine. Quite the opposite is true: jihad is a perpetual effort of self-improvement.

The authorization of the military struggle was first revealed in Medina, when the adversaries encircled the Muslims and the latter were compelled to raise arms to defend themselves and Islamic faith. The battle of Badr marked the beginning of defensive Jihad. During the second year of Hijra Allah prescribed the armed struggle: Fighting has been enjoined upon you while it is hateful to you. But perhaps you hate a thing and it is good for you; and perhaps you love a thing and it is bad for you. And Allah Knows, while you know not (sura 2, ayat 216).

Homo Religiosis or a Muslim without Religion

The rethinking of the notion of martyrdom puts a question of religiosity differently. One of the major differences Kristeva identifies as influential and problematic in Islam is the nature of the bond between its central deity and its believers. Kristeva describes this bond as tantamount to a juridical pact—which is quite different from the bond between a paternal Creator whose role is to elect (in Judaism, whose spirit, however legalistic, does not in the least suppress the creationist value that summons God's chosen people to the work of reflection and interrogation) or to love (in Christianity, even in the test of abandonment and passion).[869] Arabs still experience the feeling of guilt for the disobedience of the first couple to God. The more intensive is the feeling, the greater the inner tension and the more severe the need to sublimate. Arabs tend to work out the entire world around them into good and evil forces, which drives them to test the deepest metaphysical essences of the meaning of life.

---

[868] Ahmed Sameera, *Counselling Muslims: Handbook of Mental Health Issues and Interventions,* London: Routledge, 2012, p.11.

[869] Sutton Kyra, *Islam`s Turn on the Couch: The Psychoanalytic Theorizing of Muslim Identity in France,*Connecticut: Weyslan University, 2013, p. 53.

The Notion of Allah

Freud says that God is nothing other than an idealized father figure from whom the faithful anticipate protection and salvation. Thus the Jews call God the Father, and in Christianity God has even put forth a human Son. There is no direct line of descent between God and mankind. The Quran thus contradicts Freud's thesis[870] since in Islam Allah is not a paternal figure. Islamic faith excludes the symbolic figure of God-the-Father. Allah is beyond the logic of the son-father relation. Actually, this is Abraham, who embodies the figure of the symbolic father of Muslims (see the chapter Presence as the Absence of Father). Slavoj Žižek, in discussing and building on Benslama's text in his A Glance into the Archives of Islam, agrees with Benslama (and Kristeva) that Islam's God is outside the realm of paternal logic. "Allah is not a father, not even a symbolic one—God is one, he is neither born nor does he give birth to creatures."[871] Quran says, "God has not taken to Himself any son, nor is there any god with Him: for then each god would have taken of that which he created and some of them would have risen up over others." (sura 23, ayat 91)

Nowadays a paternal figure is often found in the persona of the President, or another ideal, where one can find a shelter from this destructive fear of castration. This might result in the appearance of somebody who adheres to the religious rituals rigidly.

Allah is a figure of transcendence, which extends beyond the conscious and the unconscious. Consciousness does not resemble anything else because it goes beyond the etymological meaning of the verb transcendere[872]. Quran narrates, "In the name of Allah, the Merciful, the Compassionate. Say (O Muhammad), He is God, the One God, the Everlasting Refuge, who has not begotten, nor has been begotten, and equal to Him is not anyone." (sura 112)

In Arabic God is translated as "rab", while Allah is the personal name. The Essence of God is equal to His Existence exactly as the Cogito in man is equal to his existence[873]. That is why the first description (wasf)

---

[870] https://en.qantara.de/content/islam-and-psychoanalysis-a-tale-of-mutual-ignorance, consulted on 01.07.2016

[871] Sutton Kyra, Islam`s Turn on the Couch: The Psychoanalytic Theorizing of Muslim Identity in France, Connecticut: Weyslan University, 2013, p. 61.

[872] Hanafi Hasan, *Islam in the modern world. Tradition, Revolution and Culture*, Cairo: Dar Kebaa Bookshop, 1995, p.138.

[873] Hanafi Hasan, *Islam in the modern world. Tradition, Revolution and Culture*, Cairo: Dar Kebaa Bookshop, 1995, p. 137.

of God is His existence. God exists (mawjud). He is perpetual (qadim), meaning that there is no starting, nor ending point (baqi) in time for His existence. God does not have one particular place (laisa fi mahal). He does not resemble anything (lya yusbihu al-hawadith). The description of the Essence of God is usually called negative theology because it marks out what God is not. In later theology (8th to 14th centuries) negative theology became a part of positive theology which describes what God is. God is Being, not nothingness, Eternal, not conditioned by events, Everlasting, not passing. Transcendent, not anthropomorphic. One not many. If the Essence of God has six descriptions (awsaf), His Attributes (sifat) are seven: Omniscience, Omnipotence, Life, Hearing, Seeing, Speaking, and Will. Each subsequent Attribute can be deduced from the preceding one. Science (knowledge) leads to potency (power) in all manifestations of life (hearing, seeing and speaking). And will means the realization of power. Each of the positive and negative theologies contained twenty attributes, six for the Essence as well as fourteen other Attributes[874]. Finally, God cannot be seen either in this world nor in the other world. God is not an object of perception, but rather a perceiving subject. The Essence of God cannot be conceived except by analogy. Like the Essence of God, man's consciousness exists Cogito ergo sum.

In Quran Allah does not say "I". Allah says, "And We have not sent you, [O Muhammad], except as a mercy to the worlds." (sura 21, ayat 107). There are known 99 names of Allah. The one, the supreme name, is excluded from mentioning. However, the total number of all names in both the Quran and the hadith actually add up to more than 99[875]. In the hadith of Sahih Muslim it is said, "Verily, Allah is Odd and He loves odd numbers." God has Attributes that are identical to His Essence. The relation between Essence and Attributes is a relation of equation (mutazilites), not of addition (asharites). The first is an option for punishment, while the second is an option for mercy.

Quran says, "He is God; there is no god but He. He is the Knower of the unseen and the visible; He is the All-Merciful, the All-Compassionate. He is God; there is no god but He. He is the King, the All-Holy, the All-Peace, the Guardian of the Faith, the All-Preserver, the All-Mighty, the All-Compeller, the All-Sublime. Glory be to God, above that they associate! He is God, the Creator, the Maker, the Shaper. To Him belong the Names Most Beautiful. All that is in the heavens and the earth

---

[874] *Ibid, p.141.*

[875] http://www.bbc.co.uk/schools/gcsebitesize/rs/god/islamrev2.shtml, consulted on 01.07.2016

magnifies Him; He is the Almighty, the All-Wise" (sura 59, ayats 22-24).The order of mentioning God`s name in Quran creates a chain of signifiers, where one signifier stems from the previous one, and amplifying the meaning of a successive one.

Ibn Arabi said that "the creation is the creator of its Creator." A phrase, which might imply certain atheism, even if Ibn Arabi was not an atheist, because he maintains that the Subject of God is at the same time the creator of God.[876]

Quran

There exist several interpretations of the word "Quran". In the first version, its root word is "qaraa", which means to compile. Prophet Muhammad received the instructions from God regarding the exact order of each ayat, sura, and their titles. "It is for us to collect and recite it" (sura 75, ayat 17). The second root word derives from "qarana" meaning unification. Imaam Sufyan Sorri affirmed that the Holy Quran was given its own special name because letters are joined to make words, words are joined to make ayats, ayats are joined to make suras and suras are joined to make the Quran. Another definition of the word "qarana" guidance, which Quran provides, "This is the book: it is guidance sure, without doubt" (sura 2, ayat 2). The third root word, "qiraathun", means to recite.

The fourth root word, "qirain", which is the plural of "qarina", denotes evidence or symbol. Quran is a word that establishes the order.

Names of the Holy Quran

The word Quran itself can be found in the scriptures: "We do relate unto you the most beautiful stories, in that We reveal to thee this (portion of the) Quran: Before this thou too was among those who knew it not" (sura12, ayat 3). Also Quran is referred to under other names, such as: al-nur the light (sura 7, ayat 157); al-hukm the judgment (sura 13, ayat 37); al-dhikr the reminder (sura 15, ayat 9); al-kitab the scripture (sura 21, ayat10); al-furqan the criterion (sura 25, ayat 1); al-tanzil the revelation (sura 26, ayat 192). The further descriptive titles include mubarak (blessing), mussadiq (confirmation of truth), mubin (explanation), hakim (wisdom), majid (glorious) and karim (honoured).

In fact, Quran does not oppose ambiguity, even though it imposes concrete prescriptions.

---

[876] http://www.jeuneafrique.com/103716/archives-thematique/les-musulmans-sur-le-divan, consulted on 21.09.2016

Promises of Quran

Quran virtuously employs the pleasure-displeasure principle in establishing the control and the limits. The Holy text uses promises to incite the righteous behaviour, and threats with punishment to prevent the opposite. Both approaches take place in the Imaginatory register. The promises of Allah to His creatures interplay at the crossroad of the Imaginary and Symbolic, which is the making of sense. The first promise of Allah, upon the creation of human souls followed: "...and be faithful to (your) covenant with Me, I will fulfill (My) covenant with you" (sura 2, ayat 40).

The Quran commences with the word: "Read", the oral transmission, which supposes the writing in the unconscious. As Lacan claims, if it can be read, then it means that it has already been inscribed in the process of writing. So, a symptom is something that does not cease from writing itself.

Judgement Day

On the Judgement Day Allah will address the jins and humans with such words : "O, you assembly of jinn and humankind! Came there not unto you messengers of your own who recounted unto you My tokens and warned you of this Day? They will say: We testify against ourselves. And the life of this world beguiled them. And they testify against themselves that they were disbelievers." (sura 6, ayat 130)

The Judgement Day can be thought of as the final and the strongest element of an attempt to make sense out of the established Quranic order, which is also regulated by the principle of receiving pleasure and avoiding pain.

PART III

MENTAL DISORDERS IN THE CONTEMPORARY ARAB WORLD

CHAPTER 16

PREVALENT MENTAL CONDITIONS

Even though there are no published data on national lifetime prevalence and treatment of mental disorders in the Arab region, this chapter will attempt to examine the most common mental illnesses by name in the descending order: from more to lesser common.

Depression (statistics)

Seven out of the top 10 countries in the world by the rank of depression in women are in MENA. Alansari found that rates of depression among women were significantly higher than for men in nine of the seventeen countries,[877] in particular: Egypt, Algeria and Morocco in North Africa, Iraq and Syria in the Levant, Oman, Qatar and Kuwait in the Gulf, and Pakistan in South Asia. The Mental Health Conference held in Dubai in 2013 revealed that 75 % of mental illness cases in UAE are linked to depression. [In Kuwait] out of the mere four million people that populate the country, 200,000 have been diagnosed with depression.[878] There was a major leap from 2010 to 2011 and rates increased by a whopping 40

---

[877] Alansari BM. Gender differences in depression among undergraduates from seventeen Islamic countries. Soc Behav Pers. 2006, 34, pp. 729–38.

[878] http://www.borgenmagazine.com/mental-illness-kuwait-rise/, consulted on 01.07.2016

percent.[879]One in five teenage students in Dubai showed symptoms of depression according to a 2013 study.[880] [In Jordan] one study suggested a prevalence of depression of greater that 30% in 493 randomly selected participants.[881] [In Oman] in May 2014, a study conducted on students by the Department of Behavioural Medicine at SQU showed that 27% had depression of varying grades.[882] Another study investigating the rate of depression among secondary school students in Oman found that 17% of the respondents showed symptoms.[883] [In Syria] 20 % have depressive disorders.[884] [In Iraq] among primary healthcare patients in Al-Nasiriyah City in 2005 prevalence rates of depression was 10.2%.[885] [In Lebanon] the most prevalent individual disorder was major depression (9.9%).[886] In Tunisia among the diagnosed patients, there are 9% with major depression.[887]

Anxiety (statistics)

Earlier studies of psychiatric morbidity among university students in Egypt showed that anxiety states were diagnosed in 36% of the study sample.[888] [In Lebanon] anxiety disorders were common (16.7%)[889] among the adults, and 18%[890] among children. This type of disorder was reported

---

[879] *Ibid*

[880] http://gulfnews.com/news/uae/health/teen-mental-health-issues-growing-in-the-uae-1.1663780

[881] https://www.y-oman.com/2015/03/changing-minds-fighting-depression/, consulted on 01.07.2016

[882] *Ibid*

[883] Afifi M., Positive health practices and depressive symptoms among high school adolescents in Oman, Singapore Med J 2006; 47(11), pp.960-967.

[884] http://applications.emro.who.int/emhj/1506/15_6_2009_1596_1612.pdf, consulted on 01.07.2016

[885] Sharma S., et al., Mental Health Policy in Iraq since 2003, a Post-Invasion Analysis, p. 3.

[886] http://www.medscape.com/viewarticle/576714_3

[887] Mental Health Atlas, World Health Organization, p.469.

[888] Okasha A., Kamel M., Sadek A. et al, Psychiatric morbidity among university students in Egypt. British Journal of Psychiatry, 131, 1977, pp.149 -154.

[889] http://www.medscape.com/viewarticle/576714_3, consulted on 01.07.2016

[890] *Ibid*

to be by contrast, significantly low 0.24% in Kuwait,[891] while in neighboring Iraq it was 3.75%[892] .

Substance Abuse (statistics)

Drug addiction rate has been recently increasing in GCC. At the mental hospital in Taif (Saudi Arabia), drug addictions (61%)[893] were among the most common inpatient diagnoses. The inpatients admitted to the Al-Amal Hospital in Dammam among the substances used, 49% injected heroin alone, 35% used heroin in combination with other drugs or alcohol, 11% used only alcohol, and an additional 20% used alcohol in combination with other drugs.[894] There is the tendency to combine cannabis (marijuana), which is the most popular drug in the region, with other stimulants. A more recent survey found out that 98% were current cigarette smokers, 40% used amphetamines, 20% alcohol, 17% heroin, 16% marijuana, and 3% cocaine or volatile substances.[895] Drug abuse disorders rose by more than 500% in the UAE in the past 20 years.[896]

---

[891] Kline, N.S., Psychiatry in Kuwait. British Journal of Psychiatry, № 109, 1963,pp. 766-74.

[892] Bazzoui, W. & Al-Issa, I. Psychiatry in Iraq. British Journal of Psychiatry, № 112, 1966, pp. 827-32.

[893] http://www.ncbi.nlm.nih.gov/pmc/articles/PMC3743653, consulted on 01.07.2016

[894] Koenig Harold, *Mental Health Care in Saudi Arabia: Past, Present and Future*, Open Journal of Psychiatry, 2014, № 4, pp. 113-130.

[895] Al-Sharqi Abdullah Mohamed et al.*Suicidal and Self-Injurious Behavior amongPatients with Alcohol and Drug Abuse.* Substance Abuse and Rehabilitation, 2012, № 3, pp.91-99.

[896] http://www.thenational.ae/uae/health/drug-use-disorders-in-uae-rises-by-more-than-500-per-cent-over-last-20-years-study, consulted on 01.07.2016

Hysteria (statistics)

In Egypt hysteria occupies a position at the top of the list of psychiatric diagnoses,[897] which involved 11.2% of the patients,[898] and 5.2% in Kuwait;[899] although hysteria did not appear in the 1966 survey from Iraq, hysterical illness was reported to be very common in its grand forms among the naive and uneducated rural inhabitants.[900] Yet, in the 1970 survey by Bazzoui, hysterical features were reported at the rate of 7.5%.

Psychotic Disorders. Schizophrenia (statistics)

In a retrospective Saudi study from the mental hospital in Taif, schizophrenia (89%)[901] was among the most common inpatient diagnoses. [In Jordan] at CMH hospital 74% of patients were diagnosed with psychotic disorders.[902][In Morocco] the patients admitted in mental hospitals are primarily diagnosed with schizophrenia (70%).[903] [In Iraq] the diagnoses of admissions to community-based psychiatric inpatient units were predominantly from schizophrenia group (69%).[904] [In Bahrain] the patients admitted to the mental hospitals belong primarily to the diagnostic groups of schizophrenia, schizotypal and delusional disorders (39%).[905] Three hundred twenty-five patients with the schizophrenic disorder were admitted between 1988 and 1996 (200 males and 125 females). Therefore,

---

897 Okasha A., Kamel M., Sadek A. et al, Psychiatric morbidity among university students in Egypt. British Journal of Psychiatry, 131, 1977, pp.149 -154.

898 Okasha, A., Kamel, M. & Hassan, A.H., Preliminary psychiatric observations in Egypt. British Journal of Psychiatry, №114, 1968, pp.949-955.

899 Kline, N.S., Psychiatry in Kuwait. British Journal of Psychiatry, № 109, 1963,pp. 766-74.

900 Bazzoui, W. & Al-Issa, I. Psychiatry in Iraq. British Journal of Psychiatry, № 112, 1966, pp. 827-32.

901 http://www.ncbi.nlm.nih.gov/pmc/articles/PMC3743653/

902 Laeth S.et al., Barriers to the Diagnosis and Treatment of Depression in Jordan. A Nationwide Qualitative Study, Journal of the American Board of family Medicine, March 1, 2005 vol. 18 no. 2, pp.125-131.

903 http://www.who.int/mental_health/evidence/morocco_who_aims_report. pdf, consulted on 01.05.2016

904 Sharma S., et al., Mental Health Policy in Iraq since 2003, a Post-Invasion Analysis, p. 4.

905 Mental health system in Kingdom of Bahrain, 2010, p.10.

---

an average annual incidence rate in Bahrain is of 1.29 per 10,000 for all ages and 2.13 for the 15 to 54 age group.[906] Schizophrenia, at 10%, was the most common form of psychotic illness across the region.[907]

PTSD (statistics)

In Iraq, 10.5% of children suffered from PTSD.[908] [In Algeria] the prevalence of posttraumatic stress disorder (PTSD) assessed using the PTSD module of the Composite International Diagnostic Interview Version 2.1 was found to be 37.4% in a community survey conducted on a sample of 653 subjects.[909]

ADHD (statistics)

Among the most common presenting symptoms of children in KSA were hyperactivity (43%), ADHD (13%), attention and concentration problems (14%).[910] An estimated 1.6 million Saudi children suffer from attention deficit hyperactivity disorder (ADHD)[911]. A study from 12 Seha hospitals in Abu Dhabi revealed that in 2013, 1,301 of children's mental illness cases received were ADHD.[912] In Lebanon, 43% of surveyed children were diagnosed with hyperactivity, whilst 13% with ADHD.[913]

---

[906] Saab Rim, Epidemiology of Schizophrenia and Related Disorders in the Arab World, The Arab Journal of Psychiatry, 2011, vol. 22, № 1, p. 2.

[907] http://kristof.blogs.nytimes.com/2014/08/01/syrias-mental-health-crisis/?_r=0, consulted on 01.07.2016

[908] Al -Jawadi A., Prevalence of childhood and early adolescent mental disorders among children attending primary health care centres in Mosul, Iraq: a cross-sectional study, BMC Public Health, 2007, № 7, p. 274.

[909] Mental Health Atlas 2005, World Health Organization, p.54.

[910] Mental Health Care in Saudi Arabia: Past, Present and Future, Open Journal of Psychiatry, 2014, 4, pp.113-130.

[911] http://www.arabnews.com/news/553851, consulted on 01.07.2016

[912] http://www.khaleejtimes.com/nation/uae-health/mental-illness-among-youth-is-not-taboo-say-uae-experts

[913] http://www.medscape.com/viewarticle/576714_3, consulted on 01.07.2016

Mental Retardation (statistics)

Based on three reports on secondary school students in KSA, between 16% and 59% have significant levels of mental [...] symptoms.[914] In Saudi Arabia over (30%) of children have diagnoses of mental retardation.[915] In Lebanon, 28% of surveyed children had delayed milestones and 30% were diagnosed with mental retardation.[916] The mental health centers in Abu Dhabi offered treatment to 329 mentally retarded schoolchildren.[917]

Autism (statistics)

In Lebanon over 13% of children have autism spectrum disorder[918].The statistics suggest that one in every 100 children in Dubai has autism[919]. Sara Ahmad Baker, head of the community service unit, Dubai Autism Centre said: "In the UAE, although no official figures are available I can tell you we are on the same track"[920] [with the world statistics, which has documented the occurrence of autism as one child in 88 births]. The Abu Dhabi`s hospitals reported for 288 young patients with autism spectrum disorders[921]. In studies conducted in KSA, over 13%[922] of children were diagnosed with autism spectrum disorder.

---

[914] Mental Health Care in Saudi Arabia: Past, Present and Future, Open Journal of Psychiatry, 2014, 4, pp. 113-130.

[915] *Ibid*

[916] Koenig Harold, *Mental Health Care in Saudi Arabia: Past, Present and Future*, Open Journal of Psychiatry, 2014,

№ 4, pp. 113-130.

[917] http://www.khaleejtimes.com/nation/uae-health/mental-illness-among-youth-is-not-taboo-say-uae-experts, consulted on 01.07.2016

[918] Koenig Harold, *Mental Health Care in Saudi Arabia: Past, Present and Future*, Open Journal of Psychiatry, 2014,

№ 4, pp. 113-130.

[919] http://www.thenational.ae/uae/health/uae-children-are-being-misdiagnosed-with-autism

[920] http://gulfnews.com/leisure/health/the-rise-of-autism-in-the-uae-1.1020114

[921] http://www.khaleejtimes.com/nation/uae-health/mental-illness-among-youth-is-not-taboo-say-uae-experts

[922] Mental Health Care in Saudi Arabia: Past, Present and Future, Open Journal of Psychiatry, 2014, 4, pp.113-130.

Suicide (statistics)

Suicide is not typical for the Arab region. However, there has also been a spate of teen suicides with about 10 students having committed suicide since 2014 in the UAE[923]. The rate of suicide in Bahrain is 8.1,[924] in Morocco 5.3,[925] in Qatar 4.31,[926] in Yemen 3.66,[927] in UAE 3.24,[928] in Tunisia 2.4,[929] in Jordan 2,[930] in Algeria 1,9,[931] in Lybia 1.8,[932] in Egypt and Iraq 1,7,[933] in Oman 1,[934] in Lebanon and Kuwait 0.9,[935] in Syria and KSA 0.4,[936] per 100,000 people per year. Only a quarter of a century ago, Egypt officially registered an annual suicide rate of 0.1 out of 100,000-- all males: No females reportedly took their own lives[937]. According to the demographics of that time, this translates to around just 24 deaths through suicide each year.[938] In Bahrain the suicide occupies the 13th place of the causes of death among the population.[939] As we can see, the Kingdom of Saudi Arabia and Syria recorded the lowest ratio among Arabs with 0.4

---

[923] http://gulfnews.com/news/uae/health/teen-mental-health-issues-growing-in-the-uae-1.1663780

[924] https://en.wikipedia.org/wiki/List_of_countries_by_suicide_rate, consulted on 01.07.2016

[925] *Ibid*

[926] http://www.worldlifeexpectancy.com/cause-of-death/suicide/by-country/, consulted on 01.07.2016

[927] *Ibid*

[928] *Ibid*

[929] https://en.wikipedia.org/wiki/List_of_countries_by_suicide_rate, consulted on 01.07.2016

[930] *Ibid*

[931] *Ibid*

[932] *Ibid*

[933] *Ibid*

[934] *Ibid*

[935] *Ibid*

[936] *Ibid*

[937] http://www.egyptindependent.com/news/egyptian-suicide-rate-rise, consulted on 01.07.2016

[938] *Ibid*

[939] http://www.worldlifeexpectancy.com/country-health-profile/bahrain, consulted on 01.07.2016

suicides per 100,000, while Sudan recorded 17.9 suicides per 100,000 among the Arabs.[940] According to Reuters, in KSA the Saudi Hospital receives around 11 cases every month of women who have failed in their suicide attempts. The report confirms that the majority of those cases fall under the categorization of drug overdose. In UAE in 2012, 274 people committed suicide across the country, 243 men and 31 women.[941]

Other (statistics)

Emotional issues. [In Syria] 31% of the population have severe emotional disorders.[942] Whereas the obsessive-compulsive behavior is mainly linked with the religious rituals.

Symptomatology (statistics)

The findings [conducted in Egypt] revealed that the most common symptoms were worrying (82%), irritability (73%), free-floating anxiety (70%), depressed mood (65%), tiredness (64%), restlessness (63%), and anergia and retardation (61%).[943] Panic attacks were present in 30%, situational anxiety in 35%, specific phobias in 37% and avoidance in 53% of the sample[944].

Comorbidity (statistics)

Moussaoui et al. conducted a study on the comorbidity between schizophrenia, depression and suicidality, using a sample of 183 patients with a schizophrenic disorder (ICD-10 criteria).[945] The authors found a prevalence of 44.3% of depressive symptoms that did not, however, warrant

---

[940] http://timesofoman.com/article/66060/Oman/Suicide-rate-in-Oman-among-lowest-in-Middle-East, consulted on 01.07.2016

[941] http://www.thenational.ae/uae/health/increased-awareness-leads-to-decline-in-uae-suicide-rate, consulted on 01.07.2016

[942] http://kristof.blogs.nytimes.com/2014/08/01/syrias-mental-health-crisis/?_r=0, consulted on 01.07.2016

[943] Okasha A., Ashour A.,Psycho-demographic study of anxiety in Egypt: the PSE in its Arabic version. British Journal of Psychiatry, 139, 1981, pp.70-73.

[944] Ibid

[945] Saab Rim, Epidemiology of Schizophrenia and Related Disorders in the Arab World, The Arab Journal of Psychiatry, 2011, vol. 22, № 1, p. 3.

a diagnosis of the major depressive disorder.[946] While 2.7% of the sample reported suicidal ideas (40% of whom had a depression or had what the authors called "a painful consciousness of their illness", that is, the patients' awareness of their illness instilled sadness in them), 5% of the sample had a specific plan to implement them.[947] The comorbidity rate of Axis I psychiatric disorders in patients with substance abuse were found to be 64.9%, using the DSM-III-R diagnostic criteria.[948] The data appears to suggest that there is strong correlation between substance abuse and rates of depression/anxiety in the Arab region.

Also, statistics attest, to the comorbidity existing between depression and addiction: 30 to 50% of depressed young people also suffer from eating disorders, alcohol, and drug abuse. With adults, the underlying depression is often present (80%) with suicide attempts, whilst the addictive behavior is present in more than 60% of depression cases.[949] In 1933 Sandor Rato described people suffering from "anxiety depression", who also have an urge to maintain artificially the euphoric self-esteem and narcissism, and use alcohol/drugs to achieve this state. Depression and addiction are interconnected, in a sense that the one turns to be the cause of the other. If depression is a bereavement of a lot object, then addiction is the denial of a loss, an attempt to preserve the lost paradise.

In conclusion, depression, anxiety, bipolar disorders, stress, schizophrenia, addiction and substance abuse are the major psychiatric disorders in MENA. Parental consanguinity, that is the marriage between close relatives, is present in 50% of cases with severe mental disorders. The recent studies conducted in GCC also showed that consanguinity leads to increased risk for schizophrenia.

Identity Crisis

A modern Arab is stuck in the deadlock of dual identity. Is he/she a Bedouin, or a westernized Muslim? Should he/she renounce from the parentally inherited identity so that to construct his/her own? Is reconciliation between the bedouin past and the Western dictated present possible? The Cambridge dictionary says that identity crisis is "a feeling of being uncertain about who or what you are." An ethnic identity implies

---

[946] *Ibid*

[947] *Ibid*

[948] *Ibid*

[949] https://www.cairn.info/revue-gestalt-2006-2-page-121.htm, consulted on 01.07.2016

a "consciousness of self within a particular group."[950] Erikson was the first psychologist, who coined a term "identity crisis". Phinney defines an "ethnic group" as one that an individual claims heritage in. The identity of modern Arabs is far more complex that that of their forefathers. Some of them were born to the Bedouin parents, raised in Muslim families, during the post-colonial time, educated in the West. And as grown-up people, most of them do not firmly know, where they exactly belong. Much of the identity problem facing the region can be traced back to imperialism and colonialism.[951] The French Muslim, the Berberic Dutch, the Israeli Arab, the Indian Arab, the Egyptian Christian...The life of a modern Muslim is still challenged with the dichotomy, even if he/she was born, raised and educated in Muslim society, he/she is living in a globalized epoch of the dominant Western civilization. The society is modernizing, while the religion remains the private matter. The common identifier is still Islam. And the identity passes through the spoken language. What particular about the identity crisis of Arabs is that, from one side, it can be called the collective identity crisis, which encompasses a whole nation. And from the other, it is a crisis between the self-identification and "the desire-to-be". The reason that Islam operates on a "repudiation of origin" crisis today, according to Benslama, is tied to Islam's own libidinal economy, which refers to the way in which desire situates and constructs identities based on the flow and distribution of desire. Both the East and the West are currently in a state of political crisis about sexuality...a permissive polysexual West and a repressive heteronormative East[952].

Identity Deficit vs Identity Crisis

Erikson's clinical observations established the connection between: (1) the image of suffocative and intrusive mothers; ambivalent fathers and (2) identity deficit crises in their children. The cultural identity deficit is developmentally caused by the rejection of parental moral standards. A subject with identity deficits lacks engagement but constantly struggles to make one. Whilst a subject with identity crisis encounters between two

---

[950] Spencer Margaret et al., Identity processes among racial and ethnic minority children in America. Child Development, 61 (2), 1990, p. 292.

[951] http://www.eden.rutgers.edu/~spath/385/Readings/Kumaraswamy%20 %20Identity%20Crisis%20in%20the%20Middle%20East.pdf

[952] Afsaneh Najmabadi, Islamicate Sexualities: Translations across Temporal Geographies of Desire. Co-edited with Kathryn Babayan. Cambridge: Harvard University Press, Middle Eastern Monographs, 2008, p.18.

strong emotional engagements too distinct and incompatible. An identity conflict may arise at any point of the lifetime.

The conflict crisis is essentially a surplus (of engagements), whilst the identity deficit, on the contrary, is a lack (of engagement). The identity conflict differs from the identity deficit in that the former has no vacuum to fill, so a new path out needs to be sought. Successful resolution of the identity crisis, either necessitates taking on a new engagement, or simply conceding to the struggle. Whereas a resolution of identity deficit requires the revision of both the issue of criterial values and the issue of behavioral implementation. The study underlines that children with current or past (resolved) identity crises perceived their parents as unstable and ambivalent. Besides, issues, connected with the identity crisis, also include such concepts as alienation vs integration, emptiness and search for meaning, rebellion and fanaticism etc. The only way out of the collective identity crisis in the Middle East is the reinvention of the Arab identity, which starts from the acceptance of one`s own origins.

Depression and Culture

In the Latin etymology *depressere* means to bring down. In psychopathology, depression entails a long-lasting impact in all three areas, which include:

- Psychic: sadness, emotional pain, aversion to life, loss of self-esteem, poor mental life;
- Somatic: sleep, appetite and sex alterations, somatic complaints, anxiety agitation or motor inhibition;
- Relational: isolation, contact difficulties, difficulty to assume emotional life. The depressed person is constantly in search of the lost loved object. In Freudian reading, it is the idealized lost object. For Melanie Klein, the depressive rupture is caused by the reactivation in the adulthood of contradictory feelings of hatred and love, which a small child lives throughout the second semester of his/her life. Jacques Lacan viewed depression as a consequence of giving up one`s own desire. Depression can be also seen as a loss of the illusion, and it is known by the absence of a desire (but for desire of nothing, the desire of death).

Depression, which has developed in the Islamic environment, is different from any other depression. Why? The explanation is that depression is highly stigmatized in the Arab world. And it tends to be considered as a lack of faith, and, therefore, as a family or group failing (and falling) rather than the individual. Most frequently an Islamic depression hides under the mask of numerous somatophorm symptoms. Evidence of the earliest accounts of depression can be found in the Islamic Holy Scripture, where depression is spoken of as "huzn" (sadness). In addition, Quran discloses six minor reasons of depression, which result from:

- Loss of the beloved one(s) or object(s). The loss is explicitly stated in the story when the mother lost her son Moses (the future Prophet Moses): "But there came to be a void in the heart of the mother of Moses .... Thus did We restore him to his mother, that her eye might be comforted, and that she might not grieve ..." (sura 28, ayats 10 and 13). A similar scene is also reflected in the case of Prophet Jacob losing his son as in this verse "And he turned away from them, and he said: how great is my grief for Joseph..." (sura 12, ayat 84).
- Oppression of the weaker person. Quran mentions the abuse of personal feelings as follows: "Let not their speech, then, grieve you..." (sura 36, ayat 76) and "We do know how your heart is distressed at what they say" (sura 15, ayat 97). Allah encouraged the Prophet as he felt great sorrow for experiencing harsh attitude from his enemies: "Perchance you may (feel the inclination to) give up a part of what is revealed unto you, and your heart feels straitened lest they say..." (sura 11, ayat 12).
- Low self-confidence. Low self-esteem makes an individual feel depressed. This is reflected in the verse "Faint not nor grieve: for you must gain mastery if you are true in faith" (sura 3, ayat 139). The sura inspires with the afflicted with sorrow Muslims to keep on, and not give up.
- Fear of challenge(s). A person may succumb to depression if his/her life is threatened, as shown in the following two verses: "And when Our Messengers came to Lut, he was grieved on their account, and felt himself powerless (to protect) them: but they said: fear not, nor grieve: we are here to save you and your kinsfolk..." (sura 29, ayat 33). "But Allah delivers the righteous to their place of salvation. No evil shall touch them, nor shall they grieve." (sura 39, ayat 61)
- Guilt feeling. Guilt is also evoked in Quran: "(He turned in mercy also) to three who were left behind; they felt guilty to such a degree that earth seemed constrained for all its spaciousness, and their (very) souls seemed straitened...." (sura 9, ayat 118). The sura

narrates the story about three people who disobeyed Allah by not fulfilling their duty of accomplishing the holy war (jihad), so the feeling of guilt consequently flooded them over. And they suffered in repentance. The guilt that stems from the wrongdoings almost always has a religious component: "But if anyone turns away from My reminder, his life will be a dark and narrow one..." (sura 20, ayat 124).

The following verse also addresses one of the possible causes of depression: "And whoever turns away from My remembrance - indeed, he will have a depressed life, and We will gather him on the Day of Resurrection blind" (sura 20, ayats 123-124). The verse above implies that whoever does not practice one's religion will suffer from depression ("a life narrowed down and dark"). However, the next verse implies that, when an individual fully grows up, he/she usually increases his/her religious devotion, which propounds the view that maturity leads to a decrease in depression. Quran says: "...when he reaches the age of full strength and attains forty years, he says, "O my Lord! Grant me that I may be grateful for Thy favour which Thou has bestowed upon me, and upon both my parents, and that I may work righteousness such as Thou mayest approve; and be gracious to me in my issue. Truly have I turned to Thee and truly do I bow (to Thee) in Islam" (sura 46, ayat 15; sura 46, ayat 15).

Indeed, a closer look at the Quranic examples enables better understanding of the Islamic model of depression. The highest levels of depression is associated with the youngest age group[953].[MENA's] women between the ages of 15–49 are said to be the most affected [by depression][954]. Moreover, the lowest rate of depression prevalence was among the older age; this result is in accordance with that of Glicken which showed that the lowest rate of depressive disorder was estimated at between 1.3% and 1.8% among individuals who were older. In Saudi Arabia, 201.000 years of life expectancy are being lost due to the destructive effects melancholy has on health.[955]

---

[953] Abdelati Naziha, Examine Islamic Perspective of Depression Causes among Libyan Muslims Adult, International Proceedings of Economics Development & Research, 2013, Vol. 73, p.56.

[954] http://blogs.worldbank.org/arabvoices/ten-facts-about-women-arab-world

[955] http://www.moroccoworldnews.com/2013/01/73164/arabs-the-most-depressed-people-in-the-world-study-3/, consulted on 01.07.2016

In the Shadow of Anxiety

Modern culture is particularly oriented towards the search of wellness at any cost, which provokes day-to-day anxiety of a Muslim, who is stuck between the traditional values and the modern life. Psychoanalysis emphasizes the archaic anxiety, the anxiety of falling down and fragmentation anxiety. Winnicott was specifically studying the separation and castration anxieties. Numerous studies have shown Muslims suffer from death anxiety more than any other religious or non-religious group.[956] The anxiety is an affect, which is felt in the body, the libidinal body. For Freud, it is a libidinal quantum of energy that was not able to be discharged because it had found out another liberating way. Not being able to get linked to the acceptable representation so that to pave the way towards satisfaction of this accumulated energy, it causes discomfort, which is located in the body. Anxiety is associated with various situations of separation, however, it actually occurs when this separation was not realized and the object was preserved by the psyche. What increases the anxiety is the inability of the subject to resolve completely in his/her favor a situation of internal conflict between the objects of the desire and those, which threaten with punishments. It is the impossibility of the subject to figure out the existing conflict. Even if he/she has a presentiment of a malaise, a sort of "accumulated ball", which distorts his/her relation with the exterior world, the subject knows that he/she suffers, however, cannot put in words, nor images the representation of his/her inner world. He/she feels bad and tries to solve the discomfort by using his/her defenses. Anxiety is a production of the internal world, its aspirations, representations and images manufactured by subject, it feeds fantasies and desires. The anxiety arises when the subject does not set the limits to one's own desire of omnipotence. Since the ancient times, the causes of anxiety have been all the same. What has changed is the objects that nourish the anxiety and the way the environment supports them. Anxiety is different from fear, which sends to a precise thing, "since anxiety is the reality of freedom, then it is possible."[957]

Consequently, in Islamic tradition, anxiety will be connected with the sin, in particular, the original sin. In such a way, the sexuality was positioned in relation to the sin. Here Kierkegaard suggests a classical theory: "Having tasted the fruit from the tree of knowledge, the difference

---

[956] https://wikiislam.net/wiki/Muslim_Statistics_-_Health_and_Disability, consulted on 01.07.2016

[957] Kierreraard Soren, Le concept d'angoisse, Paris: Gallimard, 1935, p. 62.

between the good and the evil has entered the world, but with it, the sexual difference in a form of appetite." [958] However, Kierkegaard insists that "the victory of love in a human, where the spirit is the winner to the point that the sexual is forgotten and only remembered in oblivion, is the realization of the synthesis. Thus, sensuality is sublimated and anxiety is expulsed."[959]

In the end, anxiety is the characteristic of the human liberty. The human being has a free will with all the consequences, which it entails.

Consanguinity and Psychotic Disorders

An Arabic proverb says that "only the cousin can take the bride off the horse," meaning that a bride can marry her cousin provided if nobody else is available. The word consanguineous comes from the two Latin words "con" meaning shared and "sanguis" meaning blood. Paradoxically there exists no Arabic equivalent term for consanguinity. Consanguinity (aka incest) describes a relationship between two people who share an ancestor, or common blood. In the Arab world, the first cousin unions are culturally preferred. The reason is ease of marriage decision making when the potential spouse is well-known and considered to be part of the extended family. Also, inbreeding is designed to keep the wealth and property within the tribe. And these marriages also tend to reinforce social and kin bonds from one to the next generation. The congenital costs of consanguinity have long been recognized, as has their cause: the increased risk that the offspring of an incestuous mating will get two copies of the same damaged gene, one from each parent.[960] Massive inbreeding within the Muslim culture during the last 1.400 years may have done catastrophic damage to their gene pool.[961] What are the deleterious risks of consanguineous mating? Here is a sampling: schizophrenia, congenital heart defects, pulmonary stenosis and atresia, cystic fibrosis, cystinosis, nephronophthisis, spinal muscular atrophy, albinism, achromatopsia, hearing disorders, central nervous system anomalies, congenital anomalies, physical handicaps, mental retardation, and malignancies, added risk of infant and child mortality[962].

---

[958]   Kierreraard Soren, Le concept d'angoisse, Paris: Gallimard, 1935, p. 113.

[959]   *Ibid, p.118.*

[960]   http://www.economist.com/node/1621790

[961]   http://en.europenews.dk/-Muslim-Inbreeding-Impacts-on-intelligence-sanity-health-and-society-78170.html, consulted on 01.07.2016

[962]   http://brighterbrains.org/articles/entry/cousin-marriage-70-in-pakistan-should-it-be-prohibited, consulted on 01.07.2016

Consanguineous marriages are major responsible risk factors for Bipolar disorders[963] and Down syndrome. Consanguinity is a well-known risk factor for genetic disorders, including diseases and syndromes that present with intellectual and developmental disabilities[964]. This is due to autosomal recessive disorders and also other inherited disorders. The findings of the present study are similar to findings from other studies indicating that intellectual and developmental disabilities in addition to other genetic disorders are most likely to occur among inbred offspring and the risk is significantly higher than in non-consanguineous families.[965] In Qatar, a study of 1,515 women found 54% consanguineous marriages and the most common form again between first cousins. Inbred children of these women had a significantly higher rate of asthma, intellectual disability, epilepsy, and diabetes compared with children of non-consanguineous couples.[966] In Saudi Arabia like other Middle Eastern countries, first cousin marriages account for 60 - 70% of all marriages, leading to uniquely common disorders which are either rare by Western standards or are unknown.[967] Data shows that the rate of consanguineous marriages in Oman is higher than observed in most Arab countries including Egypt (21 %), Morocco (22.8 %), Algeria (34 %), Syria (35.4 %), Lebanon (37.8 %), Tunisia (39.3 %), Bahrain (43.1 %), Yemen (44.7 %), Mauritania (47.2 %), Jordan (48.1 %), Libya (48.4 %) and the UAE (50.5 %), but lower than Qatar, Kuwait, Saudi Arabia, Iraq and Sudan.[968] The recent studies have reported an elevated parental consanguinity rate of 52% in Qatar. Among the Arab countries, where the birth deffects caused by inbreeding, prevail there are: Saudi Arabia 81.3/1000, United Arab Emirates 75.9/1000, Iraq 74.9/1000, Kuwait 74.9/1000, Oman 74.8/1000, Syria 74.3/1000,

---

[963] http://www.ncbi.nlm.nih.gov/pmc/articles/PMC2738413/, consulted on 01.07.2016

[964] *Ibid*

[965] *Ibid*

[966] *Ibid*

[967] http://english.alarabiya.net/en/life-style/art-and-culture/2015/04/04/Health-fears-question-Arab-tradition-of-cousin-marriages-.html, consulted on 01.07.2016

[968] http://www.muscatdaily.com/Archive/Oman/Consanguineous-marriages-in-Oman-higher-than-in-most-Arab-countries-241f#ixzz4AcNtvwdP, consulted on 01.07.2016

Qatar 73.4/1000, Bahrain 73.3/1000, Jordan 73.1/1000, Libya 73.0/1000, Tunisia 72.7/1000, Morocco 72.3/1000, Yemen 72.1/1000.[969]

Autism

Autism is defined as a severe psychiatric disorder of childhood marked by severe difficulties in communication and forming relationships with other people, in developing language, repetitive, and limited patterns of behaviours and obsessive resistance to small changes in the familiar surrounding.[970] Currently, autism is most frequently diagnosed between the age of 2 and 3 at average.[971] At 3 years, several characteristical traits define clearly autism. One of them is an attempt to direct the attention of an adult by pointing at the object with one's finger, as a way to express one's interest, and not to ask for it with words. A fact of using a hand of the Other, as a tool, is also an expressive feature of autism. Also, the absence of spontaneous usage of words, and with certain regularity the words-signifiers (but for papa and mama) also becomes a truthful indicator at 3 years.[972] The child cannot get separated from the Other because the Other is not a compensatory object of his/her lack, but a part of his/her libido.[973] Autist is someone who says "no" to the desire of the Other. Autism is auto(erot)ism. An autistic child procures pleasure for oneself without the Other, because the desire of the Other is dangerous. The autist forcloses on the desire of the Other, and refuses the dual relation. This is the clear refusal from staying in relations. The space of the autistic child is organized in a different from other children manner. All techniques, constructions, autistic inventions, including mimicry, serve as an attempt to artificially establish the limit, and, thus, allow a subject to avoid the feeling of being destroyed in the endless tempest. Autist accords importance to the object and to one's own inventions, where the Other would not be too

---

[969] Christianson Arnold, March of Dimes, Global Report on Birth Defects. The Hidden Toll of Dying and Disabled Children, New York, 2006

[970] Chew M., et al., Brain derived neurotropic factor and autoantibodies to neural antigens in sera of children with autistic spectrum disorders. Landau-Kleffner Syndrome, and Epilepsy, Biol Psychiatry, 2006, 59 (14), pp. 354–363

[971] https://www.cairn.info/revue-enfance-2002-1-page-21.htm, consulted on 01.07.2016

[972] *Ibid*

[973] Soler Colette, Autisme et paranoïa, Bulletin Groupe Petite Enfance, 1997, №10, pp. 22-30.

---

much present and too much intrusive. An autistic world is not capable of making distinctions, especially between the subject and object (or between "myself" and "non-myself").[974] The exterior object seems not to exist: the relation to the Other is perceived as if that with a dead ((DdA)). The real Other is always the bearer of the anguishing danger.

Annually, nearly 30 new cases of autistic disorder are diagnosed in CAPU, the only referral unit for autistic disorder in Bahrain, and referred to 3 community centres that care for autistic disorder.[975] The figure for consanguinity among the parents of autistic disorder cases seems to be high (29%).[976]

Schizophrenia

The clinic of schizophrenia is formed around three syndromic groups: 1) disorders of language and communication; 2) hallucinations and delusions; 3) behavioral disorders, which include disadaptation, stereotypical conduct, impoverishment of a thought, speech, social interactions and emotions. The functional consequences of this malady largely lead to disability. Genetic factors play a significant role in the transmission of schizophrenia.[977] Schizophrenia can be characterized by different evolutive phases, such as premorbid phase, prodromic phase, symptomatico-psychotic phase, residual phase.[978] The premorbid phase extends from the birth until the appearance of the first signs of the illness. The prodromic phase is marked by the first psychotic symptoms, which determine the onset of illness. The symptomatico-psychotic phase is generally marked by positive symptomatology with delirious ideas and references to persecution. The residual phase starts with the end of the psychotic phase. Lacan, in his seminar about psychosis, brings forward a formula: "What is excluded from the symbolic returns into the real."

---

[974] Houzel Didier,L'enfant autiste et ses espaces. Enfances & Psy. 2006, № 33, pp. 57-68.

[975] http://www.emro.who.int/emhj-vol-19-2013/9/epidemiology-of-autistic-disorder-in-bahrain-prevalence-and-obstetric-and-familial-characteristics.html, consulted on 01.07.2016

[976] *Ibid*

[977] http://www.ncbi.nlm.nih.gov/pmc/articles/PMC3721918/, consulted on 01.07.2016

[978] https://www.cairn.info/revue-adolescence-2005-2-page-225.htm, consulted on 01.07.2016

Lacan will speak about these signifiers, which give form to delusions, as of "unchained" signifiers in double senses, meaning that they have lost their symbolic anchorage, and, also, in the sense, when it says that the mother was unchained. The schizophrenia is characterized by a failure of suppression mechanism. Henri Ey considers that the schizophrenia will generate the delusions, in which the Other becomes I, which emphasizes real structural upset of I. The schizophrenic patient is alienated from I, in which I disappears as an actor of one`s own world; through delusions, I becomes the Other for oneself. The schizophrenic refuses that the phallus becomes symbolic. The schizophrenic person does not fulfill the operations of adolescence, which is passing from the imaginary to symbolic. The symbolic function of phallus is foreclosed. The schizophrenics, indeed, believe that the Other has the power. They have an impression that all the world watches them because they have phallus. They deny that the phallus is just a symbol, and think that it is the reality. They cannot tolerate when there is an appeal to this phallus. The schizophrenic thinks that he/she is a phallus in reality. When the schizophrenic speaks, it seems as if he/she speaks about everything. And this is because he/she tries to fill in the hole (with everything, which is available). Jouissance of the schizophrenic returns into the body (a phenomenon of body fragmentation, feelings of decay, agonizing experiencing of internal transformations, etc.). The clinicians claim that the treatment shall be delivered as early as possible so that to suspend the evolution at the initial stage. A study of the morbidity risk of schizophrenia to parents and siblings reported that a total of 16.4% of the schizophrenia probands had at least one first-degree relative with schizophrenia. Previous study on the prevalence of mental illness showed a high prevalence of schizophrenia in the Qatari population.[979] The [...] study shows that the high prevalence of schizophrenia among the Arab population residing in Qatar is associated with the high rate of parental consanguinity.[980]

Addiction, but, In Reality, Addiction to What?

The term "addiction" derives from the Latin word *addictus*, which refers to an ancient custom of enslavement. The English terminology gives an impression that the addicted is the slave of the single desire to escape the mental pain, the pain of existence. Addiction is primarily the quest for

---

[979] http://www.ncbi.nlm.nih.gov/pmc/articles/PMC3721918/, consulted on 01.07.2016

[980] *Ibid*

---

pleasure and not a desire to harm. Addiction is almost always a response to psychological suffering, which derive from the past (often from childhood) and, like all other psychological symptoms, it is a childish attempt to heal oneself. The emergence of addictive behavior is the interaction of three factors: the individual, his/her socio-cultural environment and the object of addiction. Joyce McDougall speaks of addictive substances/activities as substitutes for a transitional object. In this regard Winnicott considered the transitional object as universal, since it is a "universal" transition via addictive relationship to an object other than the mother, which would be the first displacement of psychic investment. Another approach to addiction suggests that it is an affectionate addiction, to a certain person, which manifests in a form of substance abuse.

Substance addiction has become a serious public health issue in the whole Arab region. So far, most published documents about substance use disorders from Arab countries were in the field of tobacco smoking and waterpipe use.[981] Predictive factors for the increase of substance abuse with the Arabian Gulf region include, but are not limited to: a lack of knowledge regarding drug use and consequences, peer influences, boredom, breakdown of family traditions, media influences, and the rapid economic growth of the GCC countries may be reasons.[982] The theory of planned behavior suggests that environmental factors, individual background, and other individual differences are some of the variables that may affect drug use and misuse.[983] Le Monde reported that between 2005 and 2010 the average consumption by the French dropped from 104.2 litres of alcohol per year to 96.7, while in the same period in the Middle East and Africa area it increased by 25%, from 11.7 billion litres to 15.2 billion.[984] Studies from Arab countries have reported a wide variety of substances and medications being abused. For example, abuse of tramadol in Egypt and other Middle

---

[981] https://substanceabusepolicy.biomedcentral.com/articles/10.1186/1747-597X-9-33, consulted on 01.07.2016

[982] Al-Harthi A., Al-Adawi S. Enemy within? The silent epidemic of substance dependency in GCC countries. SQU Journal of Scientific Research, 2002, № 4, pp.1-7.

[983] Ajzen,I., and Fishbein M. 1980. Understanding Attitudes and Predicting Social Behavior. New Jersey: Englewood Cliffs, Prentice-Hall, p. 73.

[984] https://wikiislam.net/wiki/Muslim_Statistics_-_Alcohol_and_Drugs, consulted on 01.07.2016

Eastern countries have reached an alarming limit.[985] It was reported that at least by 5% of Arab youths have been using heroin or cocaine.[986] The most popularly abused drugs in the Middle East are opium, stimulants, and marijuana.[987] Dr. Fatima Muhammad Kaaki, a psychiatric consultant at the Amal Hospital in Jedda, said most substance abusers are between 15 and 30 years old and are addicted to hashish and Captagon.[988] According to the survey results, conducted by Nora Almageni in GCC, only three (positive attitudes, perceived norms, and self-efficacy), of the five predictor variables significantly contributed to the overall variance explained in participant self-reported behavioral intentions to engaging in marijuana use.

The Eternal Hysteria: Like Mother, Like Daughter

Hysteria has been known since the time immemorial as a female illness. The ancient Egyptians had attributed it to the movements of the uterus. And later Hippocrates named it referring to this part of the body. The predisposition to hysteria is predetermined by pregenital anxiety. Freud listed nine factors that constitute the essence of the hysterical symptom: 1. The hysterical symptom is mnemonic; 2. It is a substitution of traumatic experience; 3. It is the realization of desire; 4. It is the realization of a fantasy; 5. Its purpose is sexual gratification; 6. It is the return of infantile sexual satisfaction; 7. It arises from a conflict between the opposing impulses; 8. It always has a sexual implication; 9. Last, but not the least – "a hysterical symptom is an expression, on one hand of a male fantasy and on the other, of a female fantasy, both are sexual and unconscious."[989] Hence, behind the conflict between the impulses and repression, hides a risk of psychosis in a relation with a "hysterogenic" mother, who would have perverted the reality by denying the conflict. The sexually ambivalent hysterics

---

[985] Fawzui M., Some medicolegal aspects concerning tramadol abuse: The new Middle East youth plague 2010. An Egyptian overview. Egypt Journal Forensic Science. 2011, №1 (2), pp. 99-102.

[986] http://www.ynetnews.com/articles/0,7340,L-3640272,00.html, consulted on 01.07.2016

[987] http://rehab-international.org/drug-addiction/issues-drug-abuse-middle-east, consulted on 01.07.2016

[988] http://www.arabnews.com/more-saudi-women-seeking-treatment-drug-abuse, consulted on 01.07.2016

[989] Freud Sigmund, Fantasmes hystériques et leur relation avec la bisexualité, dans Obras completas, tomo II, Madrid: Biblioteca Nueva, 1981, p. 1349.

---

want to be loved by the object and to destroy it simultaneously. In case of decompensation, hysteria would evolve into somatization or into another non-neurotic structure. Lucien Israel opposed male hysteria, which is characterized by the coexistence of the desire to be virile with the feminine maternal identification, to a hysterical woman, who knows that she is a woman, moreover, she acts as a woman, so that to get better reassurement for her bisexuality. Julia Kristeva argues that this is bisexuality, which is more explicit in women, that explains the female hysteria. Both girls and boys face the ambivalence of identification with the father and enter into rivalry with him. But whereas in men, the Oedipus complex "succumbs" to the castration anxiety in relation to the interdiction, ambivalence and resentment keep the women away from their mother without destroying the traces of identification with the primary object. However, why would the desire of a mother be denied by their daughters? This is the incestuous relation to the father, which is prohibited, and to the mother is dangerous because it erases the limits and brings the subject to violation of the self and the identity disorders. Against what does a hysteric defend herself? Freud in Inhibitions, Symptoms and Anxiety points out that the neurotic always defends oneself against the castration anxiety, because the loss of love plays there a fundamental role, which is tantamount to the threat of castration in phobias and the fear of superego in obsessional neurosis. She infers that the lack of a penis, via the phallic signification, evokes a woman`s fear of being nothing for the other (I do not have, so I am not); this approach results in the libidinal investment in her own body (or her being), as an attempt to compensate for this lack.

Arab women are expected, in accordance with traditional culture, to act hysterically under conditions of frustration and stress (e.g. death); this is also the case with males who have certain physical or kinship qualities (e.g. being born prematurely, or having a hysterical maternal uncle). Paul Boyer considered hysteria to be a physical symptom of social disease. For example, members of the Arab community may not only tolerate their hysterical behavior, but often reward it. A woman's failure to show the "correct" hysterical responses in a funeral, for example, may be interpreted in negative terms, and therefore penalized. Among Arabs, hysteria has often been reported as a predominantly female disease.[990] Also, the excessive emotionality of Arab women is often confused for hysteria. Sometimes it is the family, who plays a crucial role in encouraging

---

[990] Elsarrag, M.E., Psychiatry in the Sudan: a study in comparative psychiatry. British Journal of Psychiatry, № 114, 1968, pp. 954-948.

hysterical manifestations, thus, setting a model example for reacting to certain events.

All in all, hysteria has always remained a neurosis, it "is the expression of the fundamental conflict connected to the relations between genital love and sexuality" with its defenses against prohibited desires, repression, substitution and the importance of the fantasy life.

Families` Ties and ADHD

Attention Deficit Hyperactivity Disorder (ADHD) is one of the most common psychomotor disorders in children, and also the most studied. Its triad of symptoms, in particular: motor restlessness, impulsivity, and attention deficit disorder, is a set of disruptive elements for the subject and the environment, in which he/she develops. Corraze names the symptomatological tripod:

1. These are perceptual-motor disorders affecting different exploration functions (gnostic and perceptive aspects), action (on the physical level with the intentional motoricity), communication (especially in its non-verbal aspects) and integration of emotions, which involve the analysis of positive and negative emotions and their links with the motivation;

2. They are manifested by mild neurological signs alluding to the existence of the minimum brain dysfunction; these signs may be classified, according to Chan and Gottesman, in different sections depending on whether they affect sensorial integration (digital gnosis, stereognosis right-left confusion, extinction), motor coordination (balance, walking, jumping, finger-nose test) or inhibition mechanisms (synkinesis, Go/No Go test);

3. They are associated with psychopathological complex, which includes, first of all, emotional factors that act as triggers of problems or supporters of the problem, and, secondly, psychiatric disorders that raise the question of the associated comorbidities or disorders, and also the reaction manifestations, such as anxiety or depression that are conventional in ADHD.

The results show that 20 % of hyperactive children (versus 5 % of the children from the control group) have at least one parent, who was hyperactive in his/her childhood.[991]

The Stable Mental Retardation

IQ in inbred children (8-12 years old) is found to be lower (69 in rural and 79 in suburban populations) than that of the outbred ones (79 and 95 respectively). The onset of various social profiles like visual fixation, social smile, sound seizures, oral expression and hand-grasping are significantly delayed among the new-born inbred babies.[992] Another study shows that the risk of having an IQ lower than 70 goes up 400 percent from 1.2 percent in children from normal parents to 6.2 percent in inbred children:[993] "The data indicate that the risk for mental retardation in matings of normal parents increases from 0.012 with random matings to 0.062 for first-cousin parentage."[994] The cognitive consequences of Muslim inbreeding might explain why non-Western immigrants are more than 300 percent more likely to fail the Danish army's intelligence test than native Danes: "19.3% of non-Western immigrants are not able to pass the Danish army's intelligence test. In comparison, only 4.7% of applicants with Danish background do not pass."[995] Inability to understand and generate new information followed by low IQ rates can also explain the scarce contribution of modern Muslim scientists. "In 2003, the world average for production of articles per million inhabitants was 137, whereas none of the 47 OIC countries for which there were data achieved production above 107 per million inhabitants. The OIC average was just 13."[996] The lack of interest in science and human development in the Muslim World is also clear in the UN Arab Human Development Reports (AHDR). AHDR concludes that there have been fewer books translated into Arabic

---

[991] https://www.cairn.info/revue-la-psychiatrie-de-l-enfant-2008-1-page-275. htm, consulted on 01.07.2016

[992] http://en.europenews.dk/-Muslim-Inbreeding-Impacts-on-intelligence-sanity-health-and-society-78170.html, consulted on 01.07.2016

[993] *Ibid*

[994] *Ibid*

[995] http://nyheder.tv2.dk/article.php/id-7248606%3Anydanskere?ss=, consulted on 01.07.2016

[996] http://www.nature.com/nature/journal/v444/n7115/full/444026a.html, consulted on 01.07.2016

in the last thousand years than the amount of books translated within the country of Spain every year: "The Arab world translates about 330 books annually, one-fifth of the number that Greece translates. The cumulative total of translated books since the Caliph Maa'moun's [sic] time (the ninth century) is about 100,000, almost the average that Spain translates in one year."[997]

War Traumatism

A word "traumatism" is of Greek origins, which signifies at once the breaking and the wound, and designates the consequences of the event, whose suddenness, intensity and brutality may not only cause a psychic shock but also leave the lasting traces on the psyche of the subject, which was affected. PTSD appears in the international DSM-IV classification as an answer of the acute adaptation, brief and transitory psychotic phenomenon, which brings about the split, depersonalization, dissociation, depression, anxiety, pathological modifications of the personality, etc. Traumatism denotes the wound. Thus, traumatism results from the breaking. We certainly discover that a suppressed memory has transformed only afterwards into traumatism.[998] The traumatic is not the real event itself, but the suppressed memories, which interpret the event in question afterwards. This is the Freudian theory of the "afterwards". It says that it is only afterwards that the shock becomes trauma and produces its effects. Trauma as such suspends all capacities, all psychic activities, provocating a state comparable to the coma. According to Françoise Brette, actual traumatism may bind to the preliminary traumatism: one traumatism always hides behind another one. From Freud`s standpoint, an actual event is traumatic by its link with a previous event, which it has reactivated. In the concept suggested by Caroline Garland, the actual event is traumatic and it implies the loss of sense. Trauma is where the sense of the occurred is lost. Ferenczi was among the first to elaborate the theory of traumatogenesis, which gives an account for the radical trauma, which consists of a complete attack of the consciousness and its functions: the perception and the thought.[999] The consciousness is disconnected from the perception and realizes this

---

[997] http://en.europenews.dk/-Muslim-Inbreeding-Impacts-on-intelligence-sanity-health-and-society-78170.html, consulted on 01.07.2016

[998] Freud Sigmund, Esquisse pour une psychologie scientifique, in La naissance de la psychanalyse, Paris, P.U.F., 3e édition revue et corrigée, 1895, p.366.

[999] Ferenczi Sandor, Réflexions sur le traumatisme, in Psychanalyse, tome IV, Paris, Payot, 1982, pp. 139-147.

particular phenomenon: the traumatic perceptions are neither perceived, nor conscious. The repetition remains the only method to make at least some sense out of the series of impressions, which, despite being active, have not been processed by the conscious, nor by the thought.

Freud underlines that traumatic situations imply the extensive torn of the protective shield, which, in the end, forms the traumatism: the state of unpreparedness of the psyche. Freud noted that a traumatized person would be constantly returning to the moment, which precedes the traumatic event. And in such a way, by repetition, a traumatized subject makes an attempt to make sense out of the occurrence, and, therefore, find healing. The subject attempts to revert and bring back the time so that to get prepared for the traumatism. Freud envisages two possible destinies of traumatism: positive and organizing, which enables repetition, rememorization, and elaboration; as well as negative and disorganizing, which creates an enclave in the psyche (in Freud's words "the state inside the state"), which prevents the consequential transformation. "The afterwards" turns into a symptom, which awaits the liberating elaboration of the occurred.

Freud also approaches traumatism from the side of loss. He believes that the fundamental anxiety of a human stems from the loss (of object, love etc.) and creates the state of instability inside the psyche. Thus, traumatism produces the loss of trust in the previously stable and predictable world and in the protective function of good objects, internal and external. This loss of trust leads to the resurgence of the primitive fears, such as the cruelty and the power of bad objects.

Transgenerational Traumatism

Trauma in the Arab world is not a question of one individual, but that of the whole nation, and, sometimes, nations. The years of war, violence and loss have induced the collective disorder called accumulative traumatism. In this sense, the Arabic traumatism is much distinct from that of other peoples. A research study done by Jamil et al. (2002) showed significant evidence that there were more mental health problems found in Iraqi refugees than in other clients.[1000] The war in Muslim world is omnipresent.And sometimes Arabs lack simple awareness and psycho-emotional preparedness so that to face the traumatic consequences resiliently.

[1000] http://www.esciencecentral.org/journals/death-anxiety-ptsd-trauma-grief-and-mental-health-of-palestinians-victims-of-war-on-gaza.hccr.1000112.php?aid=21422

Civilians in the Middle East have been subjected to frequent episodes of violence, intra- and inter-group conflicts, and natural disasters. These include full-scale wars such as the Yom Kippur War (1973), the Turkey Cyprus War (1974), the Lebanese Civil War (1976-1984), the Israel-Lebanon wars (1978; 1982), the Libyan-Egyptian war (1977), the Iran-Iraq War (1980-1988), the Gulf War (1990-1991), the civil war between Kurdish factions in Northern Iraq (1994-1997), the Second Gulf War (2003), and the Israel-Hezbollah War (2006),[1001] genocidal campaign against the Iraqi Kurds (1986-1989), events 9/11, but for the ongoing Israeli-Palestinian war, the Syrian conflict and other violent insurgencies that struck the Arab region on regular basis. An examination of large, fairly representative samples of men and women age 16 or older living in Algeria, Cambodia, Ethiopia, and Gaza, de Jong et al. found high rates of PTSD in each sample (37.4%, 28.4%, 15.8%, and 17.8%, respectively).[1002] In Lebanon, it was found a 3.4% lifetime prevalence rate of PTSD in a nationally representative sample (n = 2,857) of adult Lebanese civilians.[1003] [In Lebanon] This study reported that the prevalence of major depression disorder different across these regions from 16.3% to 41.9%.[1004] In the Gaza Strip, researchers reported that the lifetime prevalence of PTSD among adults (n = 585) was 17.8%.[1005] Among Palestinian adolescents, PTSD was found to be present in 34.1% of the sample (n = 1,000) from East Jerusalem and the West Bank.[1006] [In Palestine] PTSD was diagnosed in 34.1% of the children, most of whom were refugees, males, and

---

[1001] Neria Yuval et al., Trauma and PTSD among the civilians in the Middle East, PTSD Research Quarterly, 2010, № 4, pp.2-8.

[1002] http://www.esciencecentral.org/journals/death-anxiety-ptsd-trauma-grief-and-mental-health-of-palestinians-victims-of-war-on-gaza.hccr.1000112.php?aid=21422

[1003] Neria Yuval et al., Trauma and PTSD among the civilians in the Middle East, PTSD Research Quarterly, 2010, № 4, pp.2-8.

[1004] Al-Ghzawi et al., The Impact of Wars and Conflicts on Mental Health of Arab Population, International Journal of Humanities and Social Science, Vol. 4, No. 6(1); April 2014, p.239.

[1005] Neria Yuval et al., Trauma and PTSD among the civilians in the Middle East, PTSD Research Quarterly, 2010, № 4, pp.2-8.

[1006] *Ibid*

working.[1007] Palestinians experiences variety of traumatic events: 98.1% reported hearing of shelling and bombardment of the area, 98.1% reporting hearing the sound of jetfighters, 96.4% reported watching mutilated bodies in TV, 94.2% reported saw the bombardment effect on ground, 73/1% said they left home form more safe place, 21.2% exposed to burn by bombs, and 5.8% had been arrested during incursions.[1008] In Yemen, Alyahri and Goodman (2008) reported a 0.2% PTSD lifetime prevalence rate among 7- to 10-year-old schoolchildren (n = 1,210).[1009] Overall, the general-population prevalence of PTSD in the Middle East ranges widely from less than one percent to more than a third of the sample.[1010] [In Iraq] This study revealed that PTSD was present in 60% of [...] caregivers and 87% of children.[1011]

The findings reflect that a significant proportion of Arabs, living in the war-affected areas, is suffering from serious psychological distress. Having added to this, the consequences of the secondary traumatization of the empathetically involved entire Muslim umma, we will stumble upon the phenomenon of transgenerational traumatism, which resides the collective unconscious, and passes from generation to generation.

Suicide Beyond the Dimension of Jihad

The suicide rate in Muslim countries is relatively low in comparison with the world statistics, which is also influenced by the religiosity of these nations. However, a WHO news bulletins entitled Choosing to Die-a Growing Epidemic among the Young says that Islamic countries tend to have some of the lowest suicide rates in the world, and while the figures may sometimes be low because death certificates avoid mentioning suicide,

---

[1007] Al-Ghzawi et al., The Impact of Wars and Conflicts on Mental Health of Arab Population, International Journal of Humanities and Social Science, Vol. 4, No. 6(1); April 2014, p.239.

[1008] http://www.esciencecentral.org/journals/death-anxiety-ptsd-trauma-grief-and-mental-health-of-palestinians-victims-of-war-on-gaza.hccr.1000112.php?aid=21422

[1009] Neria Yuval et al., Trauma and PTSD among the civilians in the Middle East, PTSD Research Quarterly, 2010, № 4, pp.2-8.

[1010] Ibid

[1011] Al-Ghzawi et al., The Impact of Wars and Conflicts on Mental Health of Arab Population, International Journal of Humanities and Social Science, Vol. 4, No. 6(1); April 2014, p.238

some researchers believe they are largely genuine.[1012] Historically, Donne considered religious prohibition, Durkheim proposed social integration and Stalk regarded religious commitment, especially in females, to be responsible for low suicide rates. In a Muslim country, suicide is a form of protest, which dominates, especially among the Arab youth. Among the Saudis, the suicide attempts of women prevail those undertaken by men, who in their majority, fail. The report mentions that in most cases women who overdose on a drug to end their life do not go all the way. This means that their attempts are not wholehearted and the suicide attempt might be considered a desperate cry for help. "Omani suicides are mostly linked to social and communal differences as well as financial difficulties," said the Royal Omani Police source.[1013] "The most common method of suicide in Oman is by throwing oneself off a high place or by hanging," said the source.[1014] The average age of suicide victims in the Sultanate ranges between 25 and 45 years old.[1015] There were 599 suicide cases in Oman between 2000 and 2010, according to data from the ROP forensic department.[1016] Maggie Morgan examined the issue of suicide in a Muslim country through her 2009 documentary movie called Village Suicides, which was filmed in the Egyptian village Mair, where 45 deaths by suicide were documented during the year 2008 alone. According to the filmmaker, "There are hardly any jobs in Mair. There is no industry, no entertainment, and an extremely rigid structure of social, religious, and familial control."[1017]

[1012] http://www.egyptindependent.com/news/egyptian-suicide-rate-rise, consulted on 01.07.2016

[1013] http://timesofoman.com/article/66060/Oman/Suicide-rate-in-Oman-among-lowest-in-Middle-East, consulted on 01.07.2016

[1014] *Ibid*

[1015] *Ibid*

[1016] *Ibid*

[1017] http://www.egyptindependent.com/news/egyptian-suicide-rate-rise, consulted on 01.07.2016

CHAPTER 17

DOES PSYCHOANALYSIS CONTRADICT ISLAM?

Certainly, as a therapeutic method, psychoanalysis is only beginning to evoke a genuine interest in the Arab world, even though, it still remains largely unknown and ignored. It is because of a wish to find a truly effective solution that a Muslim opts for psychoanalytic treatment. With precaution and apprehension, he/she starts the first session. Psychoanalysis has accumulated numerous prejudices around itself, which originated from fears and misunderstanding. In fact, as such, there exists no resistance of the Arab world to psychoanalysis: it is just unknown for a Muslim patient. The gap of misunderstanding extends around three main preconceptions:

1. *It is from the West, and, therefore, unsuitable in the Muslim milieu.*

Psychoanalysis deals with the most human in human – the unconscious. When Freud conceived psychoanalysis in Europe, he did not intend it to be an item of a belonging of one particular culture. Moreover, it widespread all around the globe, and marked the advancement of the whole mankind. The very essence of unconscious is that it is inherent in everyone, regardless of culture, religion or any social markers. Probably, psychoanalysis is one of those practices, which, indeed, generated in the West, but does not have for the purpose the conquest and transformation of the cultural principles of the Other. True, that the West has been feared for its eccentricity, which undermines the traditional lifestyle of non-Westerners. Well, first of all, it does not imply all practices. And, secondly, once again this is a question of dreading the unknown. It is difficult to ignore the fact that only some tens of years ago the Islamic land was oppressively colonized by Western powers, and the memory of these traces is still fresh. Also, it is hard to ignore the fact that the old generation is still reacting alarmedly to the mentioning of the word "the French", "the British", etc. And last, but not the least, the Holiest Book of Muslims refer to the Christians as to "those, who got astray from the right pathway." And Muslims, indeed, tend to look scornfully on the Westerners as on those without God. Moreover, there seems to be no compelling reason to argue that psychoanalysis is being considered seriously in the Arab clinical system. It is not surprising, with a few scholars` works remaining evidently insufficient to raise the subject to the level of critical self-questioning versus falling into the pit of stereotypes. When a patient comes into the treatment and considers the possibility of attaining relief, this already is the first intentional step to face the therapeutic resistance. Sometimes, a doubt regarding the contact with the Western serves as a pretext as not to enter the treatment. Through resistance, a patient enables the transfer, or/and reintroduces the familiar to him/her reality into the analytical setting. The interplay of "the West" is also an allusion to the Other, as well as to the personal boundaries, which were previously imposed by the Other. That is a part of personal experience, which can hide anything under the disguising formulation of "the West". The further work around the signifier "the West" could also be a part of the creation of the common space between the analysand and the analyst through the exchange. The first encounter can possibly make a beginning with an initiation to talk about the personal interpretation of the attitude towards the analytical method, which came from abroad.

2.   *It is a practice of Jewish origins, therefore, opposing the Islamic principles.*

Psychoanalysis was not invented by a Jew. Freud himself was an atheist. And this had a particular impact on the development of psychoanalysis in general, as well as the place, which was accorded in it to religion. Also, a one-way approach to religion cannot, but be criticized as a failure to tackle such a tough, but extremely provocative question of the relation between Islam and psychoanalysis. Mainly for this reason, Islam was not interrogated, and remained, purely intact under the Freud`s pen. There is no Jewishness in psychoanalysis, on the contrary, it questions all religions whether Judaism or Islam.

3.   *It is an antireligious practice, which pretends to take a place of religion.*

Psychoanalysis is not a method inspired by religion, however, this does not imply its antireligious orientation. Psychoanalysis is not the vision of the world. Freud maintained a neutral position regarding the religion. In fact, as a doctrine of psychic unconscious, psychoanalysis may contribute to the understanding of the genesis of the human civilization, along with the religion. The vision of the psychoanalysis about the religion is that of anthropogenesis; it encompasses the religion at the same time as collective destiny in the history of the culture and as a psychic function in the individual relation with the world. For Freud, the specific enigma of the religion resides in the affirmation of the God-Father, with who a man maintains a relation of desire, conviction, obedience and guilt. To its critics psychoanalysis brings three explicative elements: one of the primary process (opposition between libido as a principle of pleasure and a principle of reality), that of narcissism (origin of the idea of all-might) and that of the formation and the conservation of unconscious representations (origin of the idea of God in the image of all-mighty father)[1018].

All in all, whatever is excluded, as an excuse, it is still a pretext to avoid the dissipation of the current functioning structure of symptom. This anguishes and points at the approaching of jouissance. Joseph Schwartz said, "Nevertheless, 100 years of clinical practice have shown psychoanalysis and psychotherapy not only to be effective but to yield real understandings of the dynamics of human relationships, particularly the reality of transference—countertransference re-enactments now reformulated by our neuroscientists as right brain to right brain communication."

With some general principles, inferred from Quran, the rapport with a Muslim patient may, indeed, grow into a functioning therapeutic alliance, in particular:

a. Be genuinely warm with your clients. You are not to be neutrally detached, as the western counseling would suggest, but an involvingly empathetic.

b. Be accepting and nonjudgmental. As the Quran states, "Call to the way of your Lord with fair exhortation, and reason with them in the best manner." (sura 28, ayat 87)

c. The counseling or psychotherapeutic session is a spiritual endeavor, in which reliance upon Allah is not considered as the weakness, or treason of counseling principles, but as its main strength and motivation. In between these lines Al-Ghuniah Litalibi Tariq Alhaq said, "The conditions of good friendship are that you should be forgiving and you should accept whatever your friend says or does and to find an acceptable excuse for anything

---

[1018] http://www.islam-pluriel.net/religion/religion-et-psychanalyse

that does not look right (if it is not clearly contrary to Islamic teachings)."

The reflections delivered in this chapter give growing support to a claim that there is no incompatibility between psychoanalysis and Islam.[1019]

[1019] http://laregledujeu.org/2011/10/13/7335/il-n%E2%80%99y-a-pas-d%E2%80%99incompatibilite-entre-psychanalyse-et-islam/

CHAPTER 18

CONCLUSIONS

The traditional mores of Arab countries tend to stress on the weight of the collective good over the individual. Submission to social canons is central to the culture; accommodation to the expectations of others is highly desirable. The main principle among these is what is called "mosayara", or suppression of true thoughts and feelings so that to save the *persona*. The individual "I" is often inundated, immersed into the family "We". From one side, the Arab mentality is shaped by Bedouins values and, from the other, by Islamic principles. The Bedouin sense of honour bolsters amour-propre and aggressiveness, which are essential for the survival in the desert, whilst Islamic morals focus on altruism and compassion, as prescribed by Allah. The identity conflict, provoked by the primary repudiation of origins, strikes all levels of Muslim psyche. The preserved data suggests that the Muslims were among the first to practice psychoanalysis through dream interpretations (Prophet Muhamed), recollection of the memories from the past life to bring relief (Al-Ghazali), linking body`s suffering to mental cause (Al-Razi, Al-Kindi and others). Muslim scholars are renowned for their studies on the mind structure and its functions (ilm an-nafs), as well as the correlation between the specificities of the body constitution and the psychological predisposition of the mind (al firasa). The first mental hospitals in the world "Bimaristan" were opened in the Arabic world. It is not suprising since the Islamic law (sharia) prescribes respectful and caring attitude towards the insane. However, until the present time the mental health system of the Arab region has not been developing proportionally. And almost nothing is left from the former glory of the Golden Islamic era. Evidently, the Arab countries lack sufficient hospital infrastructure, financial resources, and qualified specialists. The descendants from North Africa and the Levantine area have been more accustomed to the psychological counseling because of war provoked endured traumas. As for their Gulf counterparts, therapy is still a relatively new concept there. However, the number of Gulf locals, who aresearching for professional help, is increasing daily.

Islam is not religion of father, nor son. It is the religion of the Absolute. In the Names-Of-Father the God`s name is excluded. The fundamental elements that constitute the conception of Arabic ethnoconciousness can be ranked within the signifiers of The Other Woman-Claim of Identity-Reliance on God-Sacrifice.

The Arabs of the XXI century are alike in their symptomatology. For instance, anxiety, depression and relationships are the most common requests addressed to the psychologist today. Frequently, patients would express their psychological symptoms in a form of physical complaints to avoid the stigma of being mentally ill. Many a time the reference to somatization, as a metaphor to disclose one`s own psychological distress is uncommonly frequently used in the GCC region. In the Muslim world, which still remains very much attached to the tradition, the scientific subject has not emerged yet. Besides, the fantasy of the magnificent past still impels some Arabs to refer back to their cultural heritage in search of the solutions to their personal hardships. Generally speaking, the development of psychoanalysis is at once tightly linked to the monotheism and the emergence of the world founded on science.[1020] The Islamization of Western secular therapeutic techniques is so vital that one really wonders why it was not done decades ago.[1021] Psychoanalysis shall be reinvented in Islamic culture so that to defy the stereotypization of its Jewishness, atheism, and sex-centredness. Moreover, psychoanalysis shall be established as an available option of mental health cure in the Islamic world. In fact, the example of Egypt shows that it is not the Islamic faith that blocks the development of psychoanalysis, but the absence of speech freedom and democracy. Clinicians have conventionally approached clients from a "faith blind" perspective, however, in the Muslim context spirituality and religion are often powerful client`s strengths. This is so because there are special disorders that cannot be treated without going into religious or local cultural issues. A psychoanalyst cannot analyze a Muslim by placing him/

[1020] http://www.jeuneafrique.com/103716/archives-thematique/les-musulmans-sur-le-divan, consulted on 21.09.2016

[1021] http://www.zeriislam.com/artikulli.php?id=987

her automatically in the mythological Greek or Latin setting since he/she belongs to the real and the symbolic, which pertain individually to him/her. So, if an analyst plunges into the singularity of the Arabo-Islamic culture (legends, myths, traditional dream interpretation), the analysis will have good chances to continue. As stated by Robert Lovinger, a deeply religious person of any personality type will need first for the therapist to demonstrate respect for his or her depth of conviction. In addition, understanding the beliefs of Muslims will enable clinicians to avoid making misdiagnoses, as in the case of a patient's mention of the presence of angels or jinns, which could be interpreted as a psychotic delusion. Quite frequently, the dual patient-doctor relation in the Muslim environment is a triad with the whole family involved in the healing process. Everything considered we may come to the conclusion that there is no incompatibility between psychoanalysis and Islam.[1022]

[1022] http://laregledujeu.org/2011/10/13/7335/il-n%E2%80%99y-a-pas-d%E2%80%99incompatibilite-entre-psychanalyse-et-islam/

References

1. Quran
2. The Old Testament, Genesis
3. Abdul-Rahman, Mohamed.2009.*The Meaning and Explanation of the Glorious Qur'an.* London: MSA Publication Limited.
4. Actes de la Fondation Européenne pour la Psychanalyse. 18.07.1994. *La formation des psychanalystes (fondation européenne pour la psychanalyse).* Paris: Point hors ligne.
5. Aertsen, Jan. 1988. *Nature and Creature: Thomas Aquinas's Way of Thought.* Leiden: Brill.
6. Afifi, Al-Akiti. 1939. *The Mystical Philosophy of Ibnul Arabi.* Cambridge: Cambridge University Press.
7. Ahmed, Ramadan et al. 1998. *Psychology in the Arab world.* Menoufia: Menoufia University Press.
8. Ahmed, Ramadan.1998. *Psychology in the Arab Countries.* In Uwe P. Gielen, Lenore A. Adler and Norman A. Milgram (eds), *Psychology in international perspective: 50 Years of the International Council of Psychologists.* Amsterdam: Swets & Zeitlinger
9. Ahmed, Ramadan et al. 1998. *Psychology in the Arab Countries.* Menoufia: Menoufia University Press.
10. Ahmed, Sameera. 2012. *Counselling Muslims: Handbook of Mental Health Issues and Interventions.* London: Routledge.
11. AlAlawna. Zeel alialyam, Islam Kotob. Cairo: Dar Almanara linashr w tawzee.
12. Al Hindi, Ali. 2005. *Kanz al umal.* Riyadh: Beyt Al Afkar.
13. Ajzen, Icek, et al. 1980. *Understanding Attitudes and Predicting Social Behavior.* New Jersey: Englewood Cliffs, Prentice-Hall.
14. Al-Abdul-Jabbar, J. et al.2000. *Psychotherapy in Islamic society.* Madison:International Universities Press.

15. Al-Adawi, Samir et al. 2001. № 7, *A survey of anorexia nervosa using the Arabic version of the EAT-26 and "gold standard" interviews among Omani adolescents.* Eating and Weight Disorders. pp.304–311.

16. Al-Azri, Khalid. 2013. *Social and Gender Inequality in Oman, The Power of Religious and Political Tradition.* London: Routledge.

17. Al-Farabi, Abu Nasr. 1985. *Mabadi ara ahl al-madinah al-fadilah (al-Farabi on the Perfect State).* Oxford: Clarendon Press.

18. Alhazen. 1972. *Opticae Thesaurus: Alhazeni Arabis Libri Septem Nunc Primum Editi, Eiusdem Liber De Crepusculis Et Nubium Asensionibus.* New York: Johnson Reprint Corp.

19. Al-Karam, Carrie et al. 2015.*Mental Health and Psychological Practice in the United Arab Emirates.*New York: Palgrave Macmillan US.

20. Al-Issa, Ihsan. 2000. *Al-Junun: Mental Illness in the Islamic World.* Madison: International Universities Press.

21. Alwishah, Ahmed. 2015. *Aristotle and the Arabic Tradition.* Cambridge: Cambridge University Press.

22. Akhtar, Mohsin. 2008. *Oracle of the Last and Final Message: History and the Philosophical Deductions of the Life of Prophet Muhammad.*Bloomington: Xlibris.

23. American Journal of Islamic Social Sciences, 16 (2), 1999. *Who is the founder of psychophysics and experimental psychology?*

24. Arberry, Arthur. 1957. *Revelation and Reason in Islam.* London: Routledge.

25. Arendt, Hannah. 1970. *On Violence.* Boston: Houghton Mifflin Harcourt.

26. Arthur M. Sackler Gallery Exposition. 2010. *Roads of Arabia: Archaeology and History of the Kingdom of Saudi Arabia.* Washington.

27. As-Sallaabee, Ali. 2005. *The Noble Life of the Prophet.* Volume 1. Houston: Darussalam.

28. Avicenna. 2005. Metaphysics of The Healing. Provo UT: Brigham.

29. Azhar, Mohamed et al. 2000. *Mental illness in the Islamic world.* Madison: International Universities Press.

30. Ayoub, Mahmoud.1984. *The Qur'an and Its Interpreters.* Volume 1. New York: State University of New York Press.

31. Badri, Malik. 1979. *The dilemma of the Muslim psychologist.* London: MWH London Publishers.

32. Badri, Malik. 2013. *Abu Zayd al-Balkhi's Sustenance of the Soul: The Cognitive Behavior Therapy of a Ninth Century Physician.* Herndon: International Institute of Islamic Thought.

33. Banna, Hassan. 1999. *The Seerah of the Final Prophet.* West Glamorgan: Awakening Publications.

34. Baker, David. 2012. *The Oxford Handbook of the History of Psychology: Global Perspectives.* Oxford: Oxford University Press.

35. Barakat, Halim. 1991.*The Arab World: Society, Culture, and State.* Berkley: University of California Press.

36. Bashier, Zakaria. 1978. *The Makkan Crucible Leicester.* Leicestershire:The Islamic Foundation.

37. Belhadj, Ali. 1993. *Le comportement sexuel féminin.* MD Thesis. Tunisia: Faculty of Medicine of Tunis.

38. Bennani, Jalil. 1996. *La psychanalyse au pays des saints.* Casablanca: Le Fennec.

39. Benslama, Fethi. 2002. *La psychanalyse à l'épreuve de l'islam.* Paris: Aubier.

40. Berfrois. 2013, May 7. *Psychoanalysis and the Veil in Islam: Rethinking Truth and Liberation.*

41. Berkey, Jonathan. 2003.*The Formation of Islam.* Cambridge:Cambridge University Press.

42. Bhawuk, Dharm. 2011.*Toward a new paradigm of psychology. In Spirituality and Indian Psychology.* New York: Springer New York.

43. Bodley, Ronald. 1946. *The Messenger: The Life of Mohammed.* New York: Doubleday Incorporated.

44. Bravmann, Max. 2009. *Spiritual Background of Early Islam.* Leiden: Brill.

45. British Journal of Psychiatry. 1981. № 139, *Psycho-demographic study of anxiety in Egypt: the PSE in its Arabic version.*

46. Brosk, Hani et al. 2000. *Technical Report "Jordan National Health Accounts" № 49.* Maryland: Partnerships for Health Reform

47. Bukhari, Sahih. 1996. *Al-Hadiths.* Alexandria: Al-Saadawi Pubns.

48. Bulletin Groupe Petite Enfance. 1997. № 10.

49. Burkert, Walter. 1983. *Homo Necans.*Berkeley: University of California Press.

50. Campbell, Donald.1926. *Arabian Medicine.*Volume 1. London: Kegan Paul, Trench, Trubner & Co. Ltd

51. Casoni, Dianne et al. 2003. *Comprendre l'acte terroriste.* Québec:Presses de l'Université du Québec.

52. Chamcham, Rouchdi. 2008. *La psychanalyse au Maroc: questions pour demain.*Casablanca: La Croisée des Chemins.
53. Chebel, Malek. 1993. *L'imaginaire arabo-musulman.* Paris: P.U.F.
54. Chittick, William.1998. *Self-Disclosure of God, The: Principles of Ibn al-'Arabi's Cosmology.* New York: State University of New York Press.
55. Chittick, William.1989. *The Sufi Path of Knowledge: Ibn Al Arabi`s Metaphysics of Imagination.*New York: SUNY Press.
56. Coates, Peter. 2002. *Ibn Arabi and Modern Thought: The History of Taking Metaphysics Seriously.* Oxford: Anqa Publishing.
57. Cook, Michael. 1983.*Muhammad.* Oxford: Oxford University Press.
58. Corbin, Henry. 1993. *History of Islamic philosophy.* London: Kegan Paul International.
59. Davidson, Herbert. 1992. *Alfarabi, Avicenna, and Averroes, on Intellect: Their Cosmologies, Theories of the Active Intellect, Theories of Human Intellect.* Oxford: Oxford University Press.
60. Derrida, Jacques. 1988.*The Ear of the Other: Otobiography, Transference, Translation.* Lincoln: University of Nebraska Press.
61. Derrida, Jacques. 1996. *Résistances.* Paris: Galilée.
62. Desomogyi, Joseph. 1996. *A Short History of Classical Arabic Literature.*Leiden: Luzac Publishing.
63. Eastern Mediterranean Health Journal. 2001. № 7. *Mental health and psychiatry in the Middle East: Historical development*, pp. 336-347.
64. Egyptian Journal Forensic Science. 2011. № 1 (2).
65. Egyptian Journal of Psychiatry. 1988. № 2, *Prevalence of depressive disorders in a sample of rural and urban Egyptian communities.*
66. El-Rakhawi, Yehia. 1972. *When Man is Denuded: Cases From A Psychiatric Clinic.* Cairo: Dar Al-Ghad.
67. Ferenczi, Sandor. 1982.*Psychanalyse.* Paris: Payot.
68. Freud, Sigmund. 1981. *Fantasmes hystériques et leur relation avec la bisexualité,* in Obras completas, tomo II, Madrid: Biblioteca Nueva.
69. Freud, Sigmund. 2010. *Moses and Monotheism.* Eastford: Martino Fine Books.
70. Freud, Sigmund. 1933. *New Introductory Lectures on Psychoanalysis.* London: Penguin Freud Library.
71. Freud, Sigmund. 2006. *Personnages psychopathiques à la scène, Résultats, idées et problèmes.* Paris: PUF.

72. Freud, Sigmund. 1991. *The Ego and the Id, On Metapsychology.* London: Penguin.
73. Freud, Sigmund. 1961. *The Future of an Illusion.*New York:W.W. Norton & Company.
74. Gabriel, Richard.2007. *Muhammad: Islam's First Great General.* Oklahoma: University of Oklahoma Press.
75. Gemmeke, Amber. 2008. *Marabout Women in Dakar: Creating Trust in a Rural Urban.*New Jersey: Transaction Publishers.
76. Ghaliongui, Paul. 1963. *Magic and medical science in ancient Egypt.* London: Hodder and Stoghton.
77. Ghanim, David. 2015 The Virginity Trap in the Middle East. New York: Springer.
78. Ghodse, Hamid. 2011. *International Perspectives on Mental Health.*London: RCPsych Publications.
79. *Global Report on Birth Defects. The Hidden Toll of Dying and Disabled Children* (by Christianson Arnold et al.) 2006. New York.
80. Goodman, Lenn. 2003. *Islamic Humanism.* Oxford: Oxford University Press.
81. Gregg, Garry. 2005. *The Middle East: A Cultural Psychology.* Oxford: Oxford University Press.
82. Haddad, Yvonne. 1991. *The Muslims of America.* Oxford:Oxford University Press.
83. Hamarneh, Sami. 1984. *Health Sciences in Early Islam: collected Papers.* Volume 2.Texas: Blanco, TX: Zahra Publications.
84. Hanafi, Hasan. 1995. *Islam in the modern world. Tradition, Revolution and Culture.* Cairo: Dar Kebaa Bookshop.
85. Hassan, Enas. 1999. *Epidemiological study of scholastic underachievement among primary school children in Alexandria: prevalence and causes.* Thesis, Faculty of Nursing. Alexandria: University of Alexandria.
86. Hassoun, Jacques.1993. *L'exil de la langue.*Paris: Point hors ligne.
87. Haykal, Mohamed. 1935. *The Life of Muhammad.* Indianapolis: American Trust Publications.
88. Healey, John. 2001. *The Religion of the Nabataeans: A Conspectus.* Leiden: Brill.
89. Hedayat-Diba, Zari. 2000. *Psychotherapy with Muslims. Handbook of psychotherapy and religious diversity.* Washington: American Psychological Association.
90. Hunt, Morton. 2009. *The story of psychology.* New York: Doubleday.

91. Ibn Ishaq. 1955. *Sirat Rasul Allah*. Oxford:Oxford University Press.

92. Ibn Khaldun. 1989. *The Muqaddimah: an introduction to history*. Volume 1. Princeton: Princeton University Press.

93. International Journal for the Advancement of Counselling. 2005. № 27, *Counseling self-efficacy and its relationship to anxiety and problem-solving in United Arab Emirates*.

94. International Journal of Humanities and Social Science. 2013. № 2.

95. International Journal of Humanities and Social Science. 2014. № 6.

96. International Journal of Psychology, 21(1-4), 1986. *What constitutes an "appropriate psychology" for the developing world?* pp. 253-267.

97. International Proceedings of Economics Development & Research. 2013. № 73.

98. Irving, Zeitlin. 2007. *The Historical Muhammad*.Cambridge: Polity

99. Iqbal, Muhammad. 2013. *The Reconstruction of Religious Thought in Islam*. Stanford: Stanford University Press.

100. Jabbour, Samer. 2012. *Public Health in the Arab World*. Cambridge: Cambridge University Press.

101. Jamaal al-Din, Zarabozo. 1999. *Hadith*.Denver: Al-Basheer Publication & Translation.

102. Jayyusi, Salma. 2012. *Classical Arabic Stories: An Anthology*. NewYork: Columbia University Press.

103. Jayyusi, Salma. 1992. *The Legacy of Muslim Spain*. Leiden: Brill.

104. Johnson, Scott. 2012. *The Oxford Handbook of Late Antiquity*. Oxford: OUP USA.

105. Johnson, Todd et al. 2013. *The World's Religions in Figures: An Introduction to International Religious Demography*. Massachusetts: Wiley-Blackwell.

106. Journal "Al-Hewar/The Arab-American Dialogue". Winter 2007.

107. Journal "Arch Gen Psychiatry". 1994. № 51.

108. Journal "American Psychologist", 32(11), 1977.

109. Journal Biol Psychiatry. 2006. № 14.

110. Journal BMC Public Health. 2007. № 7.

111. Journal "Child Development".1990. № 61 (2).

112. Journal "Comprehensive Psychiatry". 1994. № 35.

113. Journal "Enfances & Psy". 2006. № 33.

114. Journal FASEB. 2006. *Arab science in the golden age (750-1258 C.E.) and today.*
115. Journal "History of Psychiatry", 7 (25), 1996.
116. Journal "Hum Genet". 2004. № 114.
117. Journal of the American Board of family Medicine. 2005. № 2.
118. Journal of International Society of History of Islamic Medicine (JSHIM). 2006. № 5.
119. Journal of Global Religious Vision. 2001.
120. Journal "L'Evolution Psychiatrique". 1993. № 58.
121. Journal "Majalaat Ilm an-Nafs".
122. Journal "Maroc médical". 1955. № 365.
123. Journal "Middle Eastern Studies". 1984. № 3.
124. Journal "Modern Intellectual History". 2014. № 1.
125. Journal of Muslim Mental Health. 2007. № 2.
126. Journal "Neuropsychiatric Disease and Treatment". 2013. № 9.
127. Journal "Philosophical Forum". 1972. № 4.
128. Journal "Psychiatria Danubina". 2011. № 23
129. Journal Psychiatry Related Science. 2005. № 42.
130. Journal of Religion and Health. 2004. № 43.
131. Journal of Religion and Health. 2004. № 43. *Psychology from Islamic Perspective: Contributions of Early Muslim Scholars and Challenges to Contemporary Muslim Psychologists*, pp. 357-377.
132. Journal "Social Behavior and Personality". 2006. № 34.
133. Journal Social Psychiatry and Psychiatric Epidemiology. 2012. № 47.
134. Journal of Social Science. 2008. № 22.
135. Journal "Substance Abuse and Rehabilitation". 2012. № 3.
136. Journal" The Philosopher". 2002. № 2.
137. Journal "Topique". 2010. № 110.
138. Journal "UAE Psychologist", 1(2), 2011.
139. Journal "UAE University Publications". 2004. *Mental Health Care in UAE Since the Formation of Al-Itihad.*
140. Journal "Women and Health". 2001. № 34.
141. Jung, Carl.1985. *Psychologie et orientalisme.* Paris: Albin Michel.
142. Jung, Carl. 1960. *The structure and dynamics of the psyche.*Volume 8. Princeton: Princeton University Press.
143. Kafaji, Talib.2011. *The Psychology of the Arab: The Influences That Shape an Arab Life.*Bloomingthon: AuthorHouse.
144. Kamal, Ahmed. 1974. *Adil: 'ulum al-Qur'an.* Cairo:Al-Mukhtar al-Islami.

145. Kennard, Fredrick. 2015. *Thought Experiments: Popular Thought Experiments in Philosophy, Physics, Ethics, Computer Science & Mathematics.* Raleigh: Lulu.
146. Kierreraard Soren. 1935. *Le concept d'angoisse.* Paris: Gallimard.
147. La naissance de la psychanalyse. 1895. 3d edition.
148. Lacan, Jacques. 2002. *Écrits: A Selection.* New York: W. W. Norton.
149. Lancet. 2000, May 27. *Sanctions and childhood mortality in Iraq,* pp.1851-1857.
150. Lawrence, Gerstein et al. 2009. *International handbook of cross-cultural counseling: Cultural assumptions and practices worldwide.* California: SAGE Publications.
151. Leaman, Olivier et al. 2001. *History of Islamic Philosophy.* London: Routledge.
152. Lipovsky, Igor. 1996.*The Socialist Movement in Turkey: 1960-1980.* Leiden: Brill.
153. Mahmoud, Omar. 2008. *Muhammad: an evolution of God.* Bloomingthon: Author House.
154. Marenbon, John. 2012. *The Oxford Handbook of Medieval Philosophy.* Oxford: OUP USA.
155. Margoliouth, David. 2010. *Mohammed and the Rise of Islam.* New York: Cosimo Inc.
156. Meddeb, Abdelwaheb. 2012. *La maladie de l'islam.*Paris: Seuil.
157. Mental Health Atlas. 2005. WHO.
158. Mental Health System in Kingdom of Bahrain. 2010. WHO
159. Mijolla, Alain (dir.). 2013. *Dictionnaire international de la psychanalyse.* Paris: Calmann-Lévy.
160. Monthly Renaissance. 2007.№ 17. *Influence of Muslim Philosophy on the West.*
161. Mubarakpuri, Saifur. 2012. *The Sealed Nectar.*London: Darrussalam International Publications.
162. Musa, Salama. 1928. *Al-Aql al-Batin, aw Maknunat al-Nafs.* Cairo: Al-Hilal.
163. Muslim, Sahih. 2000. *Being Traditions of the Sayings and Doings of the Prophet Muhammad as Narrated by His Companions and Compiled Under the Title Al-Jamil al Sahih.* Volume 4. New Delhi: Kitab Bhavan
164. Najmabadi, Afsaneh. 2008. *Islamicate Sexualities: Translations across Temporal Geographies of Desire.* Cambridge: Harvard University Press.

165. Najmabadi, Afsaneh. 2003. *Encyclopedia of Women and Islamic Cultures*. Leiden: Brill.
166. Nahyan, Fancy. 2006. *Pulmonary Transit and Bodily Resurrection: The Interaction of Medicine, Philosophy and Religion in the Works of Ibn al-Nafīs*. Indiana: University of Notre Dame.
167. Nasr, Seyyed. 2006. *Islamic philosophy from its origin to the present: philosophy in the land of prophecy*. New York: State Univiversity of New York Press.
168. Nasr, Seyyed et al. 1996. *History of Islamic Philosophy*. London: Routledge.
169. National Report on Mental Health System and Services in Jordan. 2010. The Higher Council for Science and Technology.
170. Nicholson, Reynold. 1994. *A Literary History of the Arabs*. Volume 1. New Delhi: Kitab Bhavan
171. Nurbakhsh, Javad. 1980. *What the Sufis say*. New York: Khaniqahi - Nimatullahi Publications.
172. Okasha, Ahmed.1999. *Mental health in the Middle East: An Egyptian perspective*. Oxford: Pergamon.
173. Open Journal of Psychiatry. 2014. № 4.
174. Payeur, Bernard. 2015. *Getting to Know Allah - Legacy Edition*. Raleigh: Lulu.
175. Peters, Francis. 1994. *Muhammad and the Origins of Islam*. New York: State University of New York
176. Preminger, Alex (dir.). 1993. The New Princeton Encyclopedia of Poetry and Poetics. Princeton: Princeton University Press.
177. Proceedings of the 19th Congress of the International Association for Analytical Psychology. 2013. *100 Years On: Origins, Innovations and Controversies*. Copenhagen.
178. Psychology of Religion Newsletter, 27(4), 2002.
179. PTSD Research Quarterly. 2010. № 4.
180. Rahman, Fazlur. 1952. Avicenna's Psychology, Oxford: Hyperion Pr.
181. Razwy, Ali. 2001. *A Restatement of the History of Islam and Muslims*.Middlesex: World Federation of Khoja ShiaIthna-Asheri Muslim.
182. Report on Mental Health System in Morocco. 2006. WHO.
183. Report of Committee on Polygamous Issues. 1993. British Columbia Ministry of Women's Equality.
184. Revista Latinoamericana de Filosofía. 1990.№ 16, *La distinción entre esencia y existencia en Avicena*, pp. 183–195.

185. Revue Française de Psychanalyse. 1993. *Psychanalyse au Maroc: résistances culturelles.*
186. Revue internationale des sciences sociales (UNESCO).
187. Rosenberg, Jerry. 2012. *Aftermath of the Arab Uprisings: The Rebirth of the Middle East.*Connecticut: Hamilton Books.
188. Rosemary, Ellen Guiley et al. 2011. *The Vengeful Djinn.* Woodbury: Llewellyn Publications.
189. Rosenwein, Barbara. 2013. *Reading the Middle Ages: Sources from Europe, Byzantium, and the Islamic World.* Volume I. Toronto: University of Toronto Press.
190. Saad, Mohamed. 2001. *Kitab al-Ṭabaqat al-Kabir.* Cairo: Maktabat al-Khangi.
191. Sadik, Sabah et al. 2011. *Integrating mental health into primary health care in Iraq.* London: Radcliffe Publishing.
192. Said, Khalida. 1991. *Al mara al-arabiya: kain bi gheirihi am bi dhatihi?* Casablanca: Nashr al fanac.
193. Saudi Medical Journal. 2002. № 23.
194. Safouan, Moustapha. 1983. *Jacques Lacan et la question de la formation des analystes*, Paris: Seuil.
195. Scott, Samuel. 1904. *History of the Moorish Empire in Europe.* Philadelphia: J. B. Lippincott Company.
196. Scull, Andrew. 2014. *Cultural Sociology of mental illness, an A-to-Z Guide.* Volume 1. California: University California Press.
197. Selvik, Kjetil et al. 2011. *Stability and Change in the Modern Middle East.* Lodon: I.B.Tauris.
198. Servier, Andre. 1923. *Islam and the Psychology of the Musulman.* New York: Scribner.
199. Sharma, Sonali. 2012. *Mental Health Policy in Iraq since 2003, a Post-Invasion Analysis.* London:MedAct.
200. Shi, Leiyu. 2011.*The Nation's Health.*Burlington: Jones & Bartlett Publishers.
201. Singapore Med Journal. 2006.
202. Slattery, Dennis. 2000. *Depth Psychology - Meditations in the Field.* Einsiedeln: Daimon Verlag.
203. Smith, William. 2014. *Kinship and Marriage in Early Arabia.* Oxford: Oxford Press.
204. Social Behavior and Personality: An International Journal. 2003. № 31, *Attitudes towards seeking professional psychological help: What really counts for United Arab Emirates University Students?*
205. SQU Journal of Scientific Research. 2002. № 4.

206. Storm, Morten. 2015. *Agent Storm: My Life Inside al-Qaeda*. New York: Grove Press.
207. Sutton, Kyra. 2013. *Islam's Turn on the Couch: The Psychoanalytic Theorizing of Muslim Identity in France*. Connecticut: Weyslan University.
208. Syakir, Mahmud. 1991.*Al-Tarikh al-Islamiy Qabl al-Bi'thah*. Beirut: Al-Maktab al-Islamiy.
209. The Arab Journal of Psychiatry. 2011. №. 1.
210. The Colloquium "Culture et psychothérapies"(IV).
211. The Colloquium "Heidegger and the Contemporary Religious Situation".2008. Oxford University Faculty of Theology: Centre for Theology and Modern European Thought
212. The Conference 100 Years On: Origins, Innovations and Controversies: Proceedings of the 19th Congress of the International Association for Analytical Psychology. 2013
213. The Conferynce "Rencontres Franco-Maghrébines de Psychiatrie". 2014
214. The International Medical Journal. 2005. № 4
215. The Review of Metaphysics. 2001. № 54.
216. Tobie, Nathan. 1999. *L'influence qui guérit*. Paris: Odile Jacob.
217. Von Denffer, Ahmed. 1994. *Ulum al Qur'an: An Introduction to the Sciences of the Qur'an*.Leicester: The Islamic Foundation.
218. Wahhab, Mohamed. 1996. *Kitab At-Tauhid*.Riyadh: Dar-us-Salam Publications.
219. Wasty, Nayyar. 1962. *Muslim Contribution to Medicine*.Lahore: M. Sirajuddin & Sons Publishers.
220. Wise, Christopher. 2009. *Derrida, Africa and the Middle East*. New York: Palgrave Macmillan.
221. Yoga Journal, 1997.
222. Zarabozo, Jamal. 1998. *The World of Jinn and Devils*. Boulder: Al-Basheer Publications & Translations.
223. Zayzafoon, Lamia.2005. *The Production of the Muslim Woman: Negotiating Text, History, and Ideology*. Lenhman: Lexington Books.
224. Zdanowski, Jerzy. 2014. *Middle Eastern Societies in the 20th Century*. Cambridge: Cambridge Scholars Publishing.
225. Zeevi, Dror. 2006. *Producing Desire: Changing Sexual Discourse in the Ottoman Middle East, 1500-1900*. California: University of California Press.

ELECTRONIC RESOURCES

Academia.edu, an academic platform   www.academia.edu

Addiction Treatment Centre   www.caminorecovery.com
"Camino Recovery"

ADR Medical Recruitment   www.adr-medical-recruitment.co.uk

Al Jalila Foundation   www.aljalilafoundation.ae

AlSeef Hospital   www.alseef-hospital.com

American Mission Hospital   www.amh.org.bh

American Psychological Association   www.apa.org

American Psychological Association Divisions   www.apadivisions.org

American University of Beirut   www.aub.edu.lb

Analytical website Construction Weekonline   www.constructionweekonline.com

Arab News   www.arabnews.com

Arabic Psychological Network   http://arabpsynet.com

Bahrain Institute for Special Education   www.bised.org

Bahraini Ministry of Health   www.moh.gov.bh

Behman Hospital   www.behman.com

BioMed Central The Open Access Publisher   www.substanceabusepolicy.biomedcentral.com

BJ Psych Bulletin	http://pb.rcpsych.org
Blog Mental Illness	www.mentalillness.umwblogs.org
Borgen Magazine	www.borgenmagazine.com
Brighter Brains Institute	www.brighterbrains.org
British Broadcasting Corporation (BBC)	www.bbc.co.uk
British Council	www.britishcouncil.org
Cairn Info	www.cairn.info
Centers for Disease Control and Prevention	www.cdc.gov
Child Protection Working Group	http://cpwg.net
Cornell University Library	www.library.cornell.edu
Countries info website Chartsbin	http://chartsbin.com
Department of Halal Certification	http://halalcertification.ie
Digital Islamic Library Project Al Islam.org	www.al-islam.org
Doha News	http://dohanews.co
Economist	www.economist.com
Educational Organization Humanity in Action	www.humanityinaction.org
Egypt Independent Newspaper	www.egyptindependent.com
Emirates 24/7 News	www.emirates247.com
Encyclopedia	www.encyclopedia.com
Encyclopedia Britannica	www.britannica.com
English Al Arabiya	www.english.alarabiya.net
Eupedia	www.eupedia.com
Europe News	www.en.europenews.dk
Fawzia Sultan rehabilitation Centre	www.fsrikuwait.org
Gulf News	www.gulfnews.com
Hadiths collection	http://hadithcollection.com
Hamad Medical Corporation	www.hamad.qa
Harvard Magazine	www.harvardmagazine.com
Host Website for Author`s Artices	http://hubpages.com

Humanitarian Practice Network	http://odihpn.org
Hurriyet Daily Newspaper	www.hurriyetdailynews.com
Independent Commission for Aid Impact "ICAI"	http://icai.independent.gov.uk
Instituts français de recherche a l`etranger	www.ifre.fr
International Brain Research Organization	http://ibro.info
International Medical Corps	http://internationalmedicalcorps.org
International Network of Child and Adolescent Resilience	http://in-car.ca
International Rehabilitation Council for Torture Victims	www.irct.org
Internet Encyclopedia of Philosophy	www.iep.utm.edu
Internet Sacred Texts Archive	www.sacred-texts.com
Informative resource on Islam	www.missionislam.com
Iranian Encyclopedia	www.iranicaonline.org
Islamic fatwas collection	http://fatwa.islamweb.net
Islamic network Al Seraj	www.alseraj.net
Islamic publications Al Zahid	www.alzahid.co.uk
Islamic Research Foundation International	www.irfi.org/
Islamic resource Sultan	http://sultan.org
Islamic database	www.islam.org.uk
Islamic social network Alim	www.alim.org
Journal of Sufi	www.journalsoufi.com
Journal Nature	www.nature.com
Khaleej Times	www.khaleejtimes.com
King Hamad University	www.khuh.org.bh
Kuwait Times	http://news.kuwaittimes.net
Kuwaiti Association for Learning Differences	www.kaldkuwait.com

Kuwaiti Centre for Mental Health   http://kcmh.jimdo.com
Kuwait Psychological Medicine   www.psychiatrykuwait.com
Hospital
Lebanese Association for   http://aldep.org
Development of Psychoanalysis
(ALDeP)
Le Midi   www.lemidi-dz.com
Lebanese Ministry of Public   www.moph.gov.lb
Health
Lebanese Society of Psychoanalysis www.slp-web.org/
(SLP)
Magazine Sciences Humaines   www.scienceshumaines.com
Medical Centre Al Harub Medical   www.alharubmedical.com
Medical News Medscape   www.medscape.com
Mental Disability Advocacy   www.mdac.info
Online
Mental Health Professionals`   http://mhpal.weebly.com
Association
of Lybia
Middle East Eye   www.middleeasteye.net
Morocco World News   www.moroccoworldnews.com
Mount Lebanon Hospital   http://mlh.com.lb
Mubarak Hospital   www.mkhpsych.com
Mundus Databse   www.mundus.ac.uk
Muscat Daily Newspaper   www.muscatdaily.com
Muslim Heritage   www.muslimheritage.com
Muslim Matrimonial Website   www.naseeb.com
My Islamic Dream Database   www.myislamicdream.com
National Centre for Biotechnology   www.ncbi.nlm.nih.gov
Information
New York Times   www.nytimes.com
Nyheder TV 2 Channel   www. nyheder.tv2.dk
Noora AlHussein Foundation   www.nooralhusseinfoundation.
                                    org

Northwestern University of Qatar	www.qatar.northwestern.edu
Online articles by Shahid Athar	www.islam-usa.com
Online Journal Psychology in Africa	www.psychologyinafrica.com
Online Presentation Resource	http://slideplayer.com
Open Access Medical Journals	www.omicsonline.com
Pew Research Centre	www.pewforum.org
Prophetic Sunna	http://sunnah.com
Prophet`s Sunna	www.sunnah.org
Publisher BioMed Central Publisher	www.biomedcentral.com
Publisher Jstor	www.jstor.org
Qatari Ministry of Public Health	www.moph.qa
Qatari National Health Strategy	http://nhsq.info
Rehab International Clinic	www.rehabinternational.org
Research Gate	www.researchgate.net
Royal College of Psychiatrists	www.rcpsych.ac.uk
Rutgers University	www.eden.rutgers.edu
Scholar Works Site	www.scholarworks.iu.edu
Scientific Platform E-Science Central	www.esciencecentral.org
Sidra Hospital	www.sidra.org
Somalia Mental Health Foundation	www.somalimentalhealth.org
Stanford Encyclopedia of Philosophy	www.plato.stanford.edu
The Higher Council for Science and Technology	www.hcst.gov.jo
The Islamic Journal	http://theislamicjournal.com
The Lancet	www.thelancet.com
The Life of Prophet Muhamed	www.hadithway.com
The National	www.thenational.ae
Times of Oman	http://timesofoman.com

United Nations Development Programme	http://hdr.undp.org
United Nations Population Fund Human Development Reports	www.unfpa.org
Website about Turkish culture	www.turkishculture.org
Western Michigan University	http://scholarworks.wmich.edu
Wikipedia	https://en.wikipedia.org
Wikiislam	www.wikiislam.net
World Bank Blog	http://blogs.worldbank.org
World Bank Data	http://data.worldbank.org
World Health Organization (WHO)	www.emro.who.int
World Health Organization (WHO)	www.who.int
World Life Expectancy Site	www.worldlifeexpectancy.com
YnetNews	www.ynetnews.com
Y Oman Magazine	www.y-oman.com
Youtube	www.youtube.com
Zeri Islam	www.zeriislam.com

Index

F

Femininity
180

Freud Sigmund
130, 204, 339, 340, 355, 364, 365, 366, 371,
397, 398, 401, 402, 406, 407, 408

H

Hagar
287, 289, 313, 320

Hijab
314

Hysteria
146, 380, 397, 398, 399

I

Identity
x, xxi, 9, 28, 78, 90, 114, 150, 286, 309, 310, 313, 315, 316,
320, 331, 364, 365, 368, 370, 371, 385, 386, 387, 410

Inshallah
329, 330, 331

J

Jouissance
286, 287, 289, 312, 313, 316, 324, 331, 333, 334, 339, 395, 408

K

Kristeva Julia
371, 398

L

Lacan Jacques

N

Nashed Rafah

Neurosis

S

Schizophrenia

T

Transfer\transference

U

Unconscious

www.ingramcontent.com/pod-product-compliance
Lightning Source LLC
Chambersburg PA
CBHW020720180526
45163CB00001B/46